Healing with Art and Soul

Healing with Art and Soul:
Engaging One's Self through Art Modalities

Edited by

Kathy Luethje

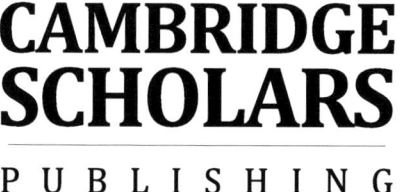

Healing with Art and Soul: Engaging One's Self through Art Modalities,
Edited by Kathy Luethje

This book first published 2009

Cambridge Scholars Publishing

12 Back Chapman Street, Newcastle upon Tyne, NE6 2XX, UK

British Library Cataloguing in Publication Data
A catalogue record for this book is available from the British Library

Copyright © 2009 by Kathy Luethje and contributors

All rights for this book reserved. No part of this book may be reproduced, stored in a retrieval system, or transmitted, in any form or by any means, electronic, mechanical, photocopying, recording or otherwise, without the prior permission of the copyright owner.

ISBN (10): 1-4438-0209-3, ISBN (13): 978-1-4438-0209-3

TABLE OF CONTENTS

Acknowledgements ix

Introduction xi

Foreword xix
Jane Goldberg

PART I: SURVEYING THE LANDSCAPE: PATHOGRAPHY TO CO-CREATION

"The Art of Healing and the Science of Art"
Carol Shore.. 2

"Healing Presence"
Julie Balzer Riley 14

"The Healing Mind"
Charles H. Ware 24

"Namaste"
Carol Yancar.. 33

"Erasing the Pain"
Kurt Fondriest.. 43

"A Letter to Chopra"
Wayne Berman 49

"Of a Different Color…"
Kathy Luethje, and Laurie Doyle 54

"Simply Being: Using Meditation and Mindful Awareness
as an Element of Change"
Rosemary J. Wentworth 80

PART II: ENGAGING SOUND:

"Therapeutic Drumming: Rhythm as a Healing Tool"
Russell Buddy Helm 92

"Toning... A Journey toward Self Discovery"
Elle Speed 100

"Sing for Your Soul"
Lauren Lane Powell.. 108

"Meta Sound: The Frequency of Love"
Rosemary Warburton 116

"A Trilogy: From Tone Deafness to Universal Music Day"
Susan Patricia Golden.. 119

"Sing and Swing: A Personal Approach to an Individual Voice"
Annette Tewes 134

"You Must Sing to be Found..."
Susan Gregory 141

PART III: ENGAGING BODY

"Meta-physical: From Movement to Magic"
Roger Millen... 152

"Circle of Dance: Meditation, Movement and Mindfulness"
Kay Plumb.. 158

"Healing, Creativity, and Transformation: A Path to the Divine"
Elijah Gary Wohlman... 165

"Laughter: Nature's Healing Refrain"
Susan M. Stewart.. 174

"Daring to Ride Our Images: Magic, Story and Movement"
Fay Wilkinson 182

PART IV: ENGAGING IMAGE

"Photo Meditation /Introspection"
Nancy Cappo 194

"As Within So Without: An Ancient Soul Map to Healing"
Christine McCullough 206

"In Search of the Soul of Image: A Cosmological Theory
for Expressive Arts Therapy"
Paula Artac 214

"Elementary, my dear, What's on tap for children & adults"
Sally Mathews 223

"Mandala: Path of Peace"
Melanie Circle 233

"A Journey Through Time"
Frances Falk 240

PART V: ENGAGING WORD

"Sometimes Words Are Not Enough"
Olive M. "Hollie" Adkins 250

"Voices from the Circle: Women's Ritual Art"
Lynn Carol Henderson 256

"Poetics of the Night: The Transformative Power of Dreams"
Kathleen M. Sands 270

"The Art of Choice Theory"
Laura JJ Dessauer 278

"The Good and the Beautiful: Aesthetic Concepts and Expressive
Arts Therapy"
Joan Forest Mage 285

PART VI: VIEWING A FIELD OF LIFELONG LEARNING

"Inner Healing: The Co-Creation of Emotional Transcendence"
Benjamin B. Keyes 298

"ArtWorks in Times of Crisis: Trauma and Troubled Teens"
Poppy Moon 309

"Sparking a Mighty Blaze: Pliant Patience Recalled"
Carol Henry 326

"Developing a Language for Trauma: Children Communicating through the Arts"
Vicki J. Morgan 338

"*Solvitur Ambulando* (It is Solved by Walking)"
Alison Morrow 346

"Expressive Arts Aren't Always Pretty: A Picture of DID"
June M. Conboy 355

"Your Daily Dose of Art—A Prescription for Healthy Aging"
Cathy DeWitt 369

"Bibliotherapy for Older Adults"
Robert Beland 378

"A Gathering of Angels"
Joan Abrahamson Voyles 386

Author Biographies 434

Index 449

ACKNOWLEDGMENTS

As editor of this book, I offer my personal gratitude to the following:

Margaret (Megan) A. Reckelhoff, our Manuscript Consultant, whose physical book this really is. She has worked tirelessly with me to put it into form.

These 'second sets of eyes,' for their time and talent to the project: (listed in alphabetical order)

Cheryl Belanger, Kathryn Bolen, Nancy Cappo, Karen Creamer, Cathy DeWitt, Susan Golden, Lynn Carol Henderson, Jon R. Luethje, Lindsay Mainland, Sally Mathews, Vicki Morgan, Steve Reckelhoff, Jacky Saeger, Kathy Sands, Rebecca Stone, Jac'line Weisgerber, and Carol Yancar..

Bayfront Medical Center, St. Petersburg, FL, home to the conference where the book project began. Doug Harrell, Chaplain and Director of Pastoral Care, who supported the Creative Expressions program at Bayfront since its beginnings in the year 2000. Dianne Arvin and Alan Schukman who were co-creators of the program. Elle Speed for her work in carrying on the music and toning programs at Bayfront. Sound Wave group for their time recording our CD.

All the contributing authors for their thought-full contributions and their patience with me on this book project. Dr. Jane Goldberg for her support in writing our forward. Dr. Sally Atkins and Dr. David Darling, both leaders in the expressive arts field, for their endorsements of the work. John Fox, CPT, for his letter of support.

Carol Koulikourdi, Amanda Millar, Nuala Coyle, & Dr. Andy Nercession, of Cambridge Scholars Publishing who were our guides in the publishing process.

Mrs. Mary Bowden, my piano teacher, who expanded one art modality into many for me when I was only six. Anona United Methodist Church, Largo, FL, and Pastor Jack Stephenson who supported me in attending the Expressive Arts Therapy classes at University of South Florida that prepared me for this work. Earlham School of Religion, Richmond, IN, who started me on this quest and taught me stillness.

INTRODUCTION

> "We are the music-makers,
> And we are the dreamers of dreams,
> Wandering by lone sea-breakers,
> And sitting by desolate streams,
> World-losers and world-forsakers,
> Upon whom the pale moon gleams,
> Yet we are the movers and shakers,
> Of the world forever, it seems."
>
> —from 'Ode' by Arthur William Edgar O'Shaughnessy 1844-1881

An amazing array of brilliantly creative minds blessed my life a few years ago. They all showed up for a conference I helped to organize. It was a nodal event for me. "Gather your people together,' had been a call from a distant dream, and I had been trying to figure out who these people were for years. I had hungered for a mentor, and when we gathered, I found not one, but many. They came to explore the use of expressive arts as healing modalities. Now, many of these artists and more have decided to join me in creating this compendium of essays to preserve in part what happened between us, and to disseminate the insights throughout the world. What we offer to the readers is not a 'how-to' book so much as a 'why-to' book, why to use art modalities in a healing practice, although there are techniques and methods within these pages. There are also stories and creative products from working with the arts for healing. Some experiences have been life changing for the authors; some have been transformative for the people within their care.

As an expressive arts practitioner, I know that having the tools of rhythm, movement, tone, color, and form to express that for which I have not yet found words, has made life rich and full of meaning. Like many writers within these pages, I believe that I have always been an expressive artist, although for years that fact went unrecognized, especially by me. Perhaps we are all born expressive artists; perhaps that quality is just what makes children so resilient. Unfortunately, unless this inborn use of the imagination and delight in the activity of making beauty is carefully cultivated in children they can soon learn to judge the products of their expressive process and find them lacking. Somewhere along the process of socialization and education they leave their 'de-Light' behind.

When we reawaken and open ourselves to the return of our Light, we allow ourselves to experience our wholeness, and therefore, our healing. It is good work. All it takes is a willingness, courage, to engage. The hope of this book is to set forth a vision for the reader of how engagement with the expressive arts can be an avenue for healing the body, mind, and soul. While many practitioners of the expressive arts have not entered this field in order to move and shake their communities, that is exactly what is happening all over the globe. It is the desire of these writers that you, the reader, will feel the passion and compassion flowing from these pages, because of our love for the expressive arts. We believe that we have found some new truths, and resurrected some old ones, about how people heal from the woundedness they receive through trauma and their everyday lives.

The arts have infiltrated traditional healing settings, and they continue to expand their influence in non-traditional settings. Those who have come to believe that the arts are healing in and of themselves are now in positions within traditional institutions, offering complementary and alternative healing avenues for people with terminal illnesses and long hospital stays. Arts practices are beginning to be a part of many individual and group therapy sessions. People from all walks of life are beginning to awaken to the use of the arts for their own well-being, some ideas that art therapists and others have known for years.

As a group of authors, we come from many different traditions and we represent a kaleidoscopic viewpoint. When we gathered a few years ago in St. Petersburg, Florida, to support, advocate for, and educate each other, most of us were at the beginning of this shared journey, although some of us had practiced our therapies and healing arts for many years. We have been the people in the trenches, the ones working directly with people who are hurting and in need of healing. Several of the people you will meet within these pages have broken away from their taught traditions and have formed innovative healing practices of their own. Their work becomes a shining example of what happens when imagination and intuition are rendered into form and action.

We consider ourselves to be both healers and artists, in the very broad sense of those terms. One of our healing tools is a compassionate companioning with our participants and clients through their own journeys; that tool is essential. We engage with our clients and students, while asking them to engage with themselves. It is the heart of the healer coming through to touch other hearts. In this way, we are co-creating with those we help, matching our tools to the other's need, and working collaboratively with them to weave a mending, a new fabric of wholeness.

Our arts take many forms; they are activated through various modalities, and are accessed through any number of the five senses. Most authors write about realizing that a sort of sixth sense, a spiritual sense, is also at play in the use of the arts for healing. When we gathered to explore the co-creation of health, we realized that most of us believe in the co-creation that happens between the therapist and the client, but also the one that happens when unseen forces move to weave the synergy that is full health. The process of coming to wholeness has been called wholistic, but also holistic, or holy, to emphasize this spiritual dimension.

What you will find in these pages is a collection of the individual voices of healing artists, and a little bit about the journey each one of them has undertaken. Most essays here are anecdotal, rather than being reports of scientific studies, but they provide evidence that there is healing power in the use of the art-making process for those in need of it. Each person writing has claimed his or her identity as a healing artist in some form, and all have taken the necessary steps to clarify for themselves what meaning such an identity has for them. Finding themselves as "music-makers" has also necessitated their being "dreamer of dreams" in order that they could break into the traditional healing settings with their work. Much of what has been done in the field to date has been done through faith, through belief in the efficacy of the work.

My own path to becoming a healing artist has included an intentional pursuit of experiences that were consciousness expanding and self-transcendent, such as zazen and hypnosis, since the 1970's. I established my career in the helping professions, hoping to relieve the hurts of the world, if even a little bit, and to help the people whom I counseled or taught to begin to realize their own innate potential. However, it is through the expressive arts process that I found the most permission to be myself and to explore what it means to be me in the most fulfilling ways. The process in the intermodal expressive arts became a way to 'fan into flames the spark' that was within me to improve the spiritual condition of the people around me. I have always wanted to help others shine forth with the light that is within them. Through the use of the arts as healing modalities, I have new tools for helping others to find the unique and beautiful in all of life. In my seminary studies, I became enamored with Process Theology, and I find that the 'process' of intermodal expressive arts resonates with this way of viewing spiritual forces as they interact with creation. There is a continual process of creating anew in life itself, and through the expressive arts, we find ourselves at the center of the creative moment.

Since it is becoming more and more essential for people to guide the process of their own healing through the maze of medical and non-traditional options, I believe that they would do well to proclaim themselves healing artists, and to begin using their imaginations and any art tools that feel right to them. Essentially, this is in order that they reach the inner parts of themselves, and begin to heal from within, "creatively integrating the inner and outer life to a life more authentically lived," in the words of Marc Ian Barasch, who believes this to be the path to healing.

> "Our bodies bear unimpeachable witness to the movements of our soul," They "speak a deeper, more spontaneous truth beyond ego's control...the body is our very presence in this world, the space only we can occupy, the place where the self's private story is given breath." (Barasch, 1993: 317)

In expressive arts, we start with the body, with what is felt inside, and express out through some sort of art form.

Barasch has also given us a definition of the word *healing*. He references Dr. Jacob Zieghelboim, saying that he views "healing as a coming into touch with the real forces of life." (1993: 318) A working definition from Wikipedia for healing is:

> "the process by which cells in the body regenerate and repair to reduce the size of a damaged area... Healing assessed spiritually, emotionally, mentally or otherwise, is a process which involves more than just the action of cells...Nature, or more specifically, the body's natural healing mechanisms, *(or the body's inborn ability to heal itself)* is the principle mechanism by which the process occurs." (http://en.wikipedia.org.2008.)

When we attempt to determine a definition for art, we enter another sort of labyrinth. There does not seem to be one all encompassing definition. Process arts are the kind of arts that focus on the art-making process rather than the art product; they may be called expressive. Expressive arts are not always 'pretty,' we are told by our author Dr. June Conboy. Perhaps this is the 'world losers/ world forsakers' part of the opening poem. My own experience of writing out what I needed to really feel, through poetry, has not been pretty; my poems have met with mixed acclaim. I am thinking about years ago, when one piece I'd written about the smells of being in bed with a person who drank too much had the sensitive private college students where I worked in an uproar that anything like that could be considered poetry. And my recent writing in a workshop by poetry therapist, teacher, and mentor John Fox about the neverland of the body was deemed "hard to listen to" by my peers. Both expressed my momentary reality.

Today, I write about a grandma waiting for the kids that never come. It won't make anybody smile. But it does help me feel better. My truth has been told. The witness, and the only one perhaps, is the piece of paper; but I still feel I have been heard. I write because I don't want these bitter ideas to live inside me. That is the reason many folks do expressive art. Although art is not always beautiful, true art usually expresses our truth.

Qualities such as visual, auditory, and kinesthetic are called modalities or 'learning or operating styles;' they are the channels through which we express. Various art-making processes employ these in terms of modality to specify which sensory pathway is being used. Expressive arts are usually movement based, since they are e-motion based; they start in the body. Then there is a weaving back and forth through different modalities, which form and inform one another to create new pathways of expression. Dr. Barbara Kazanis, founder of the provost graduate level certificate of training in the Expressive Arts at the University of South Florida, Tampa, says that this is where the aesthetic experience, the learning process, and the healing transformation form a nexus. It is a crucible for healing.

Art may not be easy to define, but there are many things we know art can do for us. Art can:

Record history   *Memorialize a person or event*

Celebrate life

Evoke thoughts or feelings

Reveal a way of life

Express who we are

Uplift and inspire us   Relax us

Stimulate our imaginations

Add to our knowledge

Excavate beliefs

Stimulate conversations

Encourage creativity and more art

There is probably much more! I have seen the arts do all of these things. That is why I believe they are so valuable to us in our quest for living balanced and vital lives.

> "Art is like faith; you either believe or you don't."
> —Loretta Benedetto Marvel

In an interesting synchronicity, several of our authors in these pages have written about the Wizard of Oz as archetypal, and our culture's formative healing myth. It is the story of coming to wholeness through an imaginative, creative path and the quest for bringing vitality home again. The body, mind, and spirit are represented in the story as heart, brain, and courage. Mircea Eliade said, "The myths preserve and transmit the paradigms, the exemplary models, for all the responsible activities in which (people) engage." (1954, p.53) They return us to what it means to be truly human. Oz is myth-making and storytelling at its best.

We hope you will resonate with our stories about healing. Each chapter is a complete entity in itself. You may select where you read. This book is not meant to be read front to back only. It is organized around the primary modalities each author uses, with the first section being mostly essays that provide an overview of the process and the work. In Engaging Sound, we learn about the intimate connection between our breath, wind, and our spirit in tone or song. We also are reminded that our bodies are vibrational, just like all substances in the world, and we re-member rhythmic patterns that affect the workings of our brains.

Engaging Body reminds us of the feeling, e-motion, and motion connection. We know ourselves to be embodied souls. We see how the body becomes the garment of the soul, and we become more aware of how our bodies express our inner nature. The section on Image offers us symbols and their meanings, and reveals a bit about how manipulating them can teach us new things about ourselves. And the chapter on Word discusses how images in art make it possible for individuals to find deeper meanings than their words can express. In the section about Lifelong Learning, we see how the arts are being used in developmental stages of life to meet people where they are. We also see how the arts can facilitate the healing of specific conditions of dis-ease...

I think you will agree with me that these authors are outstanding in their field. We hope that you will engage with this book, that you will open your mind and heart to the stories, and that you will use the tools provided here. Many of the pieces within these pages have brought me to tears. I know they will move you also. If you want to know more about the authors, there is a biography section in the back of the book. Please visit it.

I don't know if I sound more like a cheerleader, or the preacher I used to be, but I do hope you will 'catch the spirit' within the pages of this book and get involved in this work. The first time I used the expressive arts with a patient in the hospital I was told, "I forgot I had cancer while we painted." Since that moment, I was hooked. She had gone to the place of remembered wellness, a place in her consciousness where she was whole again, and I know that going there, even for a moment, changed her body in subtle ways, and changed her outlook in great ones. For some suffering people, this is enough to move them into a cycle of healing. It does not have guarantees, but what healing system does? It does have hope. That is exactly what I want to offer the people in my care.

In concluding this introduction, I would like to share with the reader an excerpt from a speech given to a group of ministers gathered at Bayfront Medical Center in St. Petersburg, Florida, in 2001, by musician and author Reed Arvin, who has given his permission for its use. He said:

> "For me, the use of the arts in healing is not fluff. When the soul spins out of control, the body spins with it; likewise, when the body turns traitor, the soul has a powerful influence on its healing. I believe this influence to be profound, and I say this after having received the most invasive and powerful treatments that technology has to offer. A diagnosis of cancer led to a surgery that removed half my lungs and more. This, combined with chemotherapy, kept me from dying. Traditional medicine did not, however, give me back my life. I had to make a new life, full of unforeseen physical compromises and opportunities. It was a process that taught me the connection between the soul and the body. They are intimately connected, like aquatic life and the ocean it inhabits.
>
> In my journey, I learned that music and meditation can be as powerful as an Ativan. I learned that journaling wasn't simply writing down my thoughts; it was giving God an opportunity to speak into my life. I learned that every day I took care of my soul my body responded, and every day I ignored it my body paid the price. The arts are invaluable here because they bring peace into chaos. They make us happy, and happiness is an energy patients desperately need to heal their bodies. But they do something deeper and more sustaining: they remind us of a life beyond our illness. Given time, they can even teach us to love our battered bodies again. Technological medicine can do none of these things. And each of these impacts our bodies as surely as a scalpel.
>
> It doesn't matter whether your language of the soul is rooted in spiritual mysticism or in the interplay of endorphins and dopamine; both are a kind of magic for those who have eyes to see. The scientist and the pastor can be allies here, as they encourage painters, poets, sculptors, and musicians to bring their healing gifts to the hospital. In so doing, they will be making a powerful statement to patients to look beyond the pill and the

knife to be made whole again. Together, we can usher in a new era of healing. "

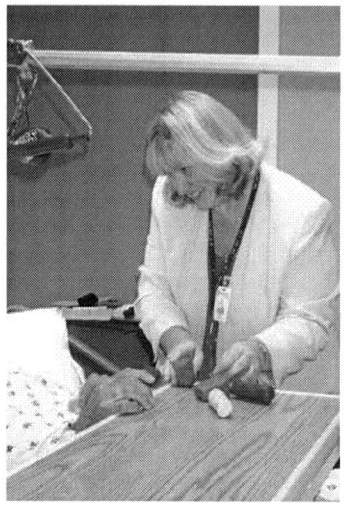

I thank Reed for this affirmation of the work of healing through the expressive arts, and I wish you, the reader, Godspeed on your own journey toward healing and toward finding your identity as a healing artist. Many of the essays in this book have touched the deep in me, and confirmed for me, again, that helping souls to find wholeness and peace is my true work here on earth. I hope they will do the same for you.

"Pay attention and your soul will live."
—Isaiah 55:63

Note: Please find all references for this introduction in the editor's essay section called "Of a Different Color…" Each author, as needed, has a 'works cited' section following his or her piece. Thank you.

FOREWORD

JANE GOLDBERG

Imagine a prolonged glimpse into the inner workings and practices of expressive arts professionals from around the world who have dedicated their lives to the service of healing those in pain and transition, and to those seeking greater fulfillment in their lives. This thoughtful publication offers you this rare opportunity.

The genesis of this wide ranging gathering of stories and methods of healing through the arts was the 18th Bi-Annual National Expressive Therapy Association (NETA) Conference in St. Petersburg, Florida in January of 2006. With the untimely death of the president of this association, Steve Ross, the conference coordinator Rev. Kathy Luethje and I took on more responsibility for the success of this conference than we had expected to. We organized groups each day to brainstorm and discuss new directions for the future. We wanted to keep the dream alive of a community of alternative expressive arts innovators. As a keynote speaker for the conference and a member of this association for 22 years, I was privileged to open the conference, to summarize the nature of our profession's innate calling and to help move us forward.

In our profession, we inspire others to open up to their own creativity and to set the stage for new beginnings or endings; to change. We nurture passions and cultivate enthusiasms for visions and dreams through the exuberance of creativity; expressing the light of imagination, and encouraging states of wonder and curiosity that call forth joy, freedom, delight and flow.
Kay Redfield Jamison, author of *An Unquiet Mind and Exuberance, The Passion for Life*, noted, "it is the infectious energies of exuberance that proclaim and disperse much of what is marvelous in life."

Absorption in the creative process *is* what heals us. Jung wrote that, "the approach to the numinous is the real therapy and inasmuch as you attain to numinous experiences you are released from the curse of pathology."

Rev. Kathy Luethje brightly welcomed all the facilitators and participants with warmth, sincerity and respect. People had come from all over the world to learn and to grow and to play. Presentations were filled with a palpable sense of heart and courage. We were ready to birth new beginnings. We were inspired to share our work. At the completion of the conference, Rev. Kathy invited workshop leaders to participate in a new undertaking, to share their wisdom and methodologies in the form of a book.

Kathy Luethje became the editor of "Healing with Art and Soul: Engaging One's Self through Art Modalities." Community members offered to share their work, ideas, stories and successes working with patients and clients over the years. Here, they have contributed their knowledge and experience in a text that provides a rich assortment of teaching stories that will help you understand and appreciate the transformational power of the expressive arts in many diverse settings. Each practitioner has been uniquely creative in designing, developing and communicating their own theories and approaches to this important work.

Earlier in their lives, each contributing practitioner had taken a risk and had stepped out to present this material in their respective settings when it wasn't the traditional choice to do so in our society at the time and they found acceptance.

It takes drive and passion to take that risk and to face the challenges inherent in bringing new material into the healthcare community. I wrote my doctoral dissertation in 1984 when the expressive arts therapies were barely recognized and respected as they are now. It was titled: "Diving Deep and Surfacing: A Creative Process Paradigm Form Change"

I proposed that the creative process, the therapeutic process and the recovery process are all parallel to each other. Isomorphic in form, they promote changes of a healing and constructive nature. I reframed the creative process as a framework for psychotherapy and revealed the 5 steps that are necessary for true and deep change. I recognized it as the archetypal pattern of change.

The synthesis of the creative process as a paradigm for change emerged in the metaphorical image of a downward-upward movement pattern entitled: Diving Deep and Surfacing. For psychotherapeutic purposes, it deals with resistance, blockages and fixations. The steps are (1) Diving In (2) Moving

Through The Waters (3) Finding The Treasure (4) Surfacing With The Treasure and (5) Sharing The Treasure. I discovered that the essence of the creative process *is* demonstrated through work and play with the expressive arts therapies

In the Fall of 1986, in light of my research, education and experience, I founded the Expressive Arts Training Institute in Newport Beach, California. We train and certify hundreds of students in our National Certification Programs, and we are delighted to see our graduates working in the world within their chosen professions. This educational/healing approach is now recognized in schools and universities, churches and synagogues, treatment centers, hospitals, individual and group psychotherapy offices, and in the community.

We all owe a great debt to the original pioneers in this Expressive Arts field, people like Shaun McNiff, Paolo Knill, Steve and Ellen Levine, and Natalie Rogers. We also wish to show our appreciation to those pioneers who listened to their own personal call, learned their skills and talents in their own way and have been out there in their own communities for years working successfully.

There are many paths to take in the creative journey to well-ness. There are many kinds of risks taken and rewards received. The number of us who have stepped forward with the vision of the healing power of creativity and the imagination, the dynamics of the creative process and the expressive arts as a catalyst for change, will definitely increase as more and more people come to accept the intrinsic value of creative and artistic approaches to healing mind, body, heart and soul.

A Course in Miracles states: "To heal is to make happy." There is no doubt in my mind that the work of the Expressive Arts will serve to make people happy, healthy and holy in ways we have not yet imagined. "Healing with Art and Soul" is filled with tools, techniques and exercises that you can immediately apply in your own work.

This book serves nonprofessionals and professionals alike. Whether you are considering entering the expressive arts field, a student or professional already in the field, a caregiver, an educator, a psychotherapist, an artist, a creative explorer and/or a lover of healing stories, I encourage you to take the time to appreciate the approaches presented in this textbook. They will give you a greater understanding of the human needs for creative self-expression and personal growth for achieving wholeness, joy and freedom as well as spark the creative process in your own life.

Jane Goldberg, Ph.D., L.M.F.T., R.E.A.T., C.E.T.
Distinguished Fellow of the National Expressive Therapy Association
Psychotherapist/Educator/Trainer
Director/Founder of The Expressive Arts Training Institute
www.ExpressiveArtsTraining.com

I: Surveying the Landscape: Pathography to Co-Creation

THE ART OF HEALING
AND THE SCIENCE OF ART

CAROL SHORE

Why are expressive arts programs being implemented in traditional healthcare settings such as hospitals? The short answer is—the arts work in ways that nothing else does, and they are cost-effective. Based on a model of wellness and human potential, of prevention and intervention, rather than a pathological model of diagnosis and cure, arts in medicine programs are "good medicine without harmful side effects."

The broader perspective sees the arts in medicine as part of an international movement toward integrative and complementary medicine that recognizes the patient as an essential partner in their medical team. Treating the whole person—body, mind, emotions and spirit—benefits healing, which is not the same as "cure."

What makes the very nature of art experiences inherently healing? This overview will outline a few basic principles of art as healing. A patient visit will document how the principles work in actual practice; however, names have been changed to protect confidentiality. Finally, an introduction into what I term the "science of art," will present key scientific discoveries that validate the positive effects of creative processes on the physiology and chemistry of healing, bridging science and art.

Art as healing is not a new idea. Since ancient times, the arts have been used to alleviate human suffering and to restore a sense of harmony, wholeness, or unity. The World Health Organization still defines "disease" in unscientific, almost poetic terms, as "a rupture in life's harmony". Cross-culturally, art has a long historical record of supporting life and health; art was a vehicle for experiencing the self as whole: body, mind, emotions, and spirit. Painting, dreams, storytelling, music and dance expressed the needs of individuals, relationships, and the collective life, and gave form to the great quests, initiations, thresholds and transformations of life that transmitted a sense of meaning, purpose or direction.

These phenomena are not rational goals, but ongoing creative life processes. Modern culture, however, has separated the individual from the creative tools by which he or she confronts the invisible needs, energies, forces and cycles of human life. The current focus in traditional medical institutions toward treating the whole person restores this basic human need for reuniting all aspects of the self for wholeness, haleness, healing. Art in medicine is integral to this revolutionary vision of what it means to heal.

The advent of arts in medicine programs in "temples of science" represents something of a paradigm shift. We live in a culture that overvalues reason, rationality, theoretical proofs and factual analysis over the soft evidence of direct experience, one's felt-sense of "knowing," or shifts in conscious awareness that transform or evolve one's very perception of reality.

A further problem exists in that the paradoxical process is not effectively communicated in words. It is best understood by direct personal experience, and those opportunities for changing personal and collective perceptions take time to develop. The arts uniquely meet a person where they are—from the need for simple diversion at one extreme, to the personal encounter with one's own living images at the other. In the short run, this diversity raises problems of stereotyping the work—seeing art in medicine as merely "arts and crafts" diversion on the one hand, or "art therapy" (viewed with guarded suspicion) on the other. These perceptions can be changed with experience and education.

The Intermodal Expressive Arts Model

The practice of arts in medicine at a specific hospital will be used as an example for this discussion. The program is based on the model of intermodal expressive arts. The term "intermodal" refers to the enhancing interplay among the arts when they are used interchangeably (Rogers, 1993:4.) Art in medicine works with creative expression in the physical, practical sense of experience, rather than theory. It creates a safe and protected environment where a person can experiment with natural, necessary expression, from which he may discover meaning in life-experiences—even challenging, fearful or life-threatening ones.

The intermodal expressive arts facilitator is not a therapist or an art teacher, but one who models entry into creative process and supports the process for others. This central concept of the creative process will be expanded in the principles that follow. Art is a dependable container that can carry the questions that we do not dare to ask without support. The creative process, not the facilitator, carries questions that are unspoken, or even beyond words. Realizing this removes the sense of burden for the artist-facilitator attending even the most burdensome images.

Art is inherently therapeutic and empowering: it does not need an intermediary. It is direct personal experience with constructive inner vision, with that which matters and gives life meaning. It gives practice in managing the powerful life energies we maneuver through us by making a container strong enough to bear with the process of change. The most therapeutic and healing effect of self-expression is that it restores this connection with self-trust, perseverance and meaning making. Attending or facilitating the person and the creative process in this way is akin to witnessing or perhaps midwifing "the image that heals," to use psychoanalyst C. G. Jung's powerful phrase. The process is inherently therapeutic, but not therapy.

The artist-facilitator sets up experiences for becoming attuned to one's own internal state and external expression, opening the possibility for the natural gradient toward healing to express itself symbolically. The artist in residence supports the living image that arrives with acceptance, curiosity and interest, modeling attitudes that respect the image, in contrast to cultural attitudes that habitually judge, compare or minimize.

This interaction between artist-facilitator and artist-participant is a rare open-ended exploration. Paolo Knill, expressive arts theorist, points out that unlike diagnostic disciplines, the creative inquiry approaches "limitations, disorders, disturbances or conflict not as things to be identified, labeled, judged or eliminated, but transformed." In its radical acceptance of what is, the expressive process invites an opening for what wants to come into being as healing potential.

The four key principles fundamental to the work of an Arts in Medicine program are:
1. **There is an artist in each of us.** We are all born with the power to create and transform our experience of life.
2. **You cannot fail.** The creative process is available to all in a safe and protected environment.
3. **Creative expression is about PROCESS rather than PRODUCT.** Engaging the creative process is the object of the work, and not the art product, performance, or outcome. The creative process is ongoing, with no final product.
4. **It is not interpretive:** Openness, freedom and safety are protected in an open studio environment, empowering each person's discovery of his/her unique potential and his/her own answers. There is no judgment, comparison, or interpretation; you may want to share or not.

The creative process is the active agent in art's restorative power. The creative process is real experience of concrete, sensuous life energies given expressive form (Kazanis, 1998.) Process is an experience of integrity that is initially beyond words, of body-mind systems working together in a state of flow. One is in contact with a different experience of time and being that is in itself restorative, and fosters resilience. In process, there is a sense of timeless being, where time is an eternal now. All tyranny of time evaporates—boredom, hurry, lateness, past and future, do not exist. There is contact with sources of deep relaxation and exhilarating energies that nourish the spirit, refresh hope and foster positive, dynamic relationship with authentic potential.

In process, one reconnects with the power of play, spontaneity and intuition, restoring the courage to feel. Creative play is discipline that is not repressive, but joyous. It has the quality of "effortless effort." Creative process expresses in images and wholes and is marked by a high tolerance for ambiguity: an attitude capable of embracing chaos and the unknown or feared thing, and letting go of goals to "play" out a paradox, while keeping in mind what is really important (Coulter, 1989.) When nothing makes sense, creating sense from playing with stimulating color or sensuous textures, can for example, express virtual emotion, or get "in touch" with intelligences beyond the rational alone.

Facilitating a person's shift into creative process benefits the mind/body/spirit in measurable ways that research is beginning to identify and validate. A model supporting resilience is an invaluable asset in a medical setting.

The term "creative process" is not synonymous with "creative product" or "art". The art product is merely a carrier of images into the world. Philosopher M. C. Richards calls art the "excrement of creative process;" that is, art is what is left over after digesting the nourishing life energies bubbling up within. An example of creative process follows.

Return from the Void

The chaplain's request for an arts in medicine visit had asked if we might do meditative movement in the patient's room, a form of gentle movement for healing in the T'ai Chi tradition. Mari was experienced in Yoga and Buddhist meditation, but in the aftermath of intense chemotherapy, she told the Rabbi, "My spirit left me." The emptiness was physical, like a hole, and she reported losing her ability to focus in meditation, her usual way of centering herself. When I knocked at the door of her room, I was surprised to be greeted by cheeriness quite out of keeping with the profound experience of loss of spirit. She was thin, almost frail, yet had a need to project this lighthearted voice as she now seemed to will the energy for moving meditation.

Afterward, I suggested painting in a circle, in the tradition of mandala sand paintings by Buddhist monks. She liked the idea. She announced, however, "I'm going to paint outside the circle. I'm painting 'being outside my body' and I'm leaving the center blank—the hole where my spirit left me." She said this now in a voice characteristic of telling a difficult truth that accompanies becoming more present to oneself, more real.

The void-empty center of her painting contrasted the surrounding colors. It was barren, cold, overwhelming. "The circle is too big," she said, reducing the size of it, when suddenly the brush accidentally slipped, making a crude orange cut into the pristine nothingness. "That's the hole in my stomach," she said, giving interpretation to the accidental. But it was clear that with one slip of the brush, her painting was taking her in directions not of her own choosing. For the first time she faltered, unsure how to proceed.

At that very moment, the arts in medicine musician knocked on the door, offering to play the harp for Mari. Sensitive to the process already underway, the musician was reluctant to interrupt, but Mari and I assured her that it was fortuitous timing. Live music might be just the inspiration to carry the moment past the place of not-knowing.

The music unfolded a sense of softness in the room—and in Mari as well—but starkly contrasted the painting's utterly empty circular center. "It needs some pink clouds," Mari sensed, and as she became absorbed with making pink to match an inner vision, no self-interpretation was superimposed on the work this time. Something more profound was taking form.

In a short time, she finished. I held the painting up at a distance so she could absorb it as a whole, and the full effect of it struck her for the first time. "It's the moon!" she exclaimed, "Surrounded by trees, like the moon peeking through the trees in my backyard! I've painted my new focus! A way to center myself in nature wherever I am!" The collaboration between moving meditation, live music and living image had supported a breakthrough, past the fearful emptiness of the trauma that is cancer, to the possibility of returning to a sense of self.

Mari's social worker was outside when I left the room, and as I listened to her concern that Mari always answered "no" when she was asked if there was anything she needed to talk about, I nodded that I understood. I had also run up against Mari's wall of protection that initially proclaimed "everything's fine." However, when words fail our truth, the arts can create an opening for authentic voice to speak in other ways.

For example, C. G. Jung points out that in a crisis of health, the natural healing function of the imagination spontaneously unfolds an image in support of the body-mind. "The image is healer," Jung says. I witness this phenomenon again and again, when like Mari's experience, The-Thing-Most-Feared flips to become the very thing that heals. Or, at the opposite extreme, when the prospects for a positive outcome are exhausted, a person's creative wrestling with fate will often galvanize a transforming awareness that heals denial and inner conflict with acceptance of a difficult truth, however unwelcome.

Finally, studies show that a traumatic event such as a diagnosis of cancer has the effect of overloading the senses. As a protective measure in crisis, the senses shut down, refusing to take in more stimulation, so that like Mari, one experiences "not being in there;" in essence, being in exile from the sensing body (Meyer, 1997.) The arts "bring us back to our senses," opening us again to feel, to express, to come alive—embodied and at one again. And research affirms the sooner, the better: unexpressed emotion is held in the body (Pert, 1999,) a stressor that can itself become symptomatic over time.

Why the Science of Art?

Mari had been open to exploring movement, painting and music as a way out of the void. But in the prevailing mindset of the culture that overvalues the literal, rational, provable, and factual—this risky, messy, unpredictable creative stuff is suspect. Until the rational mind "buys in," individuals habitually justify creative non-participation by parroting a mindless mantra that goes something like this: "I'm no artist, I'd just ruin it." "I can't draw a straight line with a ruler." "I can't carry a tune in a bucket." "I've got two left feet." In this passive model of creativity, the individual has license to abdicate self-creative powers and responsibilities, and to invest them in professionals of all kinds—"artists," but also doctors, clergy, authorities and celebrities of all stripes. Creative expression involves doing, actively involving oneself in the process of becoming, of healing, of discovery. It feels risky.

In my experience, one way to beat the rational conventional mindset is to join it. I find that if I give a person's reasoning mind a "good reason" to enjoy themselves in creative play, then they can often give themselves permission to risk opening up to creative possibility, as Mari did. It can begin by simply asking, "What is your favorite color," filling a brush with the color and inviting them to add one stroke to a community painting. And then Process often takes them over. Like eating peanuts, it's hard to have just one.

But more importantly, affirming the "science of art" can cut the cultural tape loop, opening a new conversation with the individual. Science is now discovering the positive effects of creative expression on the physiology and chemistry of healing. For example, a person whose rational attitudes defend against non-rational, non-directive creative experiences will often take down the wall when given a good reason to participate. A facilitator can say, for example, "research shows that creativity creates endorphins, improving mood and creating a sense of well being."

Given a morsel of scientific benefit, the rational mind easily gives permission for the child within each of us to come out and play. I have even observed this inner struggle acted out as a mind-body split. Just as the person is in the middle of an "I'm no artist" mantra, his hand will simultaneously reach for the brush on the table before him, and begin painting. It is as if the creative child inside, having been given safety and a good reason to assert, "but I want to do it," will not take "no" for an answer this time.

It is then that the "art of healing" ceases to be the bailiwick of the person's medical professionals, and becomes their own empowering process. Art that is personal, courageous and empowering restores a person to their internal sources of wisdom and intuition, to the knowing body's felt-sense of truth, and the living images that bubble up from below, unfolding awareness of unrealized potential.

There is a growing body of evidence in scientific research—the "science of art," so to speak—that is making it possible for people in a crisis of health to value their curative creative imagination. Science is beginning to unlock the physiology and chemistry underneath art's ancient roots in healing, making art relevant to ordinary life. Two outstanding examples highlight the growing field of research.

Brain research identifies creative expression as a function of the brain's right hemisphere. Functioning "in our right mind," so to speak, is a balancing mindset for the left hemisphere brain functions of reason and logic. It is in right hemisphere functioning that we process the mystery, wonder and awe of life, experience our aliveness. In right-mind process, we are in touch with a timeless, spacious sense of being that researcher Dr. Herbert Benson termed the "Relaxation Response," an altered state of awareness and physiologic change that can be aptly characterized as "remembered wellness" (Benson, 1975.) Cultural attitudes, however, devalue the image-making function of one-half of our information processing capability. Half a mind is a terrible thing to waste.

Linking Mind, Body and Emotions

The work of Candace Pert represents in many ways, in her words, "a convergence between what is known in ancient wisdom (traditions) and what is known in classical neuroscience" (Pert, 2000, audiotape one.) Her model shows the way in which biochemical "information molecules" such as peptides and their receptors flow and resonate, distributing information to every cell in the body simultaneously. It has unlocked the secret of how emotions literally transform our bodies—and create or disrupt our health. The role of consciousness and emotion in this "intelligence and information network" we know as the self is not to be ignored, according to Pert. Emotions are at the nexus between matter and mind, going back and forth between the two and influencing both. Consciousness—what we pay attention to—is central; it is the link between the emotions and the body.

According to Pert, mind can be understood as a constantly changing flow of molecular information in motion. The subconscious mind is the body itself; body faithfully reporting just outside conscious awareness. As we become consciously aware of this flow of information as emotions, we understand this psychosomatic network as dynamic, shifting. Pert declares:

"All of our cells are intelligent entities. Our immune system is changing moment to moment—we're much more like flickering flames than we are like hunks of meat. The emotions are key to our health—how much we flicker. That's what the alternative (complementary) medicine movement is all about... The scientific evidence is overwhelming that meditation, affirmation and visualization have been scientifically shown to alter the course of cancer...Multi-dimensional mind-body interventions work"
(Pert, 2000, audiotape two.)

In her view, expressivity is key to framing consciousness, making it possible for conscious mind to enter the network and play a deliberate and new part. Not expression as a "let it all hang out" catharsis, but as emotional integrity. Pert cites case studies of cancer patients who realized unexpressed anger and experienced spontaneous remission of tumors. "Anger can give a huge jump-start to the immune system," she says. Creative-expressive life matters. That is, it makes a material difference in immunologic strength.

Former professor of cellular biology at Stanford University and research scientist in quantum physics, Bruce Lipton states, "Biology is seventy-five years out of date. Genes do not control biology, perception controls biology" (Lipton, 2001.)

From these bridging perspectives, the role of the creative process as form-giver for our perception has biological implications. One cannot make authentic images without making positive change. Our images create the container strong enough to hold the stresses that threaten to break body, mind or spirit and make it possible to become present with the irrational and uncontrollable factors of the unknown, with the paradox, mystery and potent invisible forces of life.

One thing is clear—this is a time of creative shift in understanding—in science, in institutions, in culture, and in the individual. Could it be that art in medicine is the first tick of the pendulum in this shift back toward a new balance? Art is not separate from life; it is a living evolutionary process that strengthens life from the inside, especially in times of crisis.

Michaelina's Angel

This story is true in essential content, but names have been changed to protect patient confidentiality.

As Artist-In-Residence at a local hospital, I am often asked, "Isn't that awfully depressing work?"

That question always makes me think of working with Michaelina. She was a young woman far from her home in another country, battling a terminal cancer.

She spoke no English, and I spoke pitiful little Spanish. But the arts in medicine referral summoned me to her room anyway, to "do what you can." Standing there in the hall with watercolors, I admit that I felt foolish and more than a little inadequate.

Entering her room, I found Michaelina visibly in pain, doubled up one minute, tossing the next. "Should I come back later?" I asked in sign language. She drew me closer with a limp finger. I showed her my artist's tools and pantomimed my intention to paint for her. Unable to communicate the benefits of the process, I made a ritual of setting up to work.

Immediately her focus shifted from physical discomfort to a surprising steely determination to control even this benign activity in her territory. She stopped me with a foreign but pointed command, and if I could have excused myself and left, I would have, for then she was on the telephone, speaking with an interpreter. I sat motionless on my low painting stool during what seemed an endless exchange, even for the Spanish language.

At length, she handed the telephone to me. I explained to the translator that an arts in medicine visit can create a shift in environment—a positive field, if you will—that can have a beneficial effect on pain perception, on emotional well-being, and potentially even on immune response and healing. "With her permission, I plan to paint an angel for her."

I returned the receiver to Michaelina for the translator to relay my message in Spanish. Michaelina gave permission to proceed with a gesture that struck me as part command and part warding-off injury.

It had been an odd beginning, but I could think nothing of it then, as I entered the creative process. It is a place where everyone in the immediate environment can enter with me into the fluid state that takes us beyond ordinary awareness. It is a magical space, and as I painted, Michaelina became quiet, absorbed in the moment, as the angel emerged from the nothingness of white paper. Not like any angel seen before, but stroke by stroke, bearing more and more resemblance to Michaelina herself, raven-haired and exotic. At the bottom, I wrote the title: *Michaelina's Angel*.

When I moved to hang the painting on the back of the door, the spell was broken. Michaelina abruptly assumed control, stopping me with a pointed finger that says *not there; hang it over here!* In that moment, I became aware that the strength of her wordless command was matched by her body's command over her pain. I was witness to a remarkable change in her level of comfort, and yet as I made my way out the door, I doubted what value, if any, Michaelina herself would attach to my visit.

Several weeks later, Irma G. stopped by the arts in medicine open studio. She is a member of the psychosocial and palliative care department, and a sensitive artist herself. Irma was visibly excited as she called the team into a conference room nearby to update us on the patient we have in common.

"I have been working with Michaelina, the young woman from another country," Irma began. I nod in recognition. Irma relayed the news that Michaelina had failed her initial chemotherapy trials. This is often a negative indicator for chemotherapy outcomes, and then the social worker is called in to introduce the possibility of support services such as Hospice to the patient.

But when Irma visited Michaelina, even Irma's fluent Spanish met with communication barriers. Michaelina is an indigenous native of her country, and Spanish is her second language, not her native tongue. With great patience, slowly, Irma learned Michaelina's extraordinary story.

In her native village, Michaelina was married to a man who abused her, and so she made plans to leave him. Discovering her intention, he secretly removed some of her personal articles, took them to a native shaman and had him put a curse on her. His intention was to cause her harm, to kill her. Michaelina was convinced that her disease was a direct result of that curse, and that she was going to die.

There was nothing Irma could say to convince the girl otherwise. At a loss to know how to proceed, Irma's gaze idly fell on a patch of brilliant color on the wall facing the bed. *Michaelina's Angel*, it said.

Inspiration struck. "Michaelina," Irma said, "I am going to tell you a story. It is a story of power, the power of your very own name." Irma plunged into character—"matching wits with the shaman, engaging in a battle of words to rescue the girl's hope".

"You are named after Michael, the Archangel. It is said he is the greatest of the angels. He is the one who fights the dark forces with the power of light, and triumphs. This is the meaning of your name, Michaelina. The triumph of light over darkness."

Irma pointed to the angel on the wall. "Look. You have your own angel watching over you. She even looks like you. You do not fight this fight alone. The curse of one shaman has no power to match your heritage, your protector and namesake."

Irma admitted it was a long shot. "I felt," she said, "as if in that moment, it was *Irma Versus the Shaman*, and that Michaelina's life hung in the balance. Could I conjure up the forces of good convincingly enough to outweigh the grip of fear? The only thing in my favor was that the invisible, intangible power of the shaman was no match for the real presence of that angel right there in the room with us."

Irma took a long breath. "I came to tell you the story because Michaelina has been released from the hospital," she said.

"But what about her cancer?" we asked, almost in unison.

"She passed her remaining chemo trials with flying colors. I can hardly believe it. Against all odds, there is no trace of the cancer. She is not entirely out of the woods, but she is in remission and living with relatives in the United States.

"And she took her angel with her. I thought you'd like to know *the rest of the story*."

Artist in Residence at a hospital: is it awfully depressing work?

Not in the least!

Resources

Benson, Herbert, MD. *The Relaxation Response.* New York: Avon Books, 1975.

Coulter, Dee. *The Inner Dynamics of Creativity.* Boulder, CO: Sounds True Audio, 1989.

Jung, C. G. *Man and His Symbols.* Garden City, NY: Doubleday & Company, 1964.

Kazanis, Barbara. classroom lectures at University of South Florida, 1997.

Knill, Paolo J., Helen Nienhaus Barba, Margo N. Fuchs. *Minstrels of Soul: Intermodal Expressive Therapy.* Toronto, Ontario, Canada: Palmerston Press, 1995.

Lipton, Bruce, PhD. "Mind Over Genes." Audiotape, Lecture at the Psychology of Health, Immunity and Disease Conference, December 2001.

Meyer, Melinda. "Trauma: In Exile from the Body." Video Documentary, 1997.

Pert, Candace. *Molecules of Emotion: The Science Behind Mind-Body Medicine.* New York: Simon & Schuster, 1999.

—. "Your Body is Your Subconscious Mind." Boulder, Colorado: Sounds True Audio, 2000.

Rogers, Natalie. *Creative Connection: Expressive Arts as Healing.* Palo Alto, California: Science and Behavior Books Inc., 1993.

HEALING PRESENCE

JULIA BALZER RILEY

Healing presence...intention...moments of connection, the foundation of our work. Healing presence is the gift of holding the sacred space for the work of the expressive arts in healthcaring. Intention is the tool for setting the stage, the entrée into the work of the expressive arts in healthcaring. Moment of connection is the increment of time where the work of the expressive arts in healthcaring begins. My own work is informed by the body of work that is holistic nursing, the body of work that is psychiatric nursing and by my experience as an expressive arts facilitator in end-of-life care at a Hospice in Florida.

See what you think of this:

As I care for myself, so I care for my clients...

As I care for myself, so I care for my colleagues...

As I care for myself, so I care for my friends and family...

To be fully present for others, you must assume responsibility for your own self-care, for your own healing. In holistic nursing we say, holistic self-care is the foundation of holistic nursing.

Before you approach the bedside of a client, you must set aside your own concerns to bring your whole self to the client. A centering technique is helpful for this. See **Handout 1,** entitled, **Respirit**...bringing our selves to our work by intention: Being Fully Present. Take a few moments to read over the exercise. Close your eyes and practice this. In my hospice work, from practice, I shorten this to, "All concerns set aside; I ask that this interaction is for the greater good of the client." Then I use an imagery of placing my credentials aside, perhaps wrapped around a shrub on the way into the client's place of residence, and enter as just Julie, myself. We are setting the intention to be co-participants in the creation of the healing environment.

This work can be measured in moments, moments of connection. A client says, "I had fun today," or, " I AM an artist." Sometimes the intervention is a family intervention. I received a hospice referral for a 95-year-old man who, "Likes to talk about his days in New York as a musician. The family is looking forward to an art visit for the father." I do not have his diagnosis; because unlike my work in nursing, I am not called to spend much of my focus on details of illness except as limitations must be taken into account for successful work as client-artist. I approach each person as someone new to meet, unique. I am curious, with as little pre-judgment as possible, accepting the person as whole just as he is. Each visit is complete into itself.

To prepare for the visit, I took a CD player and music of Frank Sinatra and Tony Bennett. Intuitively, I tucked simple watercolor supplies into my art bag, a gentle introduction to expressive art making with guaranteed success once the client is willing to engage. I greeted the family and immediately focused on the client, smiling, giving direct eye contact, touching his hand. I engaged the family in setting up the music for him. I demonstrated the use of the materials, and I added color to the paper with him. After creating a watercolor on color diffusion paper (available at www.ssww.com, search keywords 'color diffusion paper,') "Just let the colors choose you and touch the brush to the paper," I said. An 85-year-old man who claimed his hands were "too stiff to paint" named his painting; "Call it a Magnificent Work of Art." After he saw the mounted piece, he exclaimed, "I AM an artist."

His daughter-in-law sent the painting, which we made into a card, gluing the small painting onto folded 8 ½ x 11" cardstock, using an envelope, 5 ¾ x 8 ¾" (purchased at Wal-Mart in a box of 50,) to his son. She said, "I will write the title on it and have him sign it. His son will be so surprised. He is a lawyer and I know he will hang it in his office. I will have Dad sign it." The stepson, who is an artist, chose the background color and enjoyed painting a card himself, never having seen the color diffusion paper. I had provided another older woman in the home who was curious with her own tin of watercolor and she painted on watercolor paper as well. I offered her stiff watercolor paper that did not require newspaper under it. I left several sheets of this paper with the stepson, who says she likes to draw fashion design and he will sketch some figures for her to paint on the next visit. While they both painted, the rest of the family sat and enjoyed the music and exclaimed that this time was the highlight of their week, so focused, usually, on full-time care giving for two family elders.

This scenario represents a rare treasure, a time for a whole family intervention. I was setting the intention for the greatest good; centering myself; bringing supplies based on initial referral information; trusting my intuition in bringing simple but engaging, elegant art materials; assessing the family as I went; going with the flow; allowing the process and intervention to unfold. In his second painting, the client painted musical instruments, told stories of his days on the road as a slide trombone player, demonstrated how he played, laughing and singing. At the end, he sang a love song to me from the 40's and I teased him, telling him, my husband was in trouble since he didn't sing to me. The daughter-in-law quipped that her neighbor says the same thing when he sings to her. The family had a good laugh together. Using gentle banter and humor reaffirms that he is still alive. Here is the opportunity to learn something new, to be in genuine contact with another person…what Martin Buber calls the I-Thou relationship, when the God in me meets the God in you. Here is healing, support, joy, and increase in self-confidence at his new status as "artist." His stories are honored by the healing presence of the arts facilitator and his family who willingly hear them again, who remind him of others to tell, and praise him for the wonderful life he has led. I thank the client and his family for the privilege of working with them. They tell me the work is a blessing to them. We agree we will sing together next time and I will bring a CD of elder sing-along songs.

In this intervention, the art is non-directed and the emphasis is on the process of the art making, not the product. He tells stories as he paints and points out a piano, mimes a piccolo, and uses gold paint to create a trombone. Paradoxically, in end-of-life care, the product of the artwork becomes valuable as legacy. My own mother was a hospice patient before this work was available. How I would have loved to have a piece of art she created with her own hands. The arts facilitator brings skills to the work to offer presentation of the art to enhance the visual appeal. In hospice care, I am looking for inexpensive, user-friendly supplies to set the client artist up to win, to produce something of value. We paint on silk, using hoops with silk stretched across them, which makes a finished piece. The cards are introduced as a place to share something left unsaid. A reluctant client may enter into a "conversation with color." First, I make a mark with color, then the client responds, and so forth until a painting is created. I ask him, "What do you see in the painting?" I ask him to "give it a name." I may bring poetry magnets for poem making. I may scribe the client's response to the activity, "My life in 25 words or less." I may scribe life stories, add digital photographs or clipart, and return typed copies for family keepsakes. I may offer clay and ask the client to simply enjoy touching it, kneading it, asking for a process of the object made or the process itself.

A natural free-flowing humor sets the tone for sacred play. The word silly comes from the Greek word, "selig," meaning blessed. I easily accept anything that goes "wrong" in the session. One of the CD's I brought skipped. The stepson got his disk cleaner and fixed it. A slow, comfortable pace; a willingness to change direction if something does not go well; an acceptance that all is well and whatever the result, it is just as it should be; these are strategies that serve me well.

The foundation for this work for me is the F.O.C.U.S.E.D.® model, which I created in response to my question, how could I teach the notion of presence to nurses and nursing students? How can I break it down into steps and a process rather than just words or assumptions that being present is something everyone intuitively understands? See **Handout 2**: F.O.C.U.S.E.D.® on Moments of Connection for this work. This model helps you stay in the moment and addresses the need for self-care and reflective time of disconnection, a letting go to return to center. This model began 37 years ago when I first studied Buber's notion of the I-Thou relationship, which I saw as the true nurse-patient relationship. This understanding of the sacred nature of moments of connection underpins my work as an expressive arts facilitator. The article by J. Watson reveals a nurse theorist who develops caring as a nursing tenet. See this influence in my **Handout 3**: Guidelines for intentional caring-healing practice, for the development of a self-practice to continue this work.

Finally, let's take a moment for you to create a plan for self-care to support your bringing you whole self, being able to be present at the bedside. Create your plan. See **Handout 4**: My plan/contract to **Re-spirit, Re-inspire, and Re-vitalize** my practice and my life.

Handout 1:
Respirit...bringing ourselves to our work by intention

Being Fully Present
Centering Technique for Healthcaring

Honor the sacred nature of your work. Take time each day to connect with your own purpose in your work. In holistic nursing, we practice centering techniques to still our minds and help us be fully present as we enter sacred space between client and nurse. Try this brief strategy:

1. Before you interact with a client, pause and take a deep breath
2. Let go of any distractions, or worries, or your "to do" list
3. Say silently to yourself, "I am here for the greater good of this client"
4. Think of someone or some situation in which you feel loved and hold onto this heart-centered feeling
5. Set the intention to be present and take another deep breath.

Dossey, B. M., L. Keegan, and C.E. Guzzetta, Holistic nursing: A handbook for practice, Sudbury, MA: Jones and Bartlett Publishers. 2005.

Zikorus, P The importance of a nurse's presence, Holistic Nursing Practice, 21:4 (2007) July/August, 208.

Centering may be a type of self-referencing biofeedback, controlling one's own heart rate. Heart rate variability changes when the emotional state changes. Research shows that when people shift their attention to their heart and feel love and appreciation, there is a greater balance between the sympathetic and parasympathetic nervous systems and their heart rates becomes coherent. When the person feels frustration, the heart rate increases in variability (McCraty et al, 1993.)

©2006 Julia Balzer Riley, RN, MN, AHN-BC, CET® Used with permission.

Handout 2:
F.O.C.U.S.E.D® on moments of connection

I. F.O.C.U.S. on moments…connections that make a difference

The I-it and I-Thou relationship (M. Buber)…looking for the sacred "What is being in the moment but being in touch with God? Who might also be called the Great Now…" (J. Cameron.)

II. **F**eel

Disconnect from personal distractions. Stay in the moment. Anticipate needs of clients, families, staff, and community. Be fully present, one thing at a time

III. **O**bserve

Look for opportunities to connect. Watch for signs of fear, anxiety, grief, confusion. Pay attention to verbal and nonverbal cues

IV. **C**onnect

Take the initiative to approach. Listen, speak, touch, share, recommend resources, offer silent prayer if appropriate, offer a private place, and offer something to drink

V. **U**nderstand

Seek first to understand before to be understood (S. Covey.) Share meaning in the illness experience. Use empathy to share your own experience, offer hope. Consider lessons you can learn.

VI. **S**hare

Share stories of moments of connection. Celebration of the connections, the gifts of intimate moments. Today and each day….making a difference in the future of healthcare. We define our practice by the stories we tell.

VII. Now…to stayed F.O.C.U.S.E.D.™…renew your commitment to life balance

VIII. **E**nergize…find ways to restore your energy.

IX.   Disconnect…take time to be alone, use inner resources

©1997, Julia Balzer Riley, RN, MN, AHN-BC, CET® Used with permission. Not to be copied without permission.

Handout 3:
Guidelines for intentional caring-healing practice

Re-spirit, Re-inspire, and Re-vitalize

This is written in nursing language. Reflect on how this applies to your own work.

1.   Begin each day with a spiritual practice such as a period of silence   and gratitude.

2.   Set the intention to be present this day and let go of things you cannot control

3.   Work to a return to the "now" during the day, framing your workplace as a sacred, healing environment.

4.   Make an effort to see the "person" behind the illness and trust the ability of people to access the healer within, in a process than cannot be rushed, fixed, or controlled by yours or others' expectations.

5.   See life experiences as lessons to grow more deeply into your own humanity.

6.   Forgive yourself for imperfections and grow in your ability to be nonjudgmental of the other person.
 End your day with gratitude for the events of the days, bless and forgive all that has entered into the sacred circle of your life and work. Let go of the day…..breathe!!!!!!!! Go play! Be with others and yourself…Energize and Disconnect (1-7 modified from Watson.) During the day take 3 minutes to ponder those things you appreciate in life.

7. Keep a journal to maintain a sense of Wonder about your work, Give yourself 5 minutes each day to answer: What surprised me today? What moved me or touched me as a human being? What inspired me today?

8. Engage in regular art-making such as a mandala journal.

©2006 Julia Balzer Riley, RN, MN, AHN-BC, CET® Used with permission

Handout 4:
My plan/contract to Re-spirit, Re-inspire, and Re-vitalize my practice and my life.

Reflect upon what you enjoy. What activity causes you to be in the flow, one in which you are so engaged that you lose the sense of the passing of time? What is fun for you? With whom can you spend time that is joyful? How can you just relax? These are the times and activities that replenish you and allow you to be F.O.C.U.S.E.D. ® on moments of connection

One thing I will do to be more fully present for my self and for my work:

_____

Signature

©2008 Julia Balzer Riley, RN, MN, AHN-BC, CET® Used with permission

References and Suggested Reading

Belitz, C., and M. Lundstrom. *The Power of Flow: Practical Ways to Transform Your Life with Meaningful Coincidences.* New York: Harmony Books, 1997.

Bolton, G. *Dying: Bereavement and the Healing Arts.* Philadelphia, PA: Jessica Kingsley Publishers, 2008.

Buber, Martin. *I and Thou.* New York: Harper & Row, 1958.

Cameron, Julia. *The Artist's Way.* Los Angeles: Jeremy P. Tarcher, Inc., 2002.

Covey, Stephen. *Seven Habits of Highly Effective People.* New York: Free Press, 1990.

Dossey, Brabara, L. Keegan, and C.Guzuetta, *Holistic Nursing: Handbook for Practice.* Sudbury, MA: Jones & Bartlett Publishers, 2005.

Ganim. Barbara. *Art and Healing: Using Expressive Art to Heal Your Body, Mind, and Spirit.* New York: Three Rivers Press, 1999.

Hawkins, AH. *Reconstructing illness: Studies in Pathography.* West Lafayette, Indiana: Purdue University Press, 1993.

Malchiodi, Cathy. A. *Expressive Therapies.* New York: The Guildford Press. 2005.

—. *The Art Therapy Sourcebook.* Los Angeles: Lowell House. 1998.

—. *The Soul's Palette: Drawing on Art's Transformative Powers for Health and Well-Being.* Boston: Shambala. 2002.

McCraty, R.M. Atkinson, and W.A. Tiller. *New Electrophysiological Correlates Associated with Intentional Heart Focus.* New York: Subtle Energies, 1993.

Nachmanovitch, S. *Free Play: Improvisation in Life and Art,* Los Angeles: Jeremy P. Tarcher, Inc. 1990.

Riley, Julia B. *Communication in Nursing.* St Louis: Mosby. 2008.

—. *From the Heart to the Hands: Keys to Healthcaring Connections,* I.M.P.S. Constant Source Seminars. 1999.

Watson, J. "Intentionality and Caring-Healing Consciousness: A Practice of Transpersonal Nursing." *Holistic Nursing Practice.* 16(4): (2002) 12-19.

Zikorus, P. "The Importance of a Nurse's Presence.", *Holistic Nursing Practice*, 21(4): (July/August 2007) 208.

THE HEALING MIND

CHARLES H. WARE

During an office visit when my children were small, our family dentist told me he had ordered a new, water-cooled drill that was going to reduce or eliminate the pain that patients experience during drilling. He explained that conventional drills and drilling generate a lot of heat and the heat is what causes the pain. He said the next time I need any drilling he would like me to consider allowing him to use no Novocain (the painkiller of choice in those days.) He assured me he would go very slowly and if I experienced any trouble, he would give me painkiller. He was a gentle man and had always treated me as if I were one of his young patients; I decided that I would go ahead with his pain management experiment.

The next time I needed drilling, we discussed the water-cooled drill, the dentist used it, and it worked! There was some sensation where he was drilling but not pain. We continued this practice of no numbing for more than ten years, ending it when my family and I moved away.

There were times when the drilling hurt. It hurt the way you would think drilling without numbing would hurt, except somewhat less severely. On those occasions, wishing to support my dentist's use of the new drill and his slow, gentle procedures, I hung on.

After moving away and finding a new dentist, I wanted to continue the practice of no numbing. For one thing, I enjoyed the idea of it and, more importantly, I experienced much less pain after the drilling stopped. This may have been because the dentist who introduced me to this idea worked more slowly than others. Later on, other dentists may have worked more slowly simply because they knew they had not given me painkiller. In any event, the dentists who worked on me were perfectly willing to adopt this practice for me; they liked it because they did not have to delay drilling until after the painkiller took effect.

Sometimes it did not work so well. It may have been because the dentist was working more quickly that day, not mindful of my situation. Or the drilling came closer to the nerve. Or I may have had a different mindset. I don't know. However, when I felt that I needed to hang on, I would "go to the beach"—that is, visualize a pleasant scene, typically a beach scene—and let go of the pain. (Resisting pain tends to intensify it.)

One particularly enlightening experience occurred when the dentist was drilling a tooth in my right lower jaw. I had trouble rising above the pain, and the drilling lasted longer than usual. I hung on. When it was over, I had a strange sensation in my jaw. The right side was numb and the left side was not! Responding to the stress of the drilling, my body had numbed the area being worked on and left the other side untouched. I had experienced these same effects on many occasions before I gave up Novocain and similar drugs. I thought I had given up numbing, but the body did the job when the need arose.

This was my introduction to the mind-body relationship and the healing mind. Now my goal is to help others find healing pathways. I intend to do that by sharing what has been experienced by others and by me.

***

Personal history

My relationship with disease and allopathic medicine has its roots in my family history. My mother, three of her sisters, and my sister were nurses. My brother-in-law was an MD, as is his son. My mother, who did not practice nursing very often, had holiday dinners that were planned around the schedules of her two sisters who did. There was a lot of talk at home about one disease or another and one patient or another. In the accounts of the struggles between disease and health, disease usually won.

Piercing this gloom was the fact that when I was eight years old I experienced double lobar pneumonia, was in a coma for seven days, consumed seven large tanks of oxygen, and fully recovered. How? With the tender, loving, round-the-clock care of my mother and two aunts and the work of the homeopathic family doctor.

Sometime during the last five years, I gave up my faith in disease. The selected readings listed at the end of this chapter have taught me that the mind is capable of letting go of tuberculosis, cancer, heart disease, and many other conditions.

Expressive Therapy

It seems to me that Expressive Therapy is rooted in the mind-body connection. The healing that comes from Expressive Therapy starts with the mind choosing healing; it is a subject beyond what I will cover here although the choice for healing is available to all of us. Having made that choice, we can then choose a modality—art, music, dance, drama—to be the medium through which we will make the mind-body connection.

Here the role of the body is not to be the vehicle for art, music, dance, or drama; it is the object of our healing. I will present some examples of the mind-body relationship to lay the groundwork for Expressive Therapy.

Pain management

A friend of mine needed major surgery. Having had a very bad experience with anesthesia in the past, she was reluctant to be anesthetized for the operation. She was experienced in the practice of self-hypnosis and taught it to clients. She decided to use self-hypnosis for pain management for what turned out to be one and a half hours of surgery. She easily found a doctor who was willing to perform the operation, the only stipulation being that an anesthesiologist must stand by. Not only did she manage the pain, but she also controlled the bleeding—there was almost none. And one of the benefits the surgeon did not foresee was her rapid recovery from the operation. By giving herself suggestions for healing quickly, my friend was back to normal in a week instead of the normal four-week period!

This friend has taught self-hypnosis for pain management to her children with great success. When her son was five years old, he fell down the stairs at home and put a large gash in his forehead. His mother heard him fall and picked him up, and upon seeing the huge white gash immediately told him to turn off the bleeding. He responded, "I don't know how". She told him, "It's easy; it's the switch next to the pain switch". To which he said, "Oh." Then she told him, "While you're at it, go ahead and turn off the pain switch as well". He only bled one drop of blood and the gash remained white. She reminded him of what he had been taught—the pain is there to alert you to the fact that you need medical attention and when that has been accomplished, it's good to turn off the pain. She assured him she was going to take care of him and get him to the hospital. When they got to the Emergency Room, it was difficult to get medical attention for the injured boy–he was not crying and or bleeding. My friend called the family physician, who came to the hospital and closed the wound with twelve stitches.

Here we see the power of the healing mind of a five-year-old boy. It suggests that this is a natural process, nothing intellectually challenging, just acting in good faith to "turn off the pain" and "stop the bleeding." It's available to you and me.

I let go of my allergy to cats

Many years ago, my wife, Sharon, and I attended a weeklong conference at the Edgar Cayce Foundation in Virginia Beach. The conference was entitled *New Dimensions in Healing* and the presenters were leaders in alternative healing. The presentation that had a profound effect on me illustrated the role forgiveness can play in healing. We were told the story of a woman who had a lymphoma in her right leg. Despite the fact that she meditated and prayed for healing, the disease progressed to the point where amputation was necessary.

The woman developed symptoms in her left leg similar to those she had experienced in her right leg. While meditating and praying for healing, an episode from her childhood came to her. She and her mother were standing on a subway platform, she was fooling around, the subway train was approaching the station, she slipped, and her mother yanked her back to safety with the words, "You're so clumsy and stupid, someday you're going to lose your (right) leg." Recalling this as an adult, her relationship with her mother came flooding back. She saw that she needed to forgive her mother as well as herself for their respective roles in that difficult relationship–forgive until the relationship was healed. This is what she did, and the symptoms in her left leg disappeared.

A few months before we attended the conference, Sharon suggested I didn't need to be allergic to cats. I completely dismissed the idea since it was clear to me I had no control over my allergic reaction. Up until then, when she and I attended a meeting in someone's home I started wheezing, I would ask if our hosts had a cat, be told they did, but be assured that the cat(s) would not bother me because it/they were outside.

Soon after *New Dimensions in Healing*, I got a flash. As a boy, eight to ten years of age perhaps, on a number of occasions my mother and two of my aunts would be chatting in our living room and the subject of Aunt Florence's cat and me would come up. When I was two years old, we were all visiting Aunt Florence's farm and her cat jumped on my back while I was on the kitchen floor; it terrified me. The telling and retelling of this story always ended with the three sisters engulfed in gales of laughter. Watching and listening to this, I felt clumsy, stupid, and embarrassed. Looking at it from the perspective of *New Dimensions in Healing*, I saw that I needed to forgive.

I forgave my mother and her two sisters for their behavior towards me in this. I forgave myself for "getting even" by exhibiting the symptoms of asthma. And I forgave the cat.

Had this enabled me to let go of my allergy to cats? I soon had a chance to find out. Ten days after the conference, Sharon and I were on Cape Cod for a mini–vacation. At the last minute, her sister and nephew decided to stay with us for one night. We had room for only one more so we asked friends on the Cape if I could stay with them. Response: of course I could.

As we reached the driveway of friends' house, we saw a cat on the front lawn: theirs. Inside was another cat in the living room. I then remembered that the last time we visited these friends I had experienced a full-blown asthma attack.

This time I was taken downstairs and told I would be staying in their daughter's room: "One cat sleeps here, and the other one sleeps over there." **I was to sleep in the cats' room!** My reaction was: Here's my chance! That evening I practiced forgiveness and drank extra water at dinner (to ease any congestion), and that night I slept well. So far, so good.

Ten days later, Sharon and I visited overnight at the home of one of my daughters and her family; they had two cats. During the previous visit, my asthma became so acute that even though I used medicine and inhalers, we had to leave around midnight to go to a motel so I could breathe. Here was another big chance! We stayed overnight, I had no asthma symptoms, and I concluded I had indeed let go of my allergy to cats. Since then we have always had cats of our own, sometimes as many as three.

This story illustrates the effects of the healing mind. There was no other intervention in my allergic reaction. In some sense, I simply changed my mind about it. Since then, I have looked to build a universal principle around this experience, but I have not succeeded. For now, I am content to enjoy my new relationships with cats and look for other ways to use my healing mind.

I let go of my allergy to almonds

Having succeeded with cats, I looked around for other allergies to let go of. I didn't have to look far: I had been allergic to nuts all my life, particularly peanuts. The nuts that gave me the mildest reaction were almonds, so I started there. I nibbled tiny pieces of almond and was keenly aware of how my body reacted. It was OK. A month or two later I attended a formal luncheon where the entrée was grape and almond salad.

Here was my chance! I ate the salad, it was delicious, and I concluded I had given up my allergy to almonds.

I have had some success with pecans but none with peanuts. These other nuts are experienced as a tingling sensation, or fear. I don't understand it, and that's OK.

Healing a series of prostate infections

Several years before my trip to Virginia Beach, I was living in Tampa, FL. I developed serious discomfort and pain, which were diagnosed as symptoms of a prostate infection. I was given some medicine and told to avoid coffee, alcohol, and spicy foods. I followed the directions carefully, and the symptoms went away. They re-occurred from time to time and each time responded to treatment.

I moved to Roanoke, VA, and there I found an urologist who explained to me that ordinary antibiotics were not very effective for treating prostate infections, I needed a sulfa drug, which is small enough to penetrate the tiny passageways to the site of the infection. I happily took the sulfa drug along with avoiding coffee, alcohol, and spicy foods. In addition, he urged me to insist on a sulfa drug if I ever was being treated by another physician.

After four years in Roanoke, we moved to Charleston, WV. In due time, I needed an urologist and went to one who was highly recommended. We had our sulfa discussion and he agreed that it was the best treatment. He gave me a prescription, I took the medicine, and my symptoms disappeared. Some time later, I again needed to see an urologist, my doctor was away, and his partner saw me. I didn't know it, but he gave me a different drug, not a sulfa drug. The symptoms did not go away. I went back to him and he explained that because I had experienced slight side effects from the sulfa drug, he had given me something else. Then he gave me a prescription for the sulfa drug I had been taking.

I was irritated by this. I don't know why, but my reaction to this was, "OK, I'll do it myself". I did not get the prescription filled; avoided coffee, alcohol, and spicy foods for the next few days, and the symptoms disappeared. Over the next thirteen years, I have had only one prostate infection, and it was successfully treated with a sulfa drug.

This is the result of the healing mind at work. Unlike letting go of my allergy to cats—a very gentle process—I became impatient and, without knowing how, switched on a healing process that worked just as well as the best available medicine.

Controlling symptoms of heart disease

I was diagnosed with heart disease several years ago. Among other things, I needed a drug (100 mg per day of Toprol were prescribed) to control "premature ventricular contractions" (PVCs.) I experienced the PVCs as skipped beats but they are actually more like double beats followed by a skip. I am averse to taking drugs, and I take as little as possible, so I immediately set out to eliminate the PVCs. I started my campaign when, on the average, I was experiencing a PVC every minute–and–a–half. I took my pulse from time to time over a period of months, each time willing fewer skips. After some progress, the cardiologist and I agreed to reduce the Toprol dose to 50 mg per day. With further progress, we reduced it to 25 mg, and with still further progress, the average time between PVCs increased to eleven minutes. This is in the normal range. In summary, the dosage was reduced fourfold and the frequency dropped sevenfold. This level has persisted for more than five years.

How did I do that? I'm not sure. I think the process is closely related to biofeedback: I willed the frequency to go down and measured my pulse rate several times a day. I have not done either of those in many years and the frequency of PVCs remains close to zero.

Staying home from school

As indicated earlier, I had a severe bout with pneumonia when I was eight years old. My mother was a nurse and very much afraid of my contracting another serious illness. Therefore, from that time on, if I had early morning cold symptoms, she would keep me home from school.

As an adult, I have explored who I am and the factors that have shaped me. When I have felt angry or upset, I have asked myself, "When is the first time I can remember feeling this way?" The answer has been hidden in some long-ago experience, and I have seen that the source of the upset can no longer reach me (an insult from another child, perhaps,) and I can let it go.

One day, about ten years ago, I was feeling early morning cold symptoms–scratchy throat and congestion, with a slight fever. I asked myself, "When is the first time I remember feeling this way?" The answer: as a child not wanting to go to school. Reflecting on this, my response was "I don't need this" and the symptoms were gone by lunchtime. I then repeated this dialogue with myself on other occasions until I was satisfied this healing was complete.

Shaping up

A thirty-something friend of mine confided in me that her body had changed its shape. As a younger woman, her cup size was "A", or more accurately, A-minus. She could have gone bra-less. In recent years, she told me, she had gained weight and consequently had filled out to a size B. When she decided to lose weight, she also decided to keep her more attractive bust line, and she did. She lost the weight she had gained but not her curves. How? By choosing her new shape. Her mind-body connection and her awareness of it made this possible.

Nothing to sneeze at

From time to time, especially when the air is loaded with allergens, I sneeze—big, loud sneezes. This is uncomfortable for me and the people around me. These sneezes are invariably preceded by light, razor-like pain inside my nose. I have often wished for soothing lotion applied to the inside of both nostrils. One day this past winter, I imagined that little people were inside my nostrils, armed with spray bottles, spraying soothing lotion all over the tender tissue. The pain went away, and I didn't sneeze. I have continued to use these little people with great effect; I call upon them to do their job. Sometimes I fail to alert them in time and I sneeze, but this occurs less frequently all the time.

The mind-body connections of multiple personalities

For me, the most dramatic results of mind-body connections are evident in some people with multiple personalities. These individuals have various names and recollections of who they are (different personal histories,) different likes and dislikes, differing temperaments, varying behavior patterns–in short, different personalities–all in the same body. The personality can change very rapidly—within a minute—and the individual's body chemistry will change just as quickly. One personality can be diabetic and the others, in the same body, not. One personality can be allergic to bee stings, and the others not. It is the most powerful illustration of the mind-body connection that I know of. It shows us what that connection can do for us, even though it doesn't show us how.

Summary

- Most of these cases involve letting go: letting go of fear, disease, concepts of pain, and bleeding.
- Others are based upon forgiveness (another form of letting go).
- All of these processes are based on using the healing mind.
- All of these processes can be aided and enhanced by Expressive Therapy–music, art, dance, drama.

There are many things we don't understand about the world we live in, and that's OK; we don't need to understand. It helps if we just look at what is: the mind can play a definitive role in healing, and Expressive Therapy can energize the mind-body connection.

Selected Reading

Achterberg, Jeanne. *Imagery in Healing: Shamanism and Modern Medicine.* Boston; New Science Library: Shambhala Publications, 1985.

Dossey, Larry, M.D. *Meaning and Medicine: Lessons from a Doctor's Tales of Breakthrough and Healing.* New York: Bantam Books, 1991.

Cousins, Norman. *Anatomy of an Illness as Perceived by the Patient: Reflections of Healing and Regeneration.* New York: Bantam Books, 1981.

Justice, Blair. *Who Gets Sick: Thinking and Health.* Derbyshire, UK: Peak Press, 1987.

Talbott, Michael. *The Holographic Universe.* New York: Harper Perennial, 1992.

NAMASTE

CAROL YANCAR

> OZ never did give nothing to the Tin Man that he didn't,
> didn't already have.
> —Song by America

Through the expressive arts, we can express all the beauty, strength, compassion, generosity, and peace, as well as the curiosity and courage each one of us carries inside. We can also express the yearning and the fear. In fact, we can use expressive arts for our entire emotional repertoire. We always have a choice, when given the opportunity to express from all of our senses, whether to allow the expressions to be blessings or burdens. I found the book by Rachael Naomi Remen, MD, *My Grandfather's Blessings*, to be astoundingly beautiful. (Speaking of beautiful, expressive art that is truly a blessing to many!) She invites us to receive all the blessings we are given, and she reminds us that some opportunities may not feel like blessings without our being willing to explore the choices they offer through all channels, through our minds, bodies and spirits.

I want to emphasize that Dr. Remen calls us to receive all the blessings we have been given, believing that we make choices about whether or not to receive, although these choices may or may not be conscious on our part. Many blessings are disguised as repressed or unresolved emotions, so that we are sometimes only aware of the anger, blame or fear we carry. Therefore, we limit ourselves to behaviors that match these feelings. Rather than receiving all things as blessings, we may simply not recognize some of our experiences at all; we push them down, away from our awareness. In so many ways, we risk limiting, rather than expanding, the abundant possibilities we all carry within.

Expression of those feelings and conditions of which we are aware is a good first step toward finding the blessings. By noticing them, we have the opportunity to expand the blessed feelings, the feel-good feelings, and the feeling of gratitude for being blessed into a compassion for the world. We see beyond the frightening and false OZ we might be in, on to the true

Light within ourselves and within each other. We move into a condition where we can truthfully say, "Namaste," offering ourselves to the world by this saying, "the Divine in me acknowledges the Divine in you."

Finding such Divine Light is done through the exploring of ourselves, and in order to do this exploration well, it is helpful to have tools that move us through all the parts of ourselves, bodies, minds, and spirits. Some of our best tools are the expressive arts. We can glory in the experience of self-expression. It can feel wonderful to get something out and away from ourselves, rather than holding it inside. Even good feelings feel better when they flow outward into the world. We also clear a path for truly listening to ourselves in this way. It can become a spiraling cycle, moving us toward more and more blessings and good feelings. As we use our inner voices, inner eyes, and inner ears, we become energized by the flow. Sometimes it takes a transcending leap out of doubt and fear.

The expressions of our Light can take the form of any of the arts, be it singing, dancing, painting, drumming, or writing. There are no limits to the way we may express the Light. We make the paradigm shift that allows us to receive affirmation from our inner knowing, to hold a better self-understanding, and then to move into the courageous creativity of external action. We can move between conscious and unconscious expression, then on to conscious fulfillment. The Tin Man from the Wizard of OZ received his heart by noticing, by attending, and then by taking action. He found his heart within himself when he realized it was him, and not the external OZ who could retrieve his heart.

We carry who we are inside us and can get very lost, confused, depressed, scared, and critical when we only look to our individual "OZ," whoever that is for us, when we need confidence, acceptance, power, wholeness, humor, compassion, approval, and love. We can get in trouble by looking only outside of our own wonderful selves for the things that we need. By using whatever modalities we choose in the expressive arts, we can touch into our own essence. When we look, listen, feel, smell, and taste with awareness, we begin, and then continue, to re-member (gathering back the scattered pieces,) explore, and notice who we are. Ralph Blum in his book, *The Runes,* mentions a still small voice within us, reminding us of who we are, that is our natural inheritance." (He may be alluding to the Biblical reference to the still small voice of God in 1 Kings 19:11-12, with which many are familiar.) When we notice, when we attend to that inner voice, we are then able to express ourselves in our own unique ways, in doing artistic activity and, subsequently, taking action in our world.

I have found it to be a blessing and a joy, one containing more than a few surprises for me, to create Mandalas for myself and to introduce to others the MARI Mandala work and the Maori Mandala work created by Angeles Arrien, PhD, and Joan Kellogg, MA, respectively. The MARI system is based on the teachings of Carl Jung, the famous psychologist, who did mandalas daily for a period of his life. He devised a system for reading these in order to gain insight into himself at a level that went deeper than his conscious mind. The Maori Mandala work came from Dr. Arrien's experience in New Zealand with the Maori people. Both of these 'modern' systems have allowed me to explore, play, and work with my intuitive/inductive self through interpretation of the drawings and card choices. I have played with different symbolic guesses/understandings from my own conscious and unconscious levels of functioning. I have enjoyed both creating my own mandalas and working with hundreds of clients as they created their mandalas to better understand themselves. Therapy at its best for me has always included some kind of intuitive process. One of the results of working with mandalas can be the excavating of personal archetypes.

I was deeply moved and experienced positive changes in my personal life, which I carried into my work with clients, through attending a workshop with Dr. Angeles Arrien. Over the course of eleven days our group danced, sang, sat in silence, drummed, rattled, rang bells, laughed, cried, and enjoyed marvelous stories. Through these artistic avenues to change, we explored living together in the Four Fold Way. In her book by that title, Dr. Arrien explores four archetypes, the Warrior, the Healer, the Visionary, and the Teacher. She teaches that we carry all four inside each of us. Each profoundly teaches us a way of expressing, then opening our hearts and bringing ourselves into alignment internally and externally. The Warrior archetype speaks of, "I Am. I make things happen, not just react to what happens, in my life," and uses the rattle to call in Dancing. The Visionary archetype uses the ability to speak one's truth without blame or judgment, and uses the bell to bring in Singing. *Dance* might include yoga and other martial arts, sculpting, cooking, or gardening as well as sports. *Singing* is the use of our voices, mouths, and fingers as we act, sing, speak and play all manner of musical instruments.

The Healer archetype, who pays attention to what has heart and meaning, uses the drum to call in Story-telling. The Teacher archetype, who stays open to outcome, yet is not attached to outcome, uses sticks or bones, to bring in Silence. *Story-telling*, as in the treasured oral tradition, honors our own personal experiences, and includes the writing of books, poetry, movies, and plays. *Silence* may be experienced as the art of true presence, and the act of listening, that brings calm and wisdom. This archetype says, "Just Be," and brings inner guidance through patience. Dr. Arrien refers to what it brings to us as a 'sweet territory' or place within where we experience silence, where we are comfortable with not knowing. When we enter this space, we experience a condition of expansion and bliss. With dancing, singing, story-telling, and silence we make space to create and transcend our conscious selves. By drawing on the power of the four archetypes, we can learn to live in harmony and balance both within and without. Because an archetype calls up the deepest mythic roots of humanity, we become a part of that heritage and tradition, one that can mend what has been fragmented from nature and begin the process of healing for ourselves and our world.

Through the above process, we all become healing artists. Although I acknowledge my artistic nature, I have a great yearning for being able to paint or draw and have my work be actually recognizable. When I make illustrations while working with a client, I pretty much have to say the name of the things I draw and laugh along with their laughter and the occasional comment, "Really Carol, that's a person?" When I don't judge the quality of my artworks, I find myself in awe. One of the reasons I am so delighted with mandala work is that I can dive into the circle, with all those interesting shapes and vivid colors, with joyful abandon. I don't have any expectations beyond the experience of the moment. This is great fun for me. There are times when I feel down, and creating a mandala is a very satisfying healing experience for me.

I have been called a visionary. The Visionary archetype is the one that brings creative joy through singing, and that is another way I have great fun. I sing when I'm alone, when I am with other people, and I sing to my adorable little dog. I used to dance along to whatever music I was playing; my legs and feet no longer cooperate with that. Thank goodness, I can tap, clap, sway with my tambourine, and visualize to the sounds and beat that so touch my soul.

Since I work with people in their need, I also know myself to be a healer. I believe we all have the ability to be healers through intention and prayer, when we are open to allowing healing energy to flow through us. The Healer brings the healing power of story to stir the imagination. Story-telling is another one of my true delights, and I am grateful for having come from a singing, story-telling family. In the stories we have told and the songs we have sung, I have found insight, inspiration, gratefulness and compassion. I also love to hear a storyteller, no matter of what genre. Listening to the beauty of putting words and experiences together from different perspectives has opened worlds of true wonder for me. I know the powerful impact of story and song "by heart;" these arts live deep within me.

Many hours of my life have been spent listening and attending to people's stories about their lives, which may be seen as a form of storytelling. We all have ways that we "tell" our stories, choosing what and how much to share. Some have had a tough time communicating. I have learned that communication is not what the speaker says but what the listener understands. Here, I give a respectful nod to Neuro Linguistic Programming (NLP) and my dear friends and mentors Maryann and Ed Reese, through whose work I learned many nuances of communication and elegant change work. In everyday conversation, not in speaking to a therapist, which is a specialized kind of conversation, we speak because we want to make a point, or perhaps express an opinion. We are more likely to be listened to, seen, heard, and attended to with respect and interest when we first sincerely give the gift of attention to another. When we develop the skill of connecting with conscious and unconscious rapport, we can honor the Light in each other—the Light in me honors the Light in you—Namaste. We are then able to practice listening to someone while sending the mostly non-verbal messages, "I see you…I hear you… You matter…We are connected…We are one in the most meaningful way." This recognition of our oneness is the beauty of Namaste.

The blessed experience of expressing myself through art in the ways discussed above have helped me to take steps toward goals in my life that I would not have otherwise been able to accomplish. I have been giving myself the gift of balance through art-making. Another way I use the arts is through the generous gifts of art in many forms and expressions that others have given me. They help to reconfirm my belief that we are all connected. I can resonate with the person who made the art through imagining myself as its creator. I can tap into this rich well of interconnectedness any time I look at beautiful art, whether the art is done professionally or created by a beginner. What is beautiful to me might not meet others' standards for beauty, but it must carry truth in some way for me. Through this kind of art appreciation, I enjoy excavating various archetypes as well.

In the OZ story, both in written and movie forms, we find an archetype of healing; it is through dependence on self, as well as through an interconnectedness, that the characters survive. Artist Alex Grey writes about this kind of interconnectedness in his poem *The Vast Expanse*, which can be found on his website. He states that our connections are endless. Nothing and nobody really acts independently. When we seek richness of spirit in another, we find it also in ourselves. There are layers of love, kindness, integrity, generosity, and compassion to explore and through which to recognize this interdependence. Sharing in this way has become essential to the survival of humanity.

The art of connecting, archetypically, following through in the spirit of self-affirmation and other-affirmation, allows me to freely tell the following vision that I had during a period in my life that was both life changing and transcendent. This has been a difficult story to tell. It happened during an extremely painful period in my life. For a long time, I did not tell anyone, although this is a very important part of my story. Fortunately, I finally came to understand it was a story to be told. I took a step into my own healing when I did. I respectfully offer this story to my reader today.

My kind, funny, gorgeous, intelligent, loving son died when he was twenty-five, having been married only eight months to an extraordinary and much loved woman, Anne. His death was devastating to me and to his extraordinary brother Greg who loved him very much. All of our family and friends felt his death to be traumatic. In the middle of my deep mourning, I had an unforgettable experience. (It was later that I learned that many people have mystical experiences during mourning; perhaps they are sent for our comfort.) The vision that follows is one I experienced; it deeply affirms to me that we truly are God's precious children and everyone is connected in ways beyond our human understanding.

I was feeling calm, sitting in a corner chair in my dining room in the middle of the day, then found myself looking out across the room, through the peach colored hibiscus at the window, past the palm trees, the huge oaks and tall pines, to my neighbor's red tile roof, and on into the vibrant blue Florida sky with large fluffy clouds gliding by. I was vaguely aware that I was now seeing the top of my neighbor's roof and was easily rising up higher and higher into clear midnight blue space. I then saw the beautiful blue, green, and white planet on which we live, the earth, spinning slowly below me.

When you see the star in the text in the following sequence, I invite you to imagine being present in each scene as it is briefly described and hearing the voice of God with me, as I experienced it, while being enveloped in the healing Presence of grace.

I heard the voice of God as each and every person in the scenes below was individually shown to me, saying, "This is my precious child whom I love."

*I heard God's rich, all-knowing, and kind voice saying this to me, indicating a Daddy and his little three or four year old girl, playing ball, laughing, in a sunny field.

* Again, God's voice spoke, lovingly, as each of a number of persons was individually shown me, saying, "This is my precious child whom I love."

Twelve or so scenes all together were shown me, one quickly following the other, with God's voice indicating each person and saying, "This is my precious child whom I love." *Please say this to yourself, or hear it with your inner ears, after visualizing each person in the following scenes. When you are finished with the scenes, say it about yourself:*

*I saw an operating room with doctors and nurses. A person on the operating table was partially covered with a white sheet...
*A man and woman walking together, arguing. Both of them were thoughtlessly flinging cruel words toward each other...
*One man was torturing another man who was helpless and in great pain...
*An elderly person was slumped in a wheelchair, alone...
*A crowd of people was cheering and smiling, each with their own joys, difficulties, and secret thoughts, while a loud colorful parade went by...
*Two people were holding each other tenderly...
*There was an office with people working at their desks, one person with a look of despair while others complained or joked...
* A lone figure in a cold, dark cell was pacing while a guard walked by...
*There was a field by a river with exhausted people wearing worn clothing walking slowly toward a large dirty yellow truck...
*On one side of a large city park, five people were holding hands in a circle and praying together at twilight...on the other side of the park, five young men were viciously fighting with each other...
*A young family was talking and laughing while traveling in a small car...
*There was a green, misty range of mountains and valleys with people scattered in groups, large and small, while others were alone, some tending to animals...

For each person, God said, "This is my precious child whom I love." We cannot hear that often enough. You are also included in God's love.

Gently, I was aware of my body again, and I felt myself moving through space, approaching the red roof, the trees, the flowers at the window, until I felt the solid wooden chair beneath me. I felt totally comfortable, completely sane, soft, strong, relaxed and deeply loved and loving.

> My boat struck something deep
> Nothing happened.
> Sound. Silence. Waves.
> Nothing happened?
> Or perhaps everything has happened
> And I am sitting in the middle of my new life
> —adapted from a South American poet by Dr. Arrien

As I came back to the present, I became aware of how this vision is linked to my life purpose of being aware of and celebrating my connection to all that is. I am grateful that I was raised in a family of service, faith, and humor. I have felt compassion, empathy and acceptance of myself and of others, more often than not. Even so, after the vision I had, above, I learned the profound difference between compassion and pity. I think of compassion as being with someone in his/her passion, holding that person in respect, acknowledging his or her pain and his or her strength, as is in, "I stand with you and I am witness to your experience." I think of pity as expressing real sorrow, yet on some level being focused on a feeling of relief that this is not happening to me.

I am grateful for this visionary experience because I feel that through it I have been able to understand acceptance and compassion on a deeper level than ever before. I came to "GROK" that God loves that person who is acting out with cruelty, prejudice, selfishness, or hatefulness just as deeply as God loves my dear children and grandchildren. This is repeatedly a glaring realization for me when I am in a situation, or hear of another's situation, or even when I contemplate the global situations that seem outrageously hurtful. I believe God grieves when God sees us hurting each other and hurting ourselves. The term "GROK" is as no other in describing a level of understanding that is truly a part of us, truly lived. The term comes from Robert Heinlein, in *Stranger in a Strange Land,* and has become a part of counseling lingo for many therapists because of its deeper layer of meaning.

After my vision ended, I awakened from my trance-like state—a state like the ones we all go in and out of everyday to some degree—and I realized that I am in real need of remembering my vision and my purpose here, remembering it every day. We always stand at the point of choice.

We may not like all the choices, yet they are present. We can choose to recognize our own Light and the Light in others. We can choose fear or love-based actions and beliefs. Just as we can receive all the blessings we are given or not, and even notice their presence or not. I choose love. "Perfect love casts out all fear" (1 John 4:18.) If we choose to love ourselves and to love others, we will choose to find ways to keep ourselves in balance. We will not have mystical experiences every day to remind us. However, we can create experiences of "re-membering" to keep us in balance.

Bringing the art of balance into our lives is a constant challenge. One way to do this is by pondering:

The art of awareness of both the internal and external reality of our daily lives.

The art of acceptance and acknowledgment of others as they are, not only as we would very much like them to be.

The art of celebrating, through daily interaction with others, feeling the genuine connection to all peoples.

The art of courageously inviting mystical as well as practical experiences.

While we are practicing these arts, we will find our Light. Sometimes that Light seems too bright to us, and we find it hard to hold onto. The words of Marianne Williamson speak to this condition:

> "Our deepest fear is not that we are inadequate. Our deepest fear is that we are powerful beyond measure. It is our light, not our darkness that most frightens us. We ask ourselves, 'Who am I to be brilliant, gorgeous, talented, fabulous?' Actually, who are you NOT to be? You are a child of God...Your playing small does not serve the world. There is nothing enlightened about shrinking so that other people won't feel insecure around you. We are all meant to shine, as children do. We were born to make manifest the glory of God that is within us. It's not just in some of us: it's in everyone. And as we let our own light shine, we unconsciously give other people permission to do the same. As we are liberated from our own fear, our presence automatically liberates others" (1992.)

There is not a finite quantity of Light or Divinity, making it an 'us or them' competition for having our Lights or Divinity shine through. My experience has allowed me to truly greet other souls, acknowledge their Light, and relish in both illuminations. There is a continual weaving together of external and internal learning that I do as I work with the expressive arts, both personally and with my clients. This weaving creates a whole fabric that holds me in one piece, and is the basis of balance in my life. We are always in need of coming back to balance mentally, physically, emotionally, spiritually, and interpersonally. I desire to focus on, and be aware of receiving, the blessings that I am given, both through me, and from others to me. I invite you to live an art-full life, one as colorful as OZ, but more true to the Light that is YOU. I reach out to you today with Namaste, the Divinity in me bows to the Divinity in you. And I celebrate all the glowing and shining Light throughout this amazing blue, green & white planet, spinning in space, all together, with you, me and the Tin Man.

Bibliography

Arrien, Angeles. *The Four-Fold Way: Walking the Path of the Warrior, Teacher, Healer, and Visionary.* San Francisco: Harper, 1993.

Blum, Ralph H. *The Book of Runes.* New York: St. Martin's Press, 1983.

Campbell, Joseph. *The Hero with a Thousand Faces.* Navato, CA: New World Library, 1968.

Campbell, Joseph and Bill Moyers. *The Power of Myth.* New York: Anchor Books/Random House, 1991.

Heinlein, Robert A. *Stranger in a Strange Land.* New York: Ace/Putnam, 1991.

Kellogg, Joan. *Mandala: Path of Beauty.* Baltimore, MD: Mandala Assessment & Research Institute, 1984.

Remen, Rachel Naomi, M.D. *My Grandfather's Blessings, Stories of Strength, Refuge, and Belonging.* New York: Riverhead Books Penguin Putnam, 2000.

Williamson, Marianne. *A Return to Love: Reflections on the Principles of A Course in Miracles.* New York: Harper Collins. 1992.

Websites

Southern Institute of NLP, Mary Ann and Ed Reese: www.intl-NLP.com
www.alexgrey.com/writings

*from http://skdesigns.com we learn that the deepest fear quote is often found incorrectly credited to Nelson Mandela from his Inauguration Speech, 1994, where he said, "As we are liberated from our own fear, our presence automatically liberates others." Copyright 1996+2008 by Shirley E. Kaiser, MA

ERASING THE PAIN

KURT FONDRIEST

"Erasing the Pain" is the name of a workshop on personal empowerment for people coping with chronic pain. The workshop was an idea I began because I felt it was long overdue; one that was a reflection of my own life lived with chronic pain. I have Fibromyalgia, a chronic muscle pain condition. The symptoms include muscle pain, fatigue, depression, anxiety, and overall body aches. As an Art Therapist and artist, I knew that I needed to express my pain through various mediums if I was going to be a survivor. I knew the role of "victim," which included a feeling of loss of identity, would be a life sentence for me. This is still a challenge and an inspiration for me as I continue to live my life as a survivor of chronic pain. It is a choice that I make.

Through expressive arts, I have come to understand the power that creativity can offer, encompassing the potential for managing one's life with chronic illness. Many who experience the workshop I facilitate have been enabled to learn techniques that foster self-care through creativity. It can alter the perception of the self to include images of survival, rather than only those of victim. The techniques from the group can be done daily at home as well as in any group setting. In my experience as an art therapist, I find that there is no limit to the amount of times one can engage in these self-healing modalities. Each time is its own unique experience.

In working with people who live with developmental disabilities of all sorts at the residential facility Misericordia Home North in Chicago, I have been able to work with 600 or more people with all levels of ability. I include here the workshop called "Erasing the Pain" in a lesson plan format, and give free reign for its use, its expansion, or transformation. I believe the exercise given can be deeply beneficial, not only to people living with chronic pain, but also for their spouses, caretakers, family members, and all who want to expand their awareness of a life lived "erasing the pain." The format for this group is deceptively simple.

Objective: To enable creative pain management for people who live with a chronic pain condition or support providers who assist these individuals.

Supplies: Erasable materials, such as:
'Zen boards' (available at art supply stores,
     use water for writing that dries)
Magic slates (my personal favorite; they remind us of childhood)
Dry erase markers and board
     Paper and pencils
     Silly putty

Considerations: A note of precaution is in order here prior to starting any workshop. In doing the workshop many times with many different populations, I have found that at times the format might need to be changed to reflect the individuals' abilities. For example, when working with people who live with Cerebral Palsy or have limited fine motor skills, I sometimes require staff assistance in the group. As in any group setting, the people involved are asked about, and agree to, a confidentiality policy.

Method: The facilitator starts by playing soft music. It is an invitation to relaxation, and should be of a meditative or ambient variety.
I then ask the participants to imagine their pain as an object.
When they have a good picture of it in their minds, I ask them what color they think takes away their pain.
I combine the two projections, asking them to again see the object in their minds.
Then they are to imagine a whole gallon of paint in the healing color.
With imaginary paintbrush in their hand, they are to paint over the object of pain.
Then I work the magic of the workshop; I pass around slips of paper and ask each person to write down the name of the pain with which they have been challenged.
I pass a hat for the papers, and then put it on my head, as all the papers fall on the floor.
This causes a round of laughter from everyone.
After using the magic hat routine, I bring out the erasable material, magic slates. This is the real magic.
The participants are instructed to either draw or write about their pain.

When they have been given time to do so, together we release and "Voila!" They simply lift the film on the slate and it is once again clear.
Sometimes, the group asks to repeat the process, and we do.

This is a creative, fun, and an emotionally healing experience. One can be truly empowered even by this simple yet profound combination of projected imagery, laughter, and relaxation. People respond to this activity with the imagination of their inner child, which is exactly who we want to join us in such activities. Practice makes perfect, and any chance we have to connect with our inner child is an opportunity for empowerment. The magic hat is terrific for this kind of transformation.

By admitting knowledge of magic slates, I may be giving away my age, although they can still be found in dollar stores and continue to delight the child in all of us. I make sure that participants in my groups have them to take back to their rooms or take home at the end of the session. I think they are wonderful tools for reflecting the process of erasing the pain.

In such a workshop, we are mainly attempting to allow the participant to be present, in the here and now. Pain can take one away from the "now." It is able to suffocate the desire to live, the hope to dream, and, basically, the overall appreciation of life. The latter is one of the most challenging bridges to cross for people living with pain.

We can find ourselves falling into a well of self-pity and a feeling of victimization. This can turn to the depths of depression. I know from firsthand experience that chronic pain is like your shadow. It is always present. On grey days, it is more subtle, not as noticeable. On sunny days, it can be harsher, in contrast. Some days are better than other days, but there is no true relief. I teach that we must find ways to embrace this pain, to own it, and to express our reactions to it, if we want to move forward.

We need support to move forward. That is another reason why the workshop format is so good for this population. We take ownership and responsibility back into our own hands when we do things to move forward. Powerful insights can combat the pain. The brush, pencil, or marker in hand to create strokes, words, or images on any surface is self-expression, and demonstrates our need to be moved, to emote.

The use of an old prescription bottle with an erasable label is another powerful prop. I have people think of an imaginary medication with a fantastic, fun name that would take away the pain forever. The person can reuse this repeatedly. Objects like these become sacred for mending the mind, body and spirit. This may merely be a way to take advantage of the placebo effect, but if it works, it is good. In fact, it can be a lifesaver. The patient becomes the doctor of the spirit, giving a symbolic prescription that has no limit on refills.

I believe we are created to reflect three elements of divine thought. These elements are the mental, spiritual, and physical. All three connect with each other to manifest within our being. I did not choose to have this pain, but the pain has become my teacher. It has enabled me to reach deeper into my creative self, and this is truly a vision for me of the divine mind.

Through the years, as a facilitator of the expressive arts, I have been reminded of the state of awe that can be created out of pain. I believe that this process is a multi-step experience. I remember when I started to transform images of pain into visual symbols. At first, they were garish, harsh and disturbing, just as I thought they should be. I was initiating a conversation with my expressive self. This was my first step into healing. It inspired me to look beyond it, and think how I might connect with others in the creative arts to express the universal sensation we know as PAIN. I went looking for an artist storefront and proposed an idea. What if artists of all disciplines, who have also lived with chronic pain, would work together on a performance piece? I did not yet have a name or even a direction. I just knew there could be a high-energy flow of expression.

My next thought was about personal images of pain. Is that what we would need to express? Something inside me kept me searching for another, deeper level of purpose. I had been writing about my own path through pain, and attending a Church of Religious Science and a Church of Christ Science. What I heard from these congregations and their viewpoints made sense to me. "Thoughts create our reality," they said, and "Change your thinking, change your life." These seemed to me to be very well grounded ideas. One minister said to me, "Put what you want into words on a paper." That was the birth of my writing on a spiritual level about pain. One Friday night, I wrote about the pain going away, and for some reason I wanted to change something about it. I erased the penciled words. And a light bulb went on in my head. That was the birth of my "Erasing the Pain" workshops.

The light bulb had gone on over my head, but the work still had to be done to bring this idea into the world. Having a show where the art was made out of erasable material would be symbolic, especially if we erased the artwork that reflected personal pain. I had to find space and people to make this happen. As people who hold chronic pain know, sometimes ideas need to be put on hold. That is what happened with my idea. The Fibromyalgia was limiting my artistic function, and I was allowing it to do so. I was going through a period of artistic flux. Working full time as a Vocational Counselor and Art Therapist in a sheltered workshop setting and taking three busses to work each day, after an hour and a half ride, I was also abusing alcohol and fighting depression. All of this left me fatigued and highly sensitive to my pain. It would not be until I faced my own need for recovery that I would re-focus on the idea for "Erasing the Pain."

I was fighting for my own spiritual identity during that time as well. I knew I had to stop using alcohol and, after many years of searching for a miracle cure, I knew my change would have to come from within myself. My own poetry reflected a powerful insight for my personal transformation. I found myself erasing images from my own past as I wrote. I was creating a new life, one image at a time. I had found a basic philosophy that could put me on the path to my own healing, the ideas of "Erasing the Pain." This path included creating images, from visual symbols to words, on paper with the aid of a helpful therapist.

The outcome of this combination of working with images in conjunction with therapy was in finding that my life was in my control. The pain was still there, yet my emotional pain had been a reaction to abuse, the abuse of substances. I had to face the fact that I was going to live with chronic pain. I was going to have to take the idea of "Erasing the Pain" and put it into practice in my daily life. That has enabled me to bear witness to the power it can really hold for individuals like myself and the challenges we face.

It has taken nearly ten years from the first light bulb of an idea to the actual materializing of doing a workshop called "Erasing the Pain." At a conference for the Healing Arts, I received encouraging responses from participants for this work. That was several years ago, and I have facilitated the workshop at the state level for art therapists as well as doing it many times in private sessions with individuals.

The power of "Erasing the Pain" is still young. I owe much to the people who have encouraged me to keep developing my insights. Such comments have enabled me to continue to focus intuitively on my own art making process. Through this work, a universal experience has come to the forefront for me. This is a way that people living with chronic pain can use creativity to manage their lives. I know that as a person with Fibromyalgia, it has been a battle for years for me against insurance companies that do not want to acknowledge the existence of my condition. However, the pharmaceutical companies have started advertising special drugs to treat it. I believe that we all must take the management of our conditions more into our own hands, and learn ways to manage that are not dependent on any larger system.

Every healing modality has a slice of the much larger pie known as healing. Medicine has its place, as does behavioral therapy, exercise, physical therapy, chiropractic, massage therapy, reflexology, and creativity/expressive arts. The label "Erasing the Pain" might be viewed as another prop. Perhaps it uses only the placebo effect, but who cares, if it works? In the workshop, each person comes up with a name of a fantasy medication that would take the pain away forever. The person can reuse it repeatedly. Such objects become sacred to the person who gets relief from them. They are sacred because they work on the level of the body as well as on the spirit.

"Erasing the Pain" can be approached in so many creative ways. Although I have written about several, I have used several more. In the right hands, the idea of erasing pain could be expanded many ways. Allow yourself to play with your imagination; it is the greatest gift we are given. Let me encourage you to take this show on the road of life yourself, for any time you, or those you help, may need it.

I still live with chronic pain, but approaching life with the use of the game I have called "Erasing the Pain" has enabled me to appreciate my journey on this path we call life.

For more information on the condition that causes my pain, you can access The National Fibromyalgia Association at www.fmaware.org.

A LETTER TO CHOPRA

WAYNE BERMAN

I wrote this letter to Deepak Chopra as a personal letter. It was not originally intended for public distribution. It will be easier to understand if you have his book entitled *The Seven Spiritual Laws of Success*. The letter below did elicit an immediate response from Deepak Chopra himself. I met with him and he connected me to a violinist friend of his from San Francisco who did work similar to my own.

November 27, 2000

Dear Deepak Chopra,

I am writing in response to your book, *The Seven Spiritual Laws of Success*. I have been using the book every day for the last five months and wonderful things have been happening. I discovered your book several months after my wife left me, and my life felt irrevocably destroyed. The fact that I am still alive is a miracle in itself. Everything around me appeared to be crumbling and my heart and mind were filled with fear and anxiety. I could find no peace, no comfort; not even in nature, which always centered and balanced me in difficult times prior to this occasion. However, your book helped me to find a quiet place in myself, where I wasn't afraid (even though I faced homelessness and personal shame.) I began to expect solutions to arise and I simply stayed alert and waited for them. All of a sudden, when things were at their very worst, help arrived from people and places I would never have even thought of before.
I am a music teacher/composer/performer. Several students just took it upon themselves to give me gifts, which I did not ask for, and did not expect. It may seem like a small token to some people, a couple of hundred dollars here and there, but it really saved my life. I was able to keep an apartment and keep my teaching position (which was in jeopardy because my life was falling apart.) Now, I feel I'm on the road to recovery and well-being. Nevertheless, this very brief personal story is only a prelude to what I would really like to share with you.

The reason I was able to relate to your book (and I have seen similar books that did not help as much) is that it resonated so directly with the work I have been doing as a composer and teacher. I am briefly going to describe a kind of music making/composing process I would guess you do not know about, although I think you may be interested. The reason you are probably unfamiliar with these practices is that this work is very obscure. Only a handful of composers have devoted themselves in this direction. And these composers tend to be isolated within the academic environment. To tell the truth, I am not sure these composers would agree with me or see the connection between their work and yours, as I see it. This work is often referred to as experimental music (a better term might be experiential expressive behavior through music) which, in this case, means any music in which you can never be sure of the outcome or product. It concentrates on a process of uncertain interaction. We call what we do "sessions," a term coined by composers J.K. Randall and Benjamin Boretz. And in many ways, these musical sessions resemble a kind of psychological group therapy more than any traditional music practices you may have encountered. Benjamin Boretz once described this music practice as personal navigation and interpersonal negotiation. Ben is a very articulate musical thinker.

This music does not begin or end; it only is documented by the tape deck being turned on or off (creating a sense of beginning, middle and end.) However, in reality, it is an on-going process. It ends when the tape runs out. We avoid discussing whether the music is "good" or "bad," or if "I like it" or "I don't like it" because these judgments cut off critical discussion of our real and direct experience. So, instead, we speak of the "isness" of the interaction; what is there to be understood and experienced. We talk of the actual reality of the people and energies present in our space. We avoid developing technique and skill as much as possible because it kills awareness. A performer learns how to use his/her skill to block out all influences present in the moment, so that they can pursue their musical score without any interference from the field of all possibilities, in an effort to keep the music fixed and unchangeable. There is no evolution in the process. If you have no technique, you must use your awareness to be present to the occasion and respond from your personally intuited ontology. Therefore, the music does not represent any larger institutions or cultural bias. Everyone comes in their own name and out of their own interests and needs, and no one is coerced to conform their own sense of expressive behavior in order to satisfy a larger institutional convention. It is not always pretty.

Usually a chaos precedes the sense of real community. Moreover, uncertainty is an absolutely essential component. Kenneth Gaburo once described composition this way, "…since at first I know little of what I am to do (this 'not knowing' is crucial)…since I prefer random processes which can reveal unlimited numbers of possible orders…(the feel of 'whatever')…the process of composing (for me) is without knowing in the so-called 'usual' way. Literally, it is a process of making sense. A profound experience…another state comes, more or less one of stayed meditation on the unknown mode: to stare: to gaze: to infer (to make the scatter in the first place is to provide a concrete occasion for profound discourse with self)…to eventually reveal that structure from a very large number of imbedded possibilities, which makes most sense to me at the time, and for which I reserve, uniquely, the expression: composition."

These are sensing compositions; they are not meant to fix and cement in undeviating purity and perfection. Even in the case of so-called improvised music, there is no real uncertainty, and hence no real personal evolution. Like in jazz, for instance, the musicians are often not really improvising. They know the language; they know what is to happen and what is not allowed to happen. They never have to be present enough to respond to truly unexpected sound. There is no real uncertainty. It always sounds like jazz. And unless you are a jazz musician, you cannot join in and play with them. You are excluded by the institutional structure of jazz music. However, in our music, no person is excluded. Anyone who is interested in sharing a genuine, person-sized sounding interaction with other real people can participate (whether or not they have ever touched a musical instrument.) It all depends on being interested and interesting (all people are interesting when they stop living by mimetic power alone and start expressing their real, true nature/self.)

There are many things between us, Deepak, but I will briefly correlate your book to my daily music practice.

1) We begin our music making process from the field of pure potentiality; anything is possible at this stage. We mediate until our impulses and intuitions direct us to some form of sounding action. We always practice non-judgment because it is the only way to keep lively attention on the object of interest. As soon as someone says, "I like something," or " I don't like something," that tends to end all discourse and take us away from the scene of our attention altogether.

2) Giving and receiving is directly experienced as a flow of thoughts, feelings, and ideas in dynamic exchange. It does not represent a larger institution (like playing a certain kind of music,) but rather

ourselves, the real actual people involved. This is truly a shared communal space created by everyone present.

3) Your book has a powerful connection to our music making practices. At every moment, there are choices to be made and the consequences of those choices can be felt as direct experience. We draw from the field of pure potentiality when making choices and we try to remind ourselves to step back after making a choice (putting a sound in the space, for instance, and witness the consequences of our choices, sounds.) We try to notice what specific responses and interactions our choices engender.

4) Acceptance is crucial if you are going to be fully present to the occasion and therefore able to respond sincerely. To benefit fully from our interaction with others, all participants must feel safe and secure enough to truly be themselves without fear of reprisal. Response-ability is the essence of what music making is all about. Listening and developing the ability to respond. When you practice an art form that is so alternative to the mainstream, you must learn defenselessness, or the pressure of the world will surely crush even the strongest person.

5) The only spiritual law that was not already a part of my music making practices may be the law about intention and desire. I believe it can be easily integrated and I am eagerly pursuing this idea. I believe that experimenting with intention during meditative music practice will yield positive results. The way this idea does already connect to our music is that we always view music making as creating reality. In this sense of creating reality, intention and desire do the same thing.

The three steps given at the end of your chapter on detachment sound like one of our musical scores. We often write or discuss these concepts as a stimulus for a sound response. Hence, I called it a musical score. A musical score is not a fixed or exact thing; it is only a stimulus that elicits a sounding response.

7) The concept of purpose is crucial to our work. In the Western high-art culture, the idea of art for art's sake is popular. We don't do art for art's sake. Our sound making is mobilized by intention and direct purpose. We feel that as we invent our music we invent ourselves and our world. Music is world-viewing, world-experiencing, and world-making.

This letter from me to you is only a brief outline of our deep connectedness. Your work (book) is crucial. It brings spirituality to issues of success (success in its most real and diverse sense.) I have struggled with poverty all my life. I believed there was no practical way to connect the spirituality or personal benefit of doing music my way (as I described above) and making money. I don't believe that anymore. I believe I need to give more and circulate more, rather than cloister up. I am the music teacher for two private schools in Tampa, Florida, and I am the current president for the Tampa Bay Composers' Forum, which is the second largest composers' forum in the world. I am very active as a composer, teacher and performer.

I believe that ultimately we are in the same business, that is, we offer the opportunity to experience health, sanity and well-being as a spiritual constant. And together as people with people, we compose ourselves and our world.

Truly your Gentle Reader,
Wayne Berman

Note: Benjamin Boretz is a composer and music theorist who edits Open Space magazine. He founded and ran Music Program Zero for 20 years. For more information, go to www.perspectivesofnewmusic.org.

Kenneth Gaburo was an electronic music pioneer and composer. For more information, go to www.angelfire.com.

Reference

Chopra, Deepak. *The Seven Spiritual Laws of Success: A Practical Guide to Fulfillment of Your Dreams.* New York: Harmony Books. 1995.

OF A DIFFERENT COLOR...

KATHY LUETHJE AND LAURIE DOYLE

Be patient toward all that is unsolved in your heart
And try to love the questions themselves...
Live the questions now.
Perhaps you will find them gradually, without noticing it,
And live along some distant day into the answer.
—Rainer Maria Rilke

An Introduction to Expressive Arts

As I paused with my brush over the tins of vibrant paint, I allowed a color to choose me, as I was instructed. These directions, given by Dr. Barbara Kazanis in Intermodal Expressive Arts classes at the University of South Florida, were purposefully ambiguous. Class members were moving about the room, following what their feet and arms "wanted to do." Music with a pronounced downbeat informed this action. Eventually, we paired up with someone whose movements matched our own, and waited, while moving in sync, to be given a new direction. That direction came, "Now, let a color choose you, and begin to paint."

It was a novel idea for me, to let myself feel the call of a color. It involved a sort of synaesthesia on my part. I wasn't sure I knew how to do this. But as I looked over the paint tin, one color jumped out, a brilliant orange, and I became "painterly" on the top of a large sheet of paper taped to the wall next to where I danced. I rode the movements onto the paper, through the brush, noticing what bounced back at me from the page. The movement became the color, and the color was power.

Then it happened. The inner dialog started. My monkey-mind started in on me. *"What is that supposed to look like?"* I heard in my head, and *"My classmates will be making beautiful pictures. They are all artists."* I managed to turn away from this frightening voice. When the next color chose me, it was a singing blue-green, and a silky, watery flow began down the paper. *"That looks like a waterfall,"* my inner voice said, *"Add some rocks at the bottom."* I was torn. How much should I listen? I should just let it flow, shouldn't I? Why am I "shoulding" on myself anyway?

Expressive arts are about "Flow," as described by Mihaly Csikszentmihalyi; they are about "Process," about learning to be "present" to what wants to happen through the senses and through the body. But when the rubber hits the road, or the paintbrush hits the canvas, decisions are made with the mind. Sometimes, the left hemisphere of my brain kicks in and tries to take over just when I need to be letting go. If I could just ride this feeling of flow, invite it, flow with it, love it, listen to it, and then give it shape to manifest its spirit into reality!

I re-focus my attention fully on the task and feel the sensation of the brush in my hand, the movement coming from deep within my body. If I can enter a state of "self-forgetting" and stay with this "not-knowing," just feeling…I then heard the voice of the philosopher/poet Rilke, *"Be patient with all that is unsolved in your heart…live the questions now…"*

I once again entered a blissful state, and began to swoop broad strokes of glitter-laden gold over the canvas, sometimes crossing colors already laid down, letting layers happen as they would. The strokes moved down, down the page. I was back in the flow. A warm yellow-grey that mixed itself on my palette then sang out to me, and I picked it up, letting it tell me what form it wanted on the page. I began making criss-cross shapes at the bottom. Until I heard the critical "I" jar me awake to its voice again. *"That's too abstract, it doesn't look like anything. I need to make it match what I've seen, or what I see in my mind's eye."* As usual, the fantasy I was having about what I was painting was much better than the reality. The voice inside won out. *"I need to make this into something that communicates, something others will recognize."* I picked up a small brush and loaded it with black, sharpening the bristles to a point, and then touched here and there, making definitive lines. *"Oh, but look, it doesn't look like I wanted it to; I am just not good enough…"*

There was no time to lament that night. Dr. Kazanis soon asked us to gather at our seats for a moment. She gave out little sticky notes to each of us. We were to take our pens and these notes to every canvas and write down our initial brief responses to each other's work…not what we thought it was, but what it evoked in us. Our words were our gifts to each person who had painted. My mood instantly brightened. Using words was fun for me. Impressions sprang from the works and I found it surprisingly easy to respond.

As for the words and phrases that I was given for my own painting, I was delighted with them. Somehow, my classmates saw what I saw in my mind's eye and more. We wrote poems from the words, another satisfying task for me since I was comfortable with words. Then we arranged the word-gifts one more time and wrote poetry again. We shared the poems, and thoughts about the process and how it felt. *"So this is intermodal expressive arts!"* I thought. (I am told that the term 'intermodal' originated with Paolo Knill, renowned author and teacher in the field.)

I took my painting home and was in for more surprises. I had been told in class to hang it up so that I could see it for a week or so, and I did. I allowed it to continue to in-form me, to resonate inside me. There was something about it that spoke to me, but I did not have the words to say what it was. One afternoon, my husband moved the picture onto its side. He had been looking at it, too. We were in a place fairly new to us, next to the sea, and had been talking about the way that being near the water was speaking to our lives. I had been telling him playfully that I was a mermaid, and bringing mermaid knickknacks into the house. "Look, it's your mermaid!" my husband said, and I saw my picture with fresh eyes. There, lying on her side was a beautiful, turquoise-tailed mermaid with long orange hair and shimmery fish scales. I had not seen her prior to this point at all…in that moment I became a believer that my subconscious was indeed at work during the "Process" of expressive arts.

Something about the way the numinous, the spiritual, and the deep unconscious moves through the expressive arts continued to intrigue me as I studied this field. I worked through an internship doing bedside art and music at a local hospital and eventually established my own arts practice of visual journaling in order to ease any compassion fatigue I felt from my work as a hospital chaplain. Using watercolor expressively after I had been present for a death or trauma became a way to harness my emotions and the zeitgeist, or spirit of the hour, to contain them on a page, and to commemorate the sentinel event that I had witnessed. I learned to turn my own "mourning into dancing" through the colors moving rhythmically across the page in my late night hours alone waiting for trauma calls.

Even though I was untrained at first in visual arts, I had been coaxed to get "painterly" through authors such as Aviva Gold in *Painting from the Source* and Michele Cassou and Stewart Cubley in *Life, Paint, and Passion*. I found myself in my office in the wee hours of the night after being at a deathbed or with a trauma family, letting the colors choose me from my small watercolor palette, losing myself and time in their mix, and forming shapes from the feelings inside my body…making commemorations, my own memorial ritual. I allowed the colors to move me, and through the freedom of movement and the beauty of the hues and shapes, I became thankful once again for life and for attachments to the earth and its people, recognizing the blessing that my work with people facing death and trauma really was for me.

With missionary zeal, I wanted to tell the world about the healing process I was personally experiencing, and witnessing others experience, through the expressive arts. I went seeking for a way to share, and a way to explain the power that can be found through this expressive "Process." "When the student is ready, the teacher will come," they say, perhaps speaking of the kind of synchronicity that psychologist C.G. Jung discovered. One day a volunteer in the hospital Pastoral Care program where I was Chaplain told me her story of learning to ride a horse. I knew her story was there to teach me, and I had found the symbolism in it that I needed in order to tell my own story and tease out its components. D.H. Lawrence once wrote, *"The horse is a symbol of potency, power, movement and action."* Perfect! The horse could become the metaphor I had been seeking for the power of the arts to heal.

There seemed to be something about the taming of a horse's raw power that spoke of the problem I was having in regards to the need for skill in the arts. Metaphors connect two differing spheres of meaning by a shared quality, according to author Joseph Jaworski in *Synchronicity* (1996.) Horsemanship and the arts share the quality of harnessing power, and concern working in collaboration for the creating of beauty. How appropriate to speak of the arts using metaphor, this metaphor, because the use of metaphor in itself, for creating and finding meaning in images, is a widely used expressive arts technique.

My Quest and its Queries:
Combing through the Wild Mane

There had always been a nag (pun intended) for me about the way in which the intermodal expressive arts process was dependent in part upon the skills of the artist. What makes the expressive arts powerful? And what does that have to do with the dependence on skill? Either there was hand-eye coordination that allowed a flow, a singing voice that kept a tonal center, a body that could move smoothly from position to position, words chosen with grace, or not. Yes, there was joy in tapping into the deep, and feeling my transcendent self come alive in the ethers that were not tied to the here and now, yet somehow lived intensely in the very moment. However, in order for me to communicate that joy, to express it outward, I felt I perhaps needed delineation; I needed some path to follow.

Without skills in this field, I was only as effective as if I were wandering around lost in a forest. I needed more direction than just open flow when I was unfamiliar with the tools of the trade and their use. Perhaps I was also overwhelmed with possibilities. In my own arts practice, when I would find myself in the middle of flowing into an art form in which I had no experience, I would freeze and could not flow. My critical mind would take hold, and I could not move into Process. I was awkward. My body "horse" was not the well-oiled "machine" of power and grace that I needed it to be. It was either a faltering old mare or a skittling colt. Neither brought much satisfaction.

I noticed that in groups or classes, those who were familiar with the particular art modality being used appeared to make smooth transitions into Process mode. They moved without hesitation; they moved with the flow, and with the power I sought. I found myself in a need-to-know position; after all, knowledge is power. I love this Process and what it has offered my life, but I wanted to know from whence came the power. I did not want to be told again to just "flow with it," at least not until I understood more about it. That is when I started studying a book called *The Power of Limits* by György Doczi (1994.)

One key to understanding the power of the arts is through Doczi's discussion of the beauty inherent in the Golden Mean, a proportion found throughout many forms of nature, in fact, nearly all forms. This proportion offers a pleasing and satisfying sensation when viewed. Human bodies, and horse bodies as well, contain Golden Mean proportions. Although I had studied harmonics and proportions in musical intervals, I had not realized that there could be a certain ratio among the parts of whole forms that looked and felt naturally beautiful to the human eye, just as certain specific intervals in music sound more harmonious to the ear.

There is a science behind the music of natural harmonics, or overtones, those that seem to sound and that our ears hear, along with what is actually sounded, a played, sung, or struck tone. When those tones actually sound together, when they become explicit, as played in harmony, we hear them as more beautiful than other pitches sounding together. They are called "perfect" intervals. While Doczi explains that this proportion used in structures also makes things strong and serviceable, the fact that they look beautiful and "right," "natural," and even "healthy" is important and speaks to my query. Beauty has power because of its ability to attract; it commands attention. The quality of being "right" or "true" is also powerful. It has an unmistakable resonance or "ring."

Proportions are parts of a whole, and therefore each are limited alone. In the preface to his work, Doczi said, "Proportions are shared limitations that create harmonious relationships out of differences" (1994.) He demonstrates this idea using the Golden Mean in the Taoist symbol for the

Yin and Yang, two fish-like swirls, held together in a circle. The "lesser," or limited part seems to yield to the "greater," fuller part in the design. While the proportions of black and white in the symbol are equal, they are designed in Golden Mean proportions and are arranged in such a way as to seem to tip over, or even to roll. It appears to me that these parts suggest that things are always in flux, always moving, just as life is never static, but continues to recreate itself. The black and white in this symbol depend on each other for forming this image, and create wholeness through the combination of the two. Without both, each is incomplete.

There are many teachings involved in the meaning of that symbol that can only be touched upon here. However, we can see how the elements of the symbol "teach us that limitations are not just restrictive, but they are also creative," when shared. (1994:139) Doczi seemed to be on a similar quest for the basics of power as I was. His model speaks of collaborative power as well as creative power. Authors Ching and Ching echo this same insight. "Creativity is a cycle of Yin and Yang," they say in *From Chi to Creativity:*

> "The right brain process often seems more exciting—exploring new wild crevices of imagination, discovery, receiving wafts of inspiration, giving them voice or form, putting them together. The left-brain task perhaps feels more tedious, yet commands respect and helps you decide what to change, to keep, and to omit. The beauty of art is that it is your soul revealed; the challenge is that it is a form of communication. The key to this relationship between right and left brain processes is separation of Yin and Yang, understanding them, working with them, and bringing them back into dialogue in a cohesive whole" (2007: 17.)

There needs to be collaboration, between all our parts, a balanced integration of wholeness, for us to experience our full power, in arts and in life. That is part of what we learn from the Yin and Yang symbol.

When we collaborate with others, sharing our limitations, we also gain power. There is the tremendous, luring power of love and power when we make any connection with others. Engaging, particularly with compassion, which literally means "feeling with" another, forms bonds that can be powerful. Perhaps it is our awareness and acknowledgement of the connectedness that is powerful, as scientists now tell us that we are all connected to everyone and everything whether we recognize it or not. Most situations would prove that two heads and two hearts are stronger, more powerful, than one.

The expressive arts practitioner moves along beside the person who is hurting or in need, and walks the path of the arts modality with them, in a gesture of companioning. It is a spiritual companioning. It touches deep places within the person that go beyond words precisely because of the metaphorical and symbolic nature of the arts. It touches the soul. And it can only truly be done with compassion. When companioned, the people involved feel that they are not alone. Doczi sees a type of sharing in the proportions of the Golden Mean, and says, "Sharing is not only a basic pattern and an art, it is also a condition of life" (1994:29.) We need one another to live, especially to live with strength and power.

I found another key to obtaining power, satisfaction and beauty through expressive arts in the making of a commitment. Prior to making that brush stroke, or writing this word, the idea has not yet been communicated. Ideas and symbols are in their morphogenic state, as scientist and author Rupert Sheldrake would tell us; they are still fields, waiting to become concrete material. They are full of possibilities. However, once a stroke of pen or brush has been committed, it becomes a form, a constant; it does not change. Yet there is an inherent freedom within this commitment. There is a sense of safety found through a known quantity, one that is unchanging. The safety becomes a strong foundation upon which the new can be built, upon which we can elaborate and become more creative.

As foundational strokes are laid down on a paper, other possibilities open up, and can build upon this fixed foundation. You may have heard it said that writing something is a thinking process; the writing process is just one example of how making a commitment opens new possibilities. In writing, as each part is made concrete, the next thoughts seem to branch, and yes, sometimes veer way off track. Without the first sentence being typed upon the page or screen, however, no further thoughts seem to come. Once a foundation is laid, momentum builds, and so does the work. But it is a paradoxical process. In the concretization of thought through the writing process, which seems to close down possibilities, with one being chosen over another, new ideas arise. So it is with the image-making process, the putting down of lines, in the visual arts. Anonda Bell, curator at Bendigo Art Gallery, has been quoted as saying, "Art is constituted by the act of choice." We cannot make art without making choices.

In his book *The Power of Commitment* (2005,) marriage and family life educator Scott Stanley tells us how this works for strong marriages. He says that in commitment, each person has given up the rabbit-trails for the sake of the main path. Each small decision's energy keeps being re-directed back into the main goal; there is a power in the couple's knowing that they are a team and counting on each other. There is a foundation of security. This power eliminates anxiety about loss so the individuals can relax into the flow of their togetherness. (How needed these words are in today's culture!)

Images and forms used as structures are powerful for building what is new in this same way. They offer a foundation upon which to turn our energy, and allow us to relax within chosen boundaries. We often use a large blank circle, or mandala form, on the paper to begin watercolor sessions at a bedside because the totally blank page can seem overwhelmingly open to possibilities. Patients, who have often been at the mercy of other people's decisions their entire stay in the hospital, are sometimes not comfortable creating something from scratch at the beginning of an arts visit. They like to have a structure on which to hang their designs. This creates a condition where both the structure is used as a boundary, offering a feeling of safety, and the flow of watery colors can happen within it, echoing the moving flow of the spirit.

> Decisions are a way of defining ourselves, they are the way to give life and meaning to words, to dreams…they are the way to let what we are…be what we want to be.
> —Sergio F. Bambaren in *The Dolphin*

Have you ever felt overwhelmed by too many choices? To alleviate that feeling, the expressive arts facilitator in visual arts will often begin with a basic form from which the participant can start their own art. When we investigate the power of limits, we learn that commitment, the making and keeping of a choice, creates a strong foundation from which free expression can flow. There are new freedoms found when choices are made. Another kind of power is found in the choosing of a name, or in finding a metaphor, or identifying a trait or state. The process of naming is similar to making a commitment. It is a closing in on multiple traits to label the named as one entity. This can seem like a confining or a closing down of what has been a living entity, in constant flux. In the Judeo-Christian tradition, the name of God was never to be spoken, because the full qualities of God cannot be captured or named. God is alive.

However, being able to name something is essential for being able to manipulate it, think about it, and control aspects of it. As a mental health therapist, one of the first things I was taught was not to label and judge someone. I have been in agreement with this ethic because I think we can close down too quickly with a label at times, and narrow the scope of possibilities we see for, and therefore communicate to, the client. We can, if you will, curtail the ability of the client to seem alive in our eyes. Clients can become objects rather than vital beings.

However, the counseling field has a whole system of defining labels through which clients and therapies are categorized called the DSM, the Diagnostic and Statistical Manuals. These labels allow therapists to communicate and to find basic tools for helping clients. This sets up a both/and, paradoxical situation for the therapist who wants to remain open to knowing who the client is as a growing and changing being, through the self disclosure of the client, as well as what can be observed. Part of my love for the expressive arts as therapy has relieved me of the tension inherent from this paradox, because through facilitating the expressive arts with a client, I am allowing the person to unfold and reveal himself or herself through the Process. Sometimes, this is the only tool that is needed for the person's healing because of its ability to tap into deep levels of the psyche and make people aware of their own inner needs. Add a little feedback, and perhaps a sprinkle of guidance and they are good to go. Unfortunately, not all therapy can be done this quickly and easily.

Once in Expressive Arts class, we made power objects, and I found that in gathering things that told my story and spoke of my unique personality I could claim more of my personal power. When I felt strongly the sense of who I am, I could move forward with more self-confidence, more self-possession, more self-efficacy, yes, and more power. It is difficult to make an impact in life if one does not know who one is. There is a thread of strength that shines through everything a person does, says, or writes, that speaks of who he or she is when a person owns him or herself. Each person must feel that empowering "I AM." In *The Soul's Code,* James Hillman wrote, "Each person bears a uniqueness that asks to be lived. A myth of the hero calls from within his acorn; it is the push of the 'oakness' in the acorn" (1996:7.) In expressive arts, we look deeply for the imprints of such an element that can be experienced as the essence of Self that we carry inside. We seek to name what we see, to give power and credibility to what is.

Our ability to name and our ability to make art may be the two characteristics that define humans apart from other species more than any other qualities. In *The World in Six Songs*, Daniel J. Levitin says:

> "What distinguishes us most is one thing no other animals do: art. It is not just the existence of art, but the centrality of it...Some of the earliest cave painting show humans dancing. (And some are horses, as in Lascaux—*my addition.)* Apart from signaling creativity and the ability to engage in abstract thinking, the development of the artistic brain allowed for the metaphorical communication of passion and emotion...Art allows us to focus another's attention on aspects of a feeling or a perception that he might not otherwise see...poetry and lyrics and all the visual arts draw

their power from their ability to express abstractions of reality...Drawings, paintings, sculpture, poems, and song allow the creator to represent an object in its absence, to experiment with different interpretations of it, and thus—at least in fantasy—to exert power over it" (2008: 20-21.)

Although the kind of power that the world is moving toward is collaborative power, rather than staying stuck in a power-over model (at least that is what I hope,) the human brain is structured to allow us to manipulate objects in this way abstractly, and therefore exert power over our surroundings. That kind of power has been needed for the survival of our species in the past.

Leonard Schlain in his *The Alphabet Versus the Goddess* (1998) reminds us that in our beginnings, prior to written language, we were able to hold things in our minds as whole and living images more easily than when we moved to the written word as our major means of communication. However, with the advent of television and movies, we have been returning to an image-based, "wholistic" way of seeing our world. Perhaps there is a correlation between this movement from word back to image and the heightened desire for collaborative power, with its lessened need for having "power over." Such a discussion of power is titillating, but goes beyond the scope of this writing about the power found through the expressive arts process.

Another form of power found in expressive arts is the power of discipline. Although I have been told all my life that "creative minds are not tidy," I have lived long enough to know the freedom and power in creating good systems of organization in my home and my paperwork, whereas chaos takes time and effort, expended over and over again. (I admit here that chaos is my more natural way of being in the world.) Only yesterday, I was working at a friend's art studio where many young Eckerd College students had gathered for a Native American medicine circle ritual for their class. During a break, one of them asked about the secrets of college success. I heard my co-author Vicki Morgan tell her "the best help ever" is to organize. We may have gone from the three ring binder to the folder system on laptops, but the basic principle for success during newfound complexity remains the same: create a system of organization and use it.

Author David L. Wilson, in *Open Your Heart with Art*, tells us that:

> "Discipline is an aspect to self-control that can be developed through a number of external training methods. In this way, discipline occurs from the outside in. That is to say that you can be taught to develop discipline...Will is from the inside...discipline and structure can formalize the effort required to reach one's goals. Structure gives discipline a

framework on which to develop....(It's) connected to art through a commitment. Through commitment, creative energy becomes art" (2007:26.)

One of my favorite author/writers is artist Julia Cameron who writes about the "horse and carriage of the typewriter" helping her to stick to the discipline of her work (Cameron, 2006.) Discipline is no stranger to the artist. It is much of the 90% perspiration that inventor Edison said makes up the lion's share of genius. Just as Leonardo DaVinci kept his Codex, we can become more familiar with the tools and processes of our art as they become more a part of who we are through discipline and practice. Discipline may seem at first a harsh concept, but it is our friend.

Who among us has not witnessed the chaotic behavior of an undisciplined child? There is a need for socialization in the beginnings of life, and the opposite need for individuation following. Children learn socialization through discipline; knowing what the culture finds acceptable does not all come naturally. They learn appropriate boundary setting by having boundaries set for them at first, then gradually being allowed to set their own. It does a child or student a disservice to throw him or her into possibilities and ambiguities prior to giving them a basis from which to survive. I believe that we do ourselves a disservice as well when we expect ourselves to thrive in chaos without a basic foundation of strength.

Surely, you have had an experience of disciplining yourself on a diet or some other kind of restrictive commitment in order to reap the reward of the practice. The discipline involved in practicing a musical instrument day in and day out, tediously, has its rewards when the skill becomes automatic and refined. A disciplined practice yields the ability to let go into flow, since trusted systems of bodily movement and mental reactions have been conditioned into place. The bodymind can be a well-trained 'horse,' if we take the time to train it.

In reading an eloquent account about the balance one must find in musical performance, between flowing spontaneity and conditioned technique, in a book by Catherine David, called *The Beauty of Gesture* (1996,) I hear how her ideas echo in the training that I had through the Music for Healing and Transition Program (MHTP) for playing music at hospital bedsides. As my experience with that program grew, the balance between flow and structure blossomed for me into finding a way to resonate from my heart with the heart of a patient through my voice. One experience during my work as a Certified Music Practitioner (CMP) in the program can provide an example:

> A woman lay dying in the ICU; she was only my age. Her daughter was having a hard time accepting how sick she was, and

insisted that the staff continue to call Code Blue when her mother's body tried to stop breathing. The daughter had prayed for a miracle. But sometimes miracles and healing come in forms we do not expect. After listening to the daughter's story, I began singing hymns that were known to the daughter, coming from her strong Christian faith. But as the MHTP program taught me, and I had practiced, I used loose rhythm and spaced out the notes so that there was no strong heartbeat feel to the music. The daughter started to cry, and I knew she was doing some needed letting go. She listened without speaking for 10-15 minutes as I continued the arrhythmic songs. Then she went to the nurse and said that she was ready to sign the papers to stop the codes. She was willing now to let her mother die. With that done, the daughter then got very close to her mother's ear and started reciting, almost chanting, the names of all the family…one by one she said their names, and after each 5, she said, "We all love you." I hummed softly the tune of a hymn, still arrhythmically, and then fell silent, bearing witness. After the daughter had said 35-40 names, she was done. Her mother took a deep sigh, which seemed somehow to be one of satisfaction, and never breathed again. It was a beautiful time. Although the mom had been in a coma, I am sure that she heard what was happening. When the rest of the family came to the bedside, I was still accompanying the daughter in her grief, and she reassured them by saying, "I told her name by name that we all loved her." Each one found some comfort knowing that this important ritual was done.

This CMP work became for me a process of finding flow through disciplined practice, as well as co-creating with another's flow. It has become quite a horse of a different color for me to study about the other side, the side that works within limits, and find a balance in the flow through a discipline that seems necessary in the expressive arts.

Many people studying this field find it difficult, or at least different, to value the openness, the flow itself. I am reminded of an art show I attended of a recently deceased local painter who could render very detailed, realistic street scenes, revealing the beautiful diversity of our city. When he began to try to paint expressively, however, his work had no focus and nothing shone through its colors to speak of his emotional life. That experience told me how difficult it is for some people, especially those who have been highly trained and have refined their skills to the point of genius, to relax into flow, and connect with the expressive Process. I personally found that I valued the openness and flow of expressive arts from the beginning, although I had trouble getting to it sometimes in practice, as I was clumsy with the tools. However, I found the other half of the story, the horse of a different color called discipline, to be just as valuable and much needed for my expressive arts practice.

Riding the Metaphor

You have heard the phrase, "horse of a different color," at least if you have been paying attention during our cultural healing myth called the Wizard of Oz (and surely you paid attention during the sing-along version!) When Dorothy and her friends enter Oz, the man at the gate and the one driving them during the process (!) remarks, "That's a horse of a different color!" as they see a horse changing from green to pink to blue before them. Frank Baum and those who turned his story into a movie used subtle wit to move us from the shades of Kansas grey, or specifically, bland sepia-tone, to the emerald Oz and all its glittering deception. Through the dancing images of the movie screen, we notice the differences between the worlds. We notice the horse of a different color, and we are told through the metaphor that we are no longer talking about the same nature of thing that we were before. The actual phrase "horse of a different color" has been around since the time of Shakespeare. It hints of a story that has yet to be told.

As with the watchwords for expressive arts, flow, Process, oeuvre, white moment, "healingspace" and still point among them, there is the other story, the horse of a different color, the one told of discipline, skill, and the power of limits, to be realized for any budding practitioner. I found that using the horse metaphor is an excellent way to write about these other necessary qualities.

> "Horses are not complicated, but neither are the deepest spiritual truths."
> "Learning about horses is learning about ourselves."
> —Tony Stromberg

What better metaphor for power could we use than the age-old one of the horse? Greek gods and Celtic goddesses have been portrayed as riding horses because of the power they possessed. No doubt, it was recognized that a rider on a horse could much more easily conquer the foe than one who was on foot. These images expand into meaning within the culture. Poseidon, king of the Gods, was envisioned as riding his horse, the strong waves of the tide, into the world. Frank MacEowen in *The Mist-Filled Path: Celtic Wisdom* reminds us that medieval chivalry was originally a mystical tradition; knights worked with horses for higher good and order.

"Horses helped the knight refine his soul, purify his heart, and elevate his character," he wrote (2002:34.)

In the Tibetan Buddhist training for the Way of the Peaceful Warrior, *Shambala*, there exists an allegory for the human soul called *windhorse*. The tradition speaks of:

> "raising the wind of power and delight, and riding on, or conquering, that energy…this wind comes as a feeling of being completely and powerfully in the present… You also feel stability…the wind principle of basic goodness is exuberant and brilliant. It can radiate tremendous power in your life… following the disciplines…particularly the discipline of letting go…in some sense, the horse is never tamed—basic goodness never becomes your personal possession. But you can invoke and promote the uplifted energy of basic goodness in your life."
> (From www.glossary.shambala.org/2008.)

The process of co-creation in expressive arts therapy speaks to us like the symbolic image of riding *windhorse* and we can also envision this in the process of *dressage* in horsemanship, which will be addressed following this story from Laurie about her experience with horses. This is the story that gave me the horse metaphor for discussion.

Laurie's Horse Tale

> "The essential joy of being with a horse is that it brings us in contact with the rare elements of grace, beauty, spirit, and fire."
> —Sharon Ralls Lemon

Twenty years ago, I was a mess. Smack in the middle of talk therapy for depression, my therapist assigned me to "find something to do that is enjoyable." Ha! Nothing was enjoyable. But from the small child's voice within me, I heard HORSES! And so began a four-year adventure that taught me a little bit about horses and a lot about myself. My therapist will never know how much his suggestion for a 'hobby' reinforced all the material we covered during our talk sessions.

It was a risk for me to call a horse barn for lessons. I was 27. Most people start riding horses as children. As luck would have it, there was an adult beginner class, and I started going. Risk. Boy, I did not like risk! Risk means possible failure and hurt; emotional and/or physical hurt. On a horse's back you are always at risk. The horse could spook, buck, roll or refuse, and you could be on the ground. And in my life, I was stuck because of fear of risk. I felt as if I was already as low as anybody could get. Job changes, personal relationships, relocation, child bearing, family...I did not want risk. I wanted perfection and guarantees. On a horse's back, as in life, nothing is guaranteed.

The first horse that threw me was not Killer or Buck. Her name was Lady, and I never saw it coming. When she threw me it was a beautiful fall day, and we were jumping. Small jumps, under control, when Lady intentionally dropped her left wither and gently bucked me into a head-over-heels fall. I still had the reins in my hands. I was shocked! I was embarrassed. I was bruised. But I was ok. And I had to get back up and do it again. Right then. For me and for the horse. The next time lady tried to throw me, I was ready. But that night I had nightmares about broken necks. Theses nightmares were mixed with my other demons that I hadn't seen coming. Infertility for one. However, I survived. Maybe perfection wasn't everything. Maybe some things are worth the risk. I continued to ride and was thrown by other horses. I came to realize that the only way to never be thrown is to never ride. And riding was fun. I was starting to think life was fun, too.

Horses hold a mystical appeal for humans. There is in us the desire to dominate something that is so beautiful yet so powerful. Little girls play "horses" on the playground and draw pictures of horses. Little boys pretend to ride charging horses in war games. In our mind's eye, the horse is a beautiful, regal creature. Intelligent, benign, affectionate. At the horse barn, I learned the awful truth about horses. They are beautiful. Sometimes. A horse is at its happiest when it has just rolled in a cool mud puddle. There are hay and briars in his main and tail. On some occasions there is snot running from his nose; his teeth are usually a pale green from grass grazing. And flatulence. A horse's digestive system is amazing for its ability to produce methane gas. A horse in its natural state was not a pretty sight. This doesn't jive with our romantic image of them. And I certainly like to hold the romantic image of things when I can.

During therapy, I had to address some of my own ugly realities. I liked to be a victim and not make choices. I liked to blame the significant other people in my life for my failures. And I liked to deny my needs and desires. At the horse barn, I realized I am in my own self-imposed stall. I was choosing very small limits out of fear, and I was living at a level that was comfortable, but not what I wanted. I was like a horse rolling in a mud puddle, serving my base needs but not pursuing anything that might take risk or discipline. Where do you get the vision for what your life could be? How do you imagine it? How do you hear the call for action? Some lucky few hear and heed the call early in life. Those people are the saints and martyrs of the ages. Most of us scramble around trying to get it right, with glimpses here and there that keep us going down the path we choose. Then some of us get stuck and need help.

There were times in therapy when I felt like my whole life had been tipped over. I questioned many of my previously held beliefs. I felt frightened, scared, and lost. It was during that time that I bought my mare, Zoe, and we met Wolfgang, a true master at horse training. Wolfgang held training clinics on weekends at the horse barn. He was a big, blond German man who was strong and imposing in body and character. However, he was so kind and gentle with the horses. He knew how a horse thought and how to bring out the best in the animals. Some trainers might have used spurs, harnesses, whips…Wolfgang used his voice, his body and sometimes a rolled up newspaper. When he was in the saddle, my wayward mare became another horse. Instead of the soft-nosed, biting, kicking mare I rode, Wolfgang rode a Zoe that arched her neck and head in beautiful balance with the forward gait he asked her to perform. Magic! Beauty! They co-created this spell. He and she made it look so easy when they melded into their beautiful horse-man dance. Ask and obey, give and take, submission and assertion, discipline and abandon. I wanted to cry when I got to watch them. And Zoe was at peace under his hand. Watching man and horse in such harmony was spiritual. As I watched, I continued to think about my life and who my master would be.

Zoe continued to develop under Wolfgang, and I started making decisions about the directions I would take. That summer Zoe was in a small dressage show where she placed first out of fifteen other contestants. I did not ride her. One of my good friends rode her, so I got to watch Zoe in her moment of glory. She seemed to know that this was her day. She was patient and gentle as we braided her main and tail and attached ribbons. Her coat shone from the bathing and currying, and her hooves were smooth and even from the work the ferrier had done. The mean, dirty half-wild horse was gone. No Cinderella could have had a more dramatic transformation than Zoe could. She carried herself so well in the ring, as all the hard work came together. Looking back over my life, this day was one of my personal best. It symbolized so much for me, and I felt that I could do anything. Dreams do come true.

My time in therapy was coming to an end as well. I had learned a lot and felt ready to say goodbye to my therapist. Relocation, a job change and a much healthier relationship with my husband were the results of my therapy. Habits are hard to break, but at least now, I had the tools to work through issues that caused me pain.

And as everyone knows, life has surprises and some of them bring pain. About six weeks after the horse show that Zoe won, there was a horrible rainstorm with lots of lightening. The rain finally stopped around 5:00 pm, feeding time for the horses. That was when the barn manager called me. Zoe had not come in for feeding, so the manager went looking for her on the 150-acre pasture. She found her on the highest hill, lying on her side, dead from being struck by lightning. When I was told, I felt like I had been struck by lightning, too. My heart hurt, and I couldn't breathe. The taste of metal was strong in the back of my mouth. How could grief be so intense? I was ashamed to admit how long I grieved my horse. As time went on, I realized that I was also grieving the lessons that Zoe and the other horses had taught me. This part of my life was over. Several months after this, we moved to an area that did not make horse life easy. And to be honest, something told me to move on and pursue other dreams and goals. The thing I did know was that what I had learned from Zoe and therapy was worth every bit of the pain they afforded me. Moreover, that knowledge gave me the courage to leap into a new life, one of passion and of joy.

> "A horse is the projection of people's dreams about themselves—strong, powerful, beautiful—and it has the capability of giving us escape from our mundane existence."
> —Pam Brown (QuoteGarden.com)

Dancing into the Distant Day

I am looking forward to Rilke's distant day when answers are found. Yet I know that part of living is learning to find balance within ambiguity. That balance creates the dance. My queries are about the power needed for transformation, for healing, found in the expressive arts. If I had to come up with a theory about what is needed in order for healing to take place and a sense of efficacy and enjoyment to be experienced, I would put the horse of a different color into the arena. I would talk about riding the flow, but with the power found through the elements of skill and discipline that allow such freedom. I would "re-member" the necessary balance to be found between free flow and choice making. I believe that only the combination of the two can bring forth a beauty and meaningfulness that is transformative. This balance, as represented by the rolling Tao symbol, as we have previously seen, is the "both/and," the ambiguity itself. It is what yields satisfaction, art-full-ness, and graceful movement within the flow. Then, in the presence of what is aesthetically pleasing, the persons involved in the expressive arts can relax into themselves, let go, and let be. That is when their physiology changes and their inborn healing capacities go to work.

In establishing an arts in medicine program at the hospital where I have worked since the year 2000, I put out a call to artists in the community to help us. We specifically wanted artists, not just willing community members with good hearts and a compassionate outlook toward others. A person with both kinds of skills is not always easy to find. We wanted artists at the bedside, those with the skill to help facilitate the process with patients and their families in such a way that there could be a result that felt pleasing and enjoyable to the person making the art. They needed knowledge of the tools. The bedside artists were guides, and often helped shape the art along with the patient.

Many of the people who joined us had already been trained in the expressive arts process, but we gave them six very full days of training, spread over a few weeks, in companioning skills and in entering process, in order to help them prepare. All in all, we taught each other, and continue to teach each other. We established a group of artists that still meet monthly to continue our education together, and we held weekly artist's rounds to discuss what was happening at the bedsides. In our program, we did whatever we could to help our arts staff to understand both how to be in Flow and how to use their skills at the bedsides. The group flourishes, and has initiated many kinds of creative "happenings" for the hospital and the community at large. We have become close friends, and feel solidified enough to call ourselves a "tribe."

During a recent trip "back home again in Indiana," I had an opportunity to meet with a lifelong friend, Jerri Orosz, and tell her about the writing I was doing about horses and the creative process. I spoke about the intuitive connection I felt, but for which I had no words. Jerri is an equestrian and she immediately, as usually is the case with her, let out a rolling stream of beautiful verbiage about horses and their riders in *dressage* that spoke perfectly to the dance of co-creation about which I wanted to write. She can have true eloquence in the moment, a condition my more studied way of approaching life seldom reaches.

It was early morning. The frost was on the pumpkin and the grandbabies were still asleep upstairs. We brought our coffee out to the front porch that overlooked the gentle hills of cornfield. In true form, I did not have a pen, and therefore could not catch what was in the moment, in this once in a lifetime performance, although I wanted to. For Jerri, it was no big deal. She was just talking about what she knows. For me, it was so like music that I wished everyone could hear it. However, I had to take myself to the computer a few days later to research (Thank you, Wikipedia!) and hear again how *dressage* is done. Now I must find a way to relate it, even if with less grace. Again, I am struck by how much experience and time with a subject can help to create Flow. Wikipedia explains *dressage* as:

> "A path and destination for competitive horse training...its fundamental purpose is to develop, through standardized progressive training methods, a horse's natural athletic ability and willingness to perform, thereby maximizing its potential as a riding horse. At the peak of a dressage horse's gymnastic development, it can smoothly respond to a skilled rider's minimal aids by performing the requested movement while remaining relaxed and appearing effortless. Dressage is occasionally referred to as 'Horse Ballet.'"

Jerri sent me a link to a YOUTUBE video of a rider named Stacy Westfall (www.westfallhorsemanship.com, 2006) to demonstrate what she told me about the riders who seem to be going *au naturel*, riding a wild horse bareback and barefoot, with no bits or bridles. Jerri pointed out that there is a tremendous amount of training for the rider that goes into such a performance. According to her, today's idea about training horses is no longer that the horse needs to be 'broken' and then will obey. Now, horses are trained according to their own temperament. The potential rider must listen to the horse and pay attention to its way of being in the world, then use the tools of training to bring out the best in the horse. It would be as if we are riding windhorse, listening to the voice of the spirit it brings, and allowing it to carry us. How very much like the creative expressive flow in the arts, especially shared to create a healing process.

When it comes to *dressage* in the ring, horse and rider are judged on rhythm, regularity, relaxation, and impulsion, the storing of the energy of engagement for thrust or power. The mind of the horse engages, focusing on the rider, allowing for a dissipation of nervous energy. There is collaborative effort, with horse and rider listening to each other. This state for horse and rider is reminiscent of the state of focused but energetic relaxation found when one is in the Process in creative expression. It is a state of being aware of everything, yet distracted by nothing. Our inner and outer selves are listening to each other. It is a paradoxical state of being in both energy and relaxation; a dynamic dance between the two conditions, it is a state in which nervous energy dissipates through "dynergic" energy, the energy that pushes and pulls at the same time in growth processes, to create Golden Mean proportions in nature, as named by Doczi (1994:3.)

I have seen this dissipation of nervous energy through centering into the point of relaxed energy in myself and in many others during expressive arts activities. Dr. Sherry Ackerman in *Dressage in the Fourth Dimension* says the "art of *dressage* means to directly experience oneness" (2008:2.) In *dressage,* there is the collaborative nature of two living beings entering the process in order to create something that shines with beauty. Who would say that this differs much from the goals of education or therapy?

Seeing *dressage* is like watching a ballet, and this *pas de deux* shows us a symbol of another, invisible grace. Doczi points out, "There is freedom and movement in ballet that appears miraculously easy. This freedom turns upon order, the order of discipline that prepares and sustains all great accomplishments. One of the secrets of this order in ballet is the support of the body's entire weight upon a single point, the center of gravity in the sacrum…growth, gravity, and grace concentrated in one point of our sacrum is the power of limits enshrined in our bones" (1994:102.) While the center of gravity in *dressage* must lie somewhere between both participating beings, the nature of support and freedom of movement with grace echoes Doczi's analysis of ballet.

Doczi has shown us how the power of limits engenders grace through sharing limitations when he speaks of the interrelatedness of all beings. All ancient wisdom and now modern cosmology tell us the same. He refers to the principles of the Kaballah, saying:

> "The divine gift of love springs from the relatedness of all that exists. There exists a deep-rooted unity below the many surface diversities of this world in a limitless order to our existence. We are split beings, living in a split world…our task in life is to restore to wholeness (and order) as many fragments as we encounter along the path of our life…one of the ways…is the pathway of Golden Mean proportions. (These proportions reveal) shared limitations (which) open the doors toward the limitless. This is the power of limits…(it) is the force behind creation…When we share our own limitations with the limitations of others, as we do in the golden (relationships) of neighbors, we complement our own and others' shortcomings, creating thereby living harmony in the art of life" (1994:139-141.)

In sharing our limitations between us, we can co-create a shared wholeness, a wholeness that does not exist when we are not in relationship.

The wholeness we seek for our relationships has a spiritual dimension. There is a placard in one of my friend's homes that says, "Bidden or unbidden, God is present." Some do not wish to name the presence as God, but still recognize an aggregate dimension, a gestalt. Ancient wisdom says, "Wherever two or three are gathered in my name, there I AM in the midst of them" (Matthew 18:20.) The "I AM" God in the gap between you and me becomes the imminent God within me touching the immanent God within you, through a golden thread, weaving us into a whole that overcomes our separateness and limitations. It is bigger than the sum of its parts. The center of gravity, however, is between both of us, neither one of us holds it alone. That center point is the place upon which all grace turns. And the wholeness found in the shared relationship is a form of healing. The words "heal" and "whole" come from the same root word in the English language. In seeking our wholeness, or oneness, we seek our healing. This can be a healing between people, or a healing within one person of a bodymind and spirit split. Shaun McNiff, renowned in the expressive arts field, reminds us, "Healing is a process that transforms conflicting forces into a new and more productive relationship...art does the same thing" (2004:272.)

Wholeness implies a peaceful existence between the parts of that whole. Who knew that in seeking healing through the expressive arts, we have also been promoting peace in the world? Perhaps, intuitively, we all have known. In creating beauty together, in allowing what is within each of us to come into the sharing, we can feel ourselves becoming more alive, and we all become more whole. There is an intimate relationship between beauty and order. As within, so without.

> "If there is righteousness in the heart,
> There will be beauty in the character,
> If there is beauty in the character,
> There will be harmony in the home.
> If there is harmony in the home,
> There will be order in the nation,
> When there is order in each nation,
> There will be peace in the world."
> —Lao-Tse 6th century

Wild horses could not pull me away from this work. Even the promise of lots more money could not keep me from its allure. My first experiences learning about the expressive arts, as recounted above, happened over 10 years ago, yet they are still rendered vividly in my memory. I can remember that part of myself well, and delight in the mythical "hippocamp," the half horse, half fish, seahorse, or mermaid, that the story evokes for me now. "Healing springs from what instinctively vivifies us, whatever sends off a glimmer of power," writes Marc Ian Barasch in *The Healing Path* (1993:314.) I have found a glimmer of power through my work with expressive arts. He also says to be whole, healed, we must find "ways to honor (our) own oddity of heart...If we do not trust what emerges from within us, we limit our aliveness "(1993:315.) Some say working with the expressive arts is an odd spin on life, an odd way of going about being in the world, and a "fringe" way of going about helping people to heal, but it is my chosen path, and I am committed to it. I find that new opportunities open to me continually along this path.

You see, I choose to live, to be alive in everything I do, and to feel alive as often as I can. I also choose to invite others to live along with me. It is the basis of my work as teacher, musician, chaplain, spiritual director and therapist. Rick Jarow in his book, *Creating the Work You Love*, says:

> "In many cases true choice is about choosing with what or whom to align ourselves...we seek to make choices that are aligned with Spirit and its power...it is up to each of us to find our own voice, to choose from our own place of clarity and power"(1995:54.)

I choose to use the work and play of expressive arts in my therapy, my chaplain work, and my teaching. I choose to add more and more of the expressive dimension to my music. I also choose to add expressive arts work to many of the times when I gather with my tribe to celebrate who we are as individuals and as a group together. Jarow also challenges me, "Will you dare to become a force in the transformation of the world?" (1995: 6.)

And my answer to that challenge is that I do not know if what I do as a therapist and teacher, or what we do as a small group of expressive arts practitioners, can make a difference in the larger world. We can only make the splash into the lake, not knowing where its ripples will touch the shore. But I am no longer afraid to dive in. My tribe keeps "moving all about," together; it may seem like the hokey-pokey to some, but it is our own authentic dance. All interaction between living beings creates this dance, just as all therapy is a dance of co-creation between the therapist and the participant. When I interact with a client as person, not as object or diagnosis, I open the dialogue for co-creation. I believe that this dialogue is essential in all of my work with people. When the dialogue is opened, there is an opportunity for the creation of art. And art, when it becomes a deep expression of someone's being, his or her essence, and his or her spirit, reveals a living relationship between the unformed spirit and its communication to the world through form.

"Making art is a rite of initiation. People change their souls."
—Julia Cameron

There remain many answers into which I yet have to dance about the expressive arts and their power; I welcome that dancing. I am thankful for the image of the horse to aide my thinking and intuitive processes. Perhaps I should make a collage to help me find some answers...Carol Shore, my peer and mentor, says that the images we create are about 6 months ahead of our conscious thinking processes.

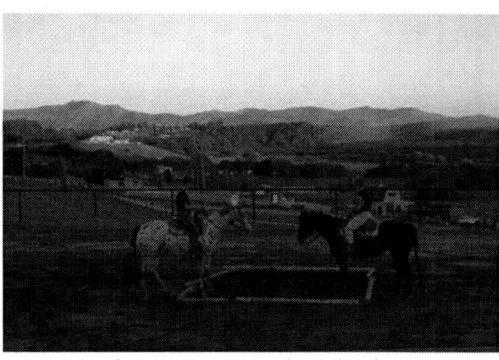

I do know some of my own answers to the queries raised here about the power for healing our troubled world. I know through my own experience, and through listening carefully to others, that there is inherent power within the process of coming forth with what lies deep within our souls. In addition, I believe that all art, when it comes to form, is about finding the balance between skillful discipline and the powerful flow of the Spirit. Perhaps, for now, that is all I need to know about the process of expressive arts, that it is a process of moving Spirit through the self, within the discipline of an art form, at the junction of the still center point. Now, I can rest there and know peace even within the dance of its mystery, within its "healingspace."

> "Except for the point, the still point, there would be no dance, and there is only the dance."
> —TS Eliot

My thanks to Elle Speed for the photograph.

Bibliography and Further Reading Possibilities:

Ackerman, Sherry. *Dressage in the Fourth Dimension*. Novato, CA: New World Library. 2008.

Apostolos-Cappadona, Diane, ed. *Art, Creativity, and the Sacred*. New York: Crossroad. 1992.

Badonsky, Jill. *The Nine Modern Day Muses*. New York: Gotham Books. 2001.

Bambaren, Sergio. *The Dolphin*. New York: Hay House. 2008.

Barasch, Marc Ian. *The Healing Path*. New York: Penguin/Arkana. 1993.

Brooke, Avery. *Healing in the Landscape of Prayer.* Boston: Cowley Publications. 1996.

Bruder, Kurt A. 'Kailash.' *Following Sound into Silence.* New York: Hay House, Inc. 2008.

Bush, Carol A. *Healing Imagery and Music.* Portland, OR: Rudra Press. 1995.

Cameron, Julia. *God Is No Laughing Matter.* New York: Jeremy P. Tarcher/Putnam. 2001.

—. *Finding Water; The Art of Perseverance.* New York; Penguin Group. 2006.

Cassou, Michele. *Point Zero.* New York: Tarcher/Putnam. 2001.

Ching, Elise Dirlam and Kaleo Ching. *Chi and Creativity.* Berkely, CA: Blue Snake Books. 2007.

Chodorow, Joan ed. *Jung on Active Imagination.* New Jersey: Princeton University Press. 1997.

Combs, Mark, and Mark Holland. *Synchronicity.* New York: Marlowe and Co. 1996.

Csikszentmihalyi, Mihaly. *Creativity, Flow, and the Psychology of Discovery and Invention.* New York: HarperCollins. 1996.

David, Catherine. *The Beauty of Gesture.* Berkeley, CA: North Atlantic Books. 1996.

Dilts, Robert, and Robert McDonald. *Tools of the Spirit.* Capitola, CA: Meta Publications. 1997.

Doczi, György. *The Power of Limits.* Boston: Shambala Publications. 1994.

Dossey, Larry, M.D. *Beyond Illness.* Boston: Shambala Publications. 1984.

Eisner, Elliot W. *The Arts and the Creation of Mind.* New Haven, CT: Yale University Press, 2002.

Enelow, Gertrude. *Body Dynamics.* New York: Information, Inc., 1960

Fox, John. *Finding What You Did Not Lose.* New York: Tarcher/Putnam, 1995.

Fox, Matthew. *Creativity.* New York: Jeremy P. Tarcher/Penguin, 2004.

Ganim, Barbara. *Art & Healing: Using Expressive Art to Heal Your Body Mind & Soul.* Novato, CA: New World Library, 1998.

Ganim, Barbara, Susan Fox. *Visual Journaling: Going Deeper than Words.* Novato, CA: New World Library, 1999.

Gold, Aviva. *Painting from the Source.* New York: Harper Perennial, 1998.

Goleman, Daniel, et. al. *The Creative Spirit.* New York: Dutton, 1992.

Graham-Pole, John, M.D., *Illness and the Art of Creative Self-Expression*. Oakland, CA: New Harbinger Publications, 2000.

Grey, Alex. *The Mission of Art*. Boston: Shambala Publications, 1998.

Hillman, James. *The Soul's Code: In Search of Character and Calling,*.New York: Warner Books, 1996.

Houston, Jean. *The Possible Human*. Los Angeles: J.P. Tarcher, 1982.

Huber, Cheri. *How you do anything is how you do everything*. Murphys, CA: Keep it Simple Books, 1988.

Institute of Noetic Sciences with William Poole. *The Heart of Healing*. Atlanta: Turner Publishing, 1993.

Jarow, Rick. *Creating the Work You Love*. Rochester, VT: Destiny Books. 1995.

Jaworski, Joseph. *Synchronicity*. San Francisco: Berrett-Koehler Publishers, 1996.

Kabat-Zinn, Jon. *Coming to Our Senses*. New York: Hyperion Books, 2005.

Knill, Paolo J., Helen Nienhaus Barba, and Margo N. Fuchs. *Minstrels of Soul: Intermodal Expressive Therapy*. Toronto: Palmerston Press, 1995.

Knill, Paolo J. *Principles and Practices of Expressive Arts Therapy*. London: Jessica Kingsley Publishers, 2005.

Kohanov, Linda. *Riding Between the Worlds: Expanding on Potential through the Way of the Horse*. Novato, CA: New World Library, 2003.

Levitin, Daniel J. *The World in Six Songs*. New York: Dutton/Penguin, 2008.

MacEowen, Frank. *The Mist-Filled Path: Celtic Wisdom for Exiles, Wanderers, and Seekers*. Novato, CA: New World Library, 2002.

Malchiodi, Cathy A. *Expressive Therapies*. New York: The Guildford Press, 2005.

McNiff, Shaun. *Art Heals*. Boston: Shambala, 2004.

—. *Art As Medicine*. Boston: Shambala, 1992.

Myss, Caroline. *Entering the Castle*. New York: Free Press, 2007.

Nimmer, Dean. *Art from Intuition*. New York: Watson-Guptill Publications, 2008.

Nuland, Sherwin B. *The Wisdom of the Body*. New York: Alfred A. Knopf, 1997.

Ornstein, Robert E. *The Psychology of Consciousness*. New York: Harcourt Brace Jovanovich, Inc, 1977.

Phillips, Rick. *Healing Communication*. New Mexico: Deva Publishing, 1996.

Progoff, Ira. *The Well and the Cathedral*. New York: Dialogue House, 1977.

Richards, M. C. *Centering*. Hanover, NH: Wesleyan University Press, 1989.

Rilke, Rainer Maria. *Letters to a Young Poet*. New York: Random House. Translated by Stephen Mitchell, 1984.

Rogers, Natalie. *The Creative Connection*. Palo Alto, CA: Science & Behavior Books, 1993.

Sacks, Oliver. *The Man Who Mistook His Wife For a Hat*. New York: Touchstone, 1998.

Schlain, Leonard, M.D. *The Alphabet Versus the Goddess*. New York: Viking/Penguin, 1998.

Sharp, Sharon, ed. *Expressive Arts Therapy*. Boone, NC: Parkway Publishers, 2003.

Sheldrake, Rupert. *A New Science of Life*, Rochester, VT: Park Street Press. 1995.

Stanley, Scott M. *The Power of Commitment: A Guide to Active, Lifelong Love,* San Francisco: Jossey-Bass. 2005.

Stewart, Ian. *Nature's Numbers*, New York: Basic Books. 1995.

Stromberg, Tony and Linda Kohanov. *Spirit Horses*, Novato, CA: New World Library. 2005.

Terruwe, Anna A., M.D. and Baars, Conrad W., M.D. *Psychic Wholeness and Healing*, New York: Alba House. 1981.

Trungpa, Chogyam. *Shambala: Sacred Path of the Warrior,* Boston: Shambala Publications. 1984.

Underhill, Evelyn. *Practical Mysticism*, Columbus, OH: Ariel Press. 1942

Wallace, Jim and The Editors of "Sojourners." *Spirit of Fire*, Washington, DC. Sojourners. 2003.

Wilson, David L. *Open Your Heart with Art: Mastering Life through Love of Everyday Creativity*, Las Vegas, Nevada. 2007.

Websites

http://snell.mystarband.net/peace_poem.htm
www.weforanimals.com/quotations
www.quotegarden.com
www.shambala.org
www.wikipedia.org
www.creativetampabay.com
www.floridaREAP.org

SIMPLY BEING: USING MEDITATION AND MINDFUL AWARENESS AS AN ELEMENT OF CHANGE

ROSEMARY J. WENTWORTH

"Changes," a twelve week, experiential group, is offered at a state prison facility and at a substance abuse residential treatment center. Mindfulness, meditation, and expressive therapy tools are integrated in order to develop skills of self-literacy, particularly distress tolerance and emotional regulation. Clients present with dual diagnosis: substance abuse and Axis 1 disorders. The same gender group is limited to twelve voluntary participants. Individuals are in either the active or the maintenance stage of motivational change and self-select for participation through reflective writing on goal changes, and a mission statement. A mindfulness attention awareness assessment, a life and satisfaction survey, along with "strengths" and "inventory of change" questionnaires help the individual highlight the direction of treatment objectives prior to committing to a journey of personal change. Clients are advised that journaling (imaging and writing,) meditation practice, mindfulness exercises, and mood logs are part of daily assignments. The client will be both observer and participant, a means to enhance self-efficacy. Clients attend a preliminary discussion about the therapeutic tools of mindfulness, meditation, and expressive arts.

Alcohol and drug use are environmental risk factors that change neural functioning that are important to problem solving, control of impulsivity, and conceptual thinking. Mindfulness, meditation, and the expressive arts can help mediate change in these same cortical operations. It is explained that these learned skills deepen self-awareness and empower already inherent personal strengths by providing a safe and non-judgmental container for self-investigation. Stories, poems, drumming and art works (masks, mandalas, dream catchers, sand paintings, photo collages, etc.) of social peers are shared, showing how an individual's history can be revealed through personal symbols: strengths, resiliencies, judging ghosts and self-clinging habits. One can become familiar with the underlying meaning of constructs, both pleasing and unlikable, and bring into play transformations through the dialogue of mindfulness and meditation. From these presentations, clients can see how "simply being" engages the healing process, mobilizing different sensations and emotions needed to release inhibitions so that further unpeeling of painful layers can be accessed (Rogers, 1993.)

"Simply being" captures the essence of the art making process, which is a concrete metaphor for mindfulness and meditative reflection. To witness is to involve oneself in a dynamic interaction. With the added components of intention and attention blended into the process of experiential inquiry in the expressive arts, further opportunities to generate new options and meanings emerge. This integral communication, accessing feeling, cognition, and sensation, makes the invisible visible, allowing for self-understanding and insight into the direction of desired change (Rogers, 1993.)

By looking at scientific research on neuroplasticity, mindfulness, art making, and meditation, one finds there are implications for subjective experience (the lived moment.) Self-literacy (a trait of positive mental health) is enhanced when these three dialogue intermodally. The expressive therapies speak the language of the unconscious. Various art modalities activate motor, somatosensory, visual, emotional, and cognitive aspects of information processing and their analogous neurobiological utilities in the brain (Lusebrink, 2004.) The acts of creating art impart information, evoke expression, and shape knowledge that can change ideas, feelings, sensations, and choices of actions to reflect the universal experience of being human.

Mindfulness, meditation, and expressive therapies are combined in a self-exploratory, experiential process. This generates a synergy that allows for communication of thoughts, emotions, and sensations without judgment and with acceptance. Basic attitudes and beliefs underlying problematic concerns can be looked at with neutrality, offering insights into understanding a current, situational experience or mood state. Negative experiences are not avoided but rather mindfully confronted and meditatively questioned from the emergence of the container of symbolic self-expression.

Mindfulness is about awareness of the present moment and accepting with openness and curiosity the current experience without attachment or expectation of a particular outcome. Meditation is focusing attention on a particular object, in this case the art product, to connect more deeply to one's personal archetypal symbology. These are the underlying premises that formed the basis of the expressive and cognitive program of "Changes".

Neuroplasticity describes these cortical re-mappings in the organizational structure and function of the brain in response to experiences (FitzGerald & Folan-Curran, 2002,) which include thinking and imagining (Cozolino, 2002.) It is what we pay attention to that allows for the increase and decrease between neurons, adding or deleting neuronal connections, which is how information is communicated through the mind and body (Cayoun, 2002.) Impulsive or addictive behaviors may be seen as examples of synaptic rewiring due to 'negative plasticity' of maladaptive behaviors. In like manner, 'positive plasticity,' developed by training, may lead to improved managing of negative emotions and moderation of immune function (Davidson et al., 2003.) Teicher's work on the neurobiology of abuse and trauma indicates that overactivation of stress may lead to conditioned patterns of emotional state dependency, such as risk taking or impulsive behaviors (Teicher, 2002.) This results in a less integrated sense of self that may be difficult to relinquish (Schiele, 1992,) and these habitual patterns of behavior are encoded in the neuronal network. Negative emotions are processed in the right hemisphere and involve the autonomic response of the release of stress producing hormones. Meditation and mindfulness encourage the release of non-stressful hormones, placing the body and mind in a more relaxed state, allowing for modification of behavior. Primary emotions such as fear, anger, or sadness are self-soothed with mindfulness and meditation techniques. Secondary emotions such as hopelessness, frustration, vulnerability, or loneliness are experienced safely within the boundaries of the art-making environment.

Therefore, one can see how the combination of mindfulness, meditation, and expressive therapy provide for a healing environment to emerge that allows the inner and outer world of the conscious and unconscious to integrate safely. The participant and the product both simultaneously witness to the unfolding of opposites and their subsequent integration into wholeness. A parallel process occurs that engages the left-brain (verbal, analytical, and sequencing) with the right brain (nonverbal, intuitive, and synergistic) in a meaningful conversation (McNamee, 2004.)

Preliminary investigation of the neural basis of mindfulness and meditation using electroencephalography (EEG,) evoked potential and cognitive event related potential (ERP) technologies, positron emission tomography (PET,) functional magnetic resonance imaging (fMRI) and spectroscopy (Baerenstein et al, 2001; Cahn & Polich, 2006) suggest alterations in neural activation patterns that seem to impact the cognitive manner of ruminative thinking and autobiographical memory as well as improved attentional and perceptual processes (Basar et al., 2001; Valentine & Sweet, 1999.) These two techniques appear to facilitate abilities of behavioral regulation, helping clients to become more fully aware of present behavior and personal belief systems, thus effectively reducing stress symptoms and mood disturbance while increasing affect regulation, trait mindfulness and perceptions of control.

Current treatment approaches, such as Dialectical Behavior Therapy (Linehan, 1993,) Mindfulness Based Stress Reduction (Kabat-Zinn, 1990) and Acceptance and Commitment Therapy (Hayes, Strosahl, & Wilson, 1999) utilize acceptance and mindfulness to help clients approach another way of knowing the world and themselves. The salient factor in all these psychological interventions is the "experiential knowing" rather than what the mind has to say about the world and the self. "Being present" not only seems to enhance more autonomous self-regulation and motivation to maintain goals, but also hinders distraction from intrusive thoughts, thus permitting greater accuracy of relevant information and decreasing habitual responding (Wenk-Sormaz, 2005) while increasing greater self-control. The creative process of art making allows one to combine the right brain's emotional intelligence with the left-brain's logical intelligence to make successful judgments (Malchiodi, 2003.) Mindfulness uncouples the habitual connections between perception, appraisal, and conditioned response, letting response rather than reaction occur, and moving one beyond stress reactivity and a survival-oriented mode of operating. The body remains the focal point where thoughts and emotions are experienced. The importance of using the body and its senses of what it has produced through creativity as a focal point engenders learning to pay attention to somatic cues as reliable emotional messages with salient information of an experience, without retreating into less effective coping strategies. One learns that if one can place the self into the stress mode, then one can easily place the self into the corresponding polarity of relaxation (Schaffer & Yucha, 2004.) The key is intention and attention. What the mind thinks, perceives, and experiences is sent from the brain to the rest of the body. This ability to capture paradox, identify difficulties, and see how one has been able to recover from ambivalence is important in forming positive self-image (Hanna, 2002) and in maintaining nonrestrictive rapport with oneself. The expressive art with its characteristic of inherent, spontaneous creativity is the natural breath of soul that moves the self from isolation to connection – "simply being."

The pain- pleasure opiate receptors (pain/pleasure,) biochemical messengers, act with aptitude throughout the body, which behaves like an unconscious mind (Pert, 1997.) Emotions knit the mind and body together. They are regulators of experiences of reality including the intangible spiritual states of awe, bliss, and consciousness. Biofeedback tells us that every change in physiology is followed by a concomitant change in the mental emotional state and vice-versa, conscious or unconscious. Furthermore, one can reach a deepened, relaxation state and allow voluntary control of physiological processes usually regarded as automatic. Pain, heart rate, tension, relaxation can be manipulated. Physiological states of stress can be deactivated and pleasurable states can be produced through meditative practices and art making.

Mindbody attention shifts are usually unconscious. However, intentional disciplines, body scanning, focusing, centering, guided imagery, or visualization aimed at increasing awareness can influence change at the cellular level. These breathing and energy based techniques influence blood flow. Oxygen and nutrients are brought to nourish and toxins are removed, thus healing can be facilitated in the bodymind (Pert, 1997.)

Healing is alchemical with the expressive arts. The expressive arts allow the unique properties and experiences of the individual to be understood as mediating variables within his/her process. The way one perceives is directly correlated with the manner in which one thinks and feels; the relationship of our visual representations speaks to the method in which our lives are patterned. This gestalt of the art experience gives insight into how things are, and makes clear the possibility of alternate choices. It is crucial to engage in, rather than ignore, the unannounced and perhaps unwelcome. These responses are means to adaptation. Therefore, skills that nurture self-awareness and intention are important adaptive processes that can facilitate awareness and creative options and uncover dormant seeds of possibility. The sanctuary where one can listen to oneself is in the experiential process of expression. Most behavior is custom, routinely arranged by core beliefs. Self-reflection of one's experiences allows for garnering insight into how this core material affects the organizing of experiences, especially how meaning and feeling are assigned to events.

The mind-body-soul's natural language of communication is through images. By attending to images and symbols of the inner reality, a connection can manifest itself with outer reality. Art making fits this framework, offering the needed flexibility to reduce stress, enhance positive interactions, and recognize and manage difficulties. The strength-based application of expressive arts allows inherent resilience to manifest itself, nurturing the distinctive creation of its maker. Art by its very nature is about growing and remaking into new. It can be a safe and natural container to express strong emotions. Past actions and feelings can be communicated, not suppressed, at the pace of the participant's comfort level. As a universal language, art speaks to the creator in a non-direct and transpersonal manner. The emotions become connected to the experience so that they can be discussed in other modalities. By reconciling, and integrating one's mythology as a response to ongoing self-actualization, insight illuminates the characteristic patterns and strategies that have been layered to organize skill. Evoking experience within the mindful awareness lowers the noise, so that awareness can gather information about itself and work through emotional release, become integrated and thus transformed. This allows the being to move into becoming, and enter into a new chosen way of being.

Art is like a bridge between the known and unknown. The experiential process lets personal symbols and images emerge and link with the Self. Knowing through art offers a phenomenological porthole into redefining the meaning and connection within the status of change. Images are symbols from the unconscious and can be healing agents, which move the creator to greater spiritual and psychological health.

Loss of social support and the ability to share and express feelings is distressing. Individuals who have trouble with expressing their loss in words find the use of art materials a beneficial tool for the manifestation of feelings non-verbally. It is a natural way to derive intuitive insight and it transcends time and space. The images and symbols of the inner self are heard and heeded, creating connection. The physical transformation of space moves one beyond the confines of conventional three dimensions. Forms and colors become players in a space that begins at the surface, but then extends into a spectator-participant relationship with its creator-explorer. Lines become movements in time and space. It is a structuring of perspective that allows the eye to see "I" and the other simultaneously.

Negative and fearful emotions block the body, mind, and spirit, interfering with the ability to feel, to learn, and to be in the universe. When difficult emotions are expressed in color, shape, form, design, texture, and movement (externalized,) positive physiological benefits accrue. The immune system is strengthened and there is an increase in anti-stress neurotransmitters, moving the body/mind to homeostasis. The energy that is in the emotion informs the substance utilized. The released energy is no longer held within and is expressed in a harmless way that unblocks the resistance. This release communicates new learning, and as the insights are understood, they are internalized into new visualizations.

In conclusion, healing work that comes from the challenge of pain and confusion can lead to resolution and reconstruction, moving a committed individual to a more integrated Self by encoding a coping mechanism that adapts to change. This is based on strengthening the inherent resiliency within, between the conscious and unconscious processes. The expressive arts allows for the natural unfolding of that which is hidden but seeking to be known and recognized, bringing *"dark matter into the light"* not unlike the process of natural creation (Keith, 2003.)

Some of the participants describe their encounters with meditation, mindfulness and the expressive arts in the "Changes" program below. All feedback by the artists is used with permission. Clients are asked to comment on, "What has been the Transformative Piece for you in this Process?"

> "I've been able to connect my physical ailments with my emotions. I've learned to know what to expect, what my feelings mean. I have become open to awe and wonder again. What is important is what I think about myself, not that my family has given up on me and sees me as the big screw up, never going to be anything but a black sheep to them. They'll change when they see and watch that I've changed. I'm not mad about it. It just is the way things are. The one I have to please is myself. I want to like to live within my skin and not try to live up to other people's expectations" D.I.

> "I have been able to see common recurring themes in my life. I am beginning to understand the body-mind-soul connection, and that it is all related to each other. I have changed my focus. I am less judgmental. I have a problem with anger and rage. I didn't want to try the anger management classes because I thought they were sissy stuff but now I know that I hurt myself more with my anger and that I can learn about how not to be out of control. I've learned that I am teachable. I was always told I was unteachable." R.D.

> "I'm learning to use my tools in relationships, asking the questions I need to ask for myself. What am I doing? Is this right for me? If it feels wrong, paying attention to my intuition. I feel more at ease within, inside myself, dealing with the anxiety and ambiguity. I'm getting insight into how other people behave and why. I'm getting better at making decisions. I've learned to observe my own internal dialogue. I can have a sense of wonder about life." W.S.

> "When I first started this class I did not like it, but I came back the third time. I started participating more and really getting into it. You know how some programs tell you this is right and this is wrong but don't tell you how to use the tools. The first thing I got was a journal and you have to write down your thoughts and feelings twice a day and you are taught how

to relax your body how to breathe properly, and even how to relax your mind, and use parts of your brain and skills that you never knew you had. How to deal with your feelings that you have hidden. I never used to talk about my personal feelings and now I talk in class. You can actually notice you are changing and making progress and you're so proud you want everyone to know. It shows you a part of yourself that you never knew existed." P.W.

"I now know the quiet inside and how to relax when doing something. Time used to chase me. Time used to be one of my fears, especially being locked up. I'm facing things more, I'm not running or trying to prevent stuff from happening. Time is on my hands, or should I say my time is in my hands. Time to learn has come, and here I am learning to breathe, crawl, walk and run. Time is funny and I'm learning to laugh sometimes." J.S.

"I came with a very negative attitude. I was very cocky, brash and didn't think I would ever change. I sat in for the first couple of classes and thought 'What am I getting myself into?' Well with some time and effort and some insight. I can honestly say my life has changed. It started to help me to start focusing on the big picture, take into account the things that really matter to me. It also taught me how to deal with everyday stress. I never imagined myself meditating or keeping a journal. The things I've learned so far have taken me to greater heights in my personal life. I don't get angry as easily anymore. I've learned how to deal with problems, take the moment and breathe into the gap, that moment just before the adrenalin hits, so it doesn't." A.P.

"I have more clarity through the mixed emotions. I did a lot of Inner Child imagery work and I am learning about why I do things the way I do them. I'm not as hard on myself about always messing up. I'm better able to anticipate my reaction to things, and so when the anger comes I can deal with it before it explodes. I'm not great at reading the cues but I'm more aware of them. I'm learning how to slow down and be aware. I thought this drawing and breathing right would be sissy stuff, but not now. I know that I hurt myself more with my anger and that I can learn about how not to be out of control." S.R.

A case can be made for integrating mindfulness, meditation, and expressive arts as a multidimensional and holistic approach to modify perceptions and expectations, thus encouraging empathy and open-mindedness, leading to significant therapeutic change of affective development, i.e., identification of feelings, increased awareness of inner experience of emotions and external expression of emotions. The expressive arts allows for the safe and empathic relationship of emotional and neurobiological reorganization. This evocative medium offers an enriched and stimulating environment for fluent growth of new ways of perceiving oneself and the world.

References

Baerenstein, K.B., N.V. Hartwig,, H. Stodkilde-Jorgensen, and J. Mammen. "Onset of meditation explored with fMR.." *NeuroImage* 13:6, Suppl.1(2001) 297.

Basar, E., C. Basar-Eroglu,, S. Karakas, and M. Schurman. "Gamma, Alpha, Delta and Theta Oscillations Govern Cognitive Processes." *International Journal Psychophysiology"* 39 (2001) 241-248

Cahn, B. R., and J. Polich. "Meditation States And Traits: EEG, ERP And Neuroimaging Studies" *Psychological Bulletin*; 132 (2006) 180-211.

Cayoun, B. A. "From Co-Emergence Dynamics to Human Perceptual Evolution: The Role of Neuroplasticity During Mindfulness Training." *Keynote at 2005 National Conference of New Zealand Psychological Society,* Otago University, Dunedin, New Zealand. 2005.

Cozolino, D. *The Neuroscience of Psychotherapy: Building and Rebuilding the Human Brain,* New York: W.W. Norton, 2002.

Davidson, R. J,, J. Kabat-Zinn, J. Schumacher, et al. "Alterations In Brain And Immune Function Produced By Mindfulness Meditation." *Psychosomatic Medicine* 2003; 65 (2003) 564-570.

FitzGerald, M. J. T., and J. Folan-Curran, *Clinical Neuroanatomy and Related Neurosciences* (4th Ed.). London: Saunders. 2002.

Hanna, F.J. "Therapy With Difficult Clients: Using The Precursor Model To Awaken Change," Washington, DC: American Psychological Association. 2002.

Hayes, S.C., K. Strosahl, and K. G. Wilson. *Acceptance and Commitment Therapy: An Experimental Approach to Behavior Change.* NY: Guilford Press. 1999.

Kabat-Zinn, J. "Full Catastrophe Living: The Program of The Stress-Reduction", Clinic at the University Of Massachusetts Medical Center. New York: Delta. 1990

Keith, J. " The Art of Healing: Noting the Ongoing Positive Impact of Arts in the Clinical Setting, Hospital Administrators, Artists, Consultants, Architects, Designers, Physicians, and Patients Work Together to Ensure a Healthful, Uplifting Environment." *Art Business News.* Sept. 2003.

Linehan, M. *Cognitive-behavioral treatment of borderline personality disorder.* New York: Guilford Press. 1993.

Lusebrink, V. B. "Art Therapy And The Brain: An Attempt To Understand The Underlying Processes Of Art Expression In Therapy". *Art Therapy: Journal of the American Art Therapy Association,* 21(3): (2006) 125-135.

Malchiodi, C. A. *Handbook of Art Therapy.* New York: Guilford Press. 2003.

McNamee, C.M. "Using Both Sides Of The Brain: Experiences That Integrate Art And Talk Therapy Through Scribble Drawings." *Art Therapy: Journal of the American Art Therapy Association,* 21(3): (2004) 136-142.

Pert, C. *Molecules of Emotion*, New York: Scribner. 1997.

Rogers, N. *Creative Connection: The Expressive Arts as Healing.* Palo Alto: Science & Behavior Books. 1993.

Schaffer, S.D. and C. B. Yucha. "Relaxation and Pain Management: The Relaxation Response Can Play a Role in Managing Chronic and Acute Pain." *American Journal of Nursing* 104(8): (2004) 75-82.

Schiele, D. R. "The Neuropsychobiology of Addiction, Trauma and Dissociation" Paper presented at 5th Annual Western Clinical Conference on Multiple Personality & Dissociation, Costa Mesa, CA, April 10-12, 1992.

Teasdale, J. D., Z. V. Segal, and J. M. G. Williams. "How Does Cognitive Therapy Prevent Depressive Relapse And Why Should Attentional Control (Mindfulness) Training Help?" *Behavior Research and Therapy,* 33: (1999) 25-39.

Teicher, M. H. "Scars that Won't Heal: The Neurobiology of Child Abuse". *Scientific American.* March: (2002) 68-75.

Valentine, E.R., and P. L. G. Sweet. "Meditation and Attention: A Comparison Of The Effects Of Concentrative And Mindfulness Meditation On Sustained Attention." *Mental Health Religious Culture* 2: (1999) 59-70.

Wenk-Sormaz H. "Meditation Can Reduce Habitual Responding.". *Alternative Therapies* 11(2): (2002) 42-58.

II. ENGAGING SOUND

THERAPEUTIC DRUMMING:
RHYTHM AS A HEALING TOOL

RUSSELL BUDDY HELM

New insights into how the brain, the body and our minds work have given us a unique tool for healing. This is not a new tool-but the way we can use it is modern. This tool is our sense of rhythm.

By using both hands in a mirrored, coordinated back and forth repetitive groove, our brain lobes talk to each other in a focused manner that occupies our conscious mind just enough to access our deeper psychological issues. This was initially developed where a patient passed a ball back and forth- from hand to hand. Drumming is like this with the added mythic elements of a heroic personal journey as the deep resonance vibrates in our bodies. It has a very positive sense memory. Drumming is musical and creative, giving the patient an instant sense of accomplishment, insight, beauty and control. It can also become for the person an accompaniment and the psychological armor for the hero's journey upon which we all must embark.

Slowing down the tempo allows people to enter trance state. In this self-induced mindset, the person can rhythmically reprogram his or her belief system and personal operating system. One session is often enough to change a person's behavior permanently. Rhythm is effective in either a steady state groove or intentionally slowing down incrementally to absolute slowness. As a blues musician, I had to learn the subtleties of a "laid-back" groove; i.e. late to the metronome. Delaying the notes just enough to relax into the pocket. "Back in the pocket" is where most rhythmic players strive to be. It is a state of alert relaxation and joyful state of grace.

We are rhythmic animals. We entrain or synch-up to environmental rhythms as part of our ancient survival system. This tendency may be hard-wired into our systems. Often we are not aware of the effects of rhythm on our psychology or our health. We can use this tendency to entrain to heal, but most of the time we are not aware of how rhythmically sensitive we really are.

Advertising and media have used our rhythmic suggestibility for decades. Film composers manipulate our feelings with predictable results. We believe what we are rhythmically persuaded to believe. Certain tempos have proven to be optimal for selling products. Research funded by major advertising agencies, started in the early nineteen sixties, has progressed to an exacting science, whereby specific tempos are used to enhance product desirability by entrancing the audience. Pulsing music in malls, grocery stores, and restaurants is designed to get us to spend money. Introducing anxious rhythms, those programming them put us into an anxious feeling state. Anxiety can be reduced by rhythm also. This is a basis for soundtrack marketing strategies.

Rhythm can also heal. By using our tendency to go into rhythmic trance, we can insert commands into our operating system as effectively as programming a computer, freeing us from trauma, and destructive/obsessive behavior. We can acquire tools for anger management, depression, cancer survival, stress relief, posttraumatic delayed stress, grief, attention deficit disorder, and many other conditions, as well as accessing enhanced joy. Applied grooves provide quality of living, far beyond what was hoped for by many people in therapy.

Monitoring the rhythms of our environment has been a part of our survival system far back into our ancestral memory. Tempos give us clues as to whether we are safe or in danger. If the tempo speeds up, the survival mind assumes from experience that there is possible danger in the environment so adrenaline is pumped into the system, fight or flight responses are engaged. If the tempo slows down, then there is a signal to the survival operating system that the environment is relatively safe. As a result of this rhythmic decision, chemical components change in the human organism. Instead of adrenaline, endorphins are secreted. Blood pressure drops, T-cell count changes, muscle tension reduces, and respiration deepens. Brain frequencies change. A healing environment is created. All this can be triggered by merely dropping the tempo of a steady groove pulse from about 80 beats a minute to below 30 beats a minute in a graceful curve.

The person is actively involved in the rhythmic reprogramming therapy, compatible with the belief that "If I do the work, I deserve to heal." They do not need to have any musical training or ability. Through rhythmic diagnosing, their history can be seen. Our unconscious uses rhythm to communicate what needs to be addressed. The client needs only to hit the downbeat in the middle of the drumhead with alternating hands while the practitioner reduces tempo. Simple rhythms are used. Nothing too complicated is needed. The patient and the practitioner are sharing the groove, each playing a drum together-preferably a djembe, the African style drum that is tuned lower to get a deep heartbeat tone with little effort. This differs from conventional therapy where the patient passively verbalizes and becomes entrenched in jargon. This physical activity creates a moving model of coping where acceptance comes with movement through the trauma memory into an integrated forward-looking insight. By feeling the sensations of a soothing groove, the patients heal themselves. This is a physical tool with concrete predictable effects on the human organism. It does an end-run around the intellect and addresses the operating system directly, rhythmically re-patterning learned responses to anger, love, fear, doubt, distraction and other mindsets. Confidence grows quickly and body chemistry improves as the over-stimulated survival mind is persuaded to slow down. A rhythmic healing tool is created for individuals to use on their own, which updates when the unconscious decides it needs a new rhythmic mantra.

"I believe in myself" and "Thank-you to my body" are examples of generic phrases that are spoken while hitting the downbeat on each important syllable or word. This reinforces the intention, with pleasant, confident physical encoding. Slowing down is important to release the emotional charge on the programming phrase. Most therapies do not take into account the importance of tempo in their modalities. Speeding up can create a negative anxiety charge on the learning experience. Even when tempos creep up gradually in speed, the brain must constantly recalibrate so the body never gets a chance to relax and just enjoy the experience, it is always trying to catch up.

The challenge in our culture is to relearn how to relax. By learning how to slow down our tempos, we change our psychologies. We can "drum-in" potent new commands into our systems, overriding older less life enhancing beliefs that are neither healthful nor true.

Consistently repeating affirmations or release phrases for prolonged periods of time gently implants the concept. For instance, "I am a miracle" drummed and spoken for long periods of time has shown great effect on cancer survivors when using my slowing tempo Helmtone Protocols technique. The necessity to name this process stems from the various emerging "healing drum therapies," and a need to distinguish this process as unique and not just "healing drums". My concern is based on over twenty years of field research and a lifetime of music training of all types from Classical to the Blues. Extensive psychological investigation with reputable academics combined with powerful anecdotal evidence shows that we can be our own healers by using rhythmic programming techniques that can mechanically be learned and applied, regardless of musical ability. Ethical standards are very important when accessing a person's belief system. This is another reason that I brand name this process, so as the keep a high level of integrity.

By using his or her own sense of rhythm, the trained practitioner is personally involved. This approach is unique. This puts the practitioner in the same arena of healing as the patient. Our sense of rhythm reveals truths about ourselves. Many people are insecure about their sense of rhythm. Why is this? Cultural intimidation or personal trauma can play roles in this rhythmic insecurity. Rhythmic diagnostics can reveal a person's history quicker than words can tell their story. Rushing the downbeat or a randomly tapping foot are examples of "rhythmic indicators" whereby the subconscious communicates directly without being filtered by the intellect. The drum therapist is a detective finding clues expressed by the body wisdom of the client, strewn along the trail of the groove. I suggested one patient use this process with her own therapist but she said that she could not depend on her therapist to be steadily constant on the downbeat. We are all suffering from traumatic effects that trick us into speeding up. It is a condition of our modern culture.

In pre-industrial times, we entrained to the slower cycles of nature like the seasons, equinox, solstice, and lunar, annual, and tidal pulses. When the human organism was in-synch with these natural rhythms, survival was possible. This rhythmic imperative became part of the survival structure for the human animal. On a very deep level of our being, we are feeling the tempo of each event in our lives and determining if we are safe or in danger. By consciously using this tendency, we can release and heal trauma. If we are not in-synch, our survival system warns us. Our ancient survival sense of rhythm is stressed beyond our comprehension today. Modern society is so fast that we are unaware of the individual pulses. It is no coincidence that Freud defined neurosis at the beginning of the Industrial Revolution. As technological rhythms began to overwhelm our sense of organic rhythms we felt inadequate in keeping up with unforgiving machine rhythms.

Everything rhythmic affects us more than we would like to admit- windshield wipers, car alarms, jackhammers, digital clocks, turn signals, and the ubiquitous drum machine. Electronic drums have been dictating a mechanical landscape for over thirty years and its toll on the human psyche is showing. Feelings of edginess, inadequacy, feeling like "damaged goods," low self-esteem, explosive anger, depression, the list is endless. The drum machine is not a real drum. The vibrations are different when people put hand on drumhead. I suspect that the current interest in drumming by non-drummers is nourishment of a need that is not being met by culture. One specific danger for drumming therapists to avoid is unconsciously inserting their own rhythmic neurosis into a healing drum session. This was another reason I decided to certify practitioners. That is why I make a distinction as to the type of drumming that we use for healing. It is non- aggressive, non-dramatic, non-musical and non-intellectual. Yet it reprograms behavior and body mechanics according to the needs of the person.

Rhythmic dysfunction is felt on a cellular level and affects physical and emotional health. Healing can be initiated by using positive, specific life-enhancing rhythmic vocabulary. We are surrounded by technological rhythmic saturation. We decide not to be driven by panic or fear, but by self-nurturing awareness of our own strong rhythms. Rhythm is a language without words, and is understood by our intuition, our instincts, our body and our heart. We take control of our rhythmic environment and the result is a sense of well-being.

In this type of drumming, there are no wrong notes. There are only clues. The body responds rhythmically to life. Those learned responses appear when stress has been introduced. Drumming is a safe way to investigate these stress loops. The groove is a repetitive massage that can break the dysfunctional loop of repetitive behavior. The patient quickly learns to use the continuous groove as protection from paralyzing remembrances. The therapist can see that the groove is a mysterious protective cocoon of empowerment. Just keep the groove going and the patient will find their own way through and out of the morass of emotional distractions in the unconscious. This changes the emotional charge on what had previously been a debilitating loop. The impact of past events is diminished by the desire to play and enjoy the continuing downbeat groove. This overrides the original trauma memory with a new emotional charge.

Some drum instructors inadvertently instill trauma into their patients/students as a result of their own unresolved history. There is a history of tough drum teachers. The drumming student is in a very suggestible state that should be respected by the teacher. Many people come to the drum to heal- not necessarily to play traditional African, Afro Cuban, belly dancing, Celtic, Native American or Brazilian or any other kind of specialized drumming art form. The simple desire to use rhythm to integrate our beings is as old as the dance. "Let your backbone slip" is a lyric by one of my musical collaborators, Big Joe Turner. He instinctively knew that dancing was a method of healing.

Through the science of chiropractics, we have come to understand that gentle movement of the spine in a rhythmic manner releases subluxations along the meningeal envelope. This in turn reduces the impediments of the electrical signal moving up and down through the saline solution within the spinal envelope. This increased electrical potential is one reason that yogi's refer to the white light of insight that results from years of yogic exercise to loosen up the kundalini energy. By releasing these areas along our spine through rhythmic healing, we integrate sections of our past that have been cut off from the flow of nurturing acceptance. The slowing downbeat creates a safety net that reinforces acceptance of whatever the patient is experiencing. Grief resolution is one area where this process is useful. Learning rhythm from a forgiving point of view is essential for a healing experience.

Our sense of rhythm is a survival tool just as important as any of our other senses. However, we have been tricked into disregarding it, even being ashamed of it, because of certain cultural restrictions dating back to the middle Ages in European culture. When the Roman legions crossed northern Europe, they wiped out all ethnic tribal rhythms and replaced them with liturgies in Latin, sung without a rhythmic pulse. Anyone drumming and praying to original tribal deities was burned at the stake. Mythic tribal grooves are a basic form of security and race identity. Other cultures such as African, American Indian, some Irish, Muslim, Far East, South American and various other tribes do not have this schism and have retained their organic cultural rhythms. But the lack of rhythm can have unfortunate consequences in the evolution of culture. There are accounts of Crusaders losing their sense of balance and falling off their horses when they heard the mesmerizing tempos of the Saracen battle drummers. Many cultures use the latter basic six beat pattern to go into specific types of trance. John Phillip Sousa used it to create stirring military brass band songs. The six beat has a driving power regardless of dialectic. Paradoxical rhythm patterns that were overlaid in the six beat rhythms confused the inner ears of the Crusaders because they had no experience with the groove. They had no rhythmic vocabulary to match it.

This same mysterious overlay of six beat rhythms is also used in Santeria, a form of voodoo, to induce specific trances that invoke their deities; it is also used in the Native American Ghost Dance. The lack of tribal ethnic grooves explains to "primitive societies" why the great white onslaught of concrete is so personal. The empire's men had no groove and were not about to allow anyone else to feel a groove either. We are in need of rediscovering our sense of rhythm in order to feel and survive. If we can feel, then we can heal.

However, healing is just the first step. Evolving is really where rhythm is essential. As we become more digitized, we need a "humanity truth detector." Our intellect is constantly being fooled; rhythm gives us a language to evaluate our environment, and it is this gyroscope that gives us stability in the swirling virtual world of tomorrow. It can tell us what is real, but the language it uses is feelings. The great martial arts teacher Guro Dan Inosanto has been studying with me for ten years and likes this aspect of drumming. Rhythmic sensing is quicker and more accurate than thinking, many times.

Drumming is a form of empowerment that transcends logic and rational thought. The mind cannot dance. Rhythm is the domain of the body and it awakens body wisdom. This is a form of enlightenment that has no words. The drum was invented before the word. It articulates a language that has existed since the beginning of time. There are basic rhythmic patterns that all cultures use which have been the same and will be the same until the end of time. These are the rhythms we use to heal our culture and ourselves. Rhythm is a language and a form of energy that is essential to life. Without rhythm, there is no life. With rhythm, life can flow with purpose, integrity, joy, creativity, success and health.

Using the groove as a carrier wave enables us to apply sophisticated psychological concepts into our operating system without struggling to convince the intellect that it is a good idea. "Drumming-in" a good thought or specific intention is as exacting as typing a computer command line. It operates in the same manner.

In therapy, the action of hitting the drum is also a truth or lie detector. The patient finds a slow tempo that they can speak with even when they have never hit a drum before. They find something comforting in hitting a drum while they recall events in their lives. The steady beat is an indicator; if the beat speeds up while the client is relating to their past, then one could make a good bet that they are having strong feelings about that event. They continue to drum while relating and eventually they come to a form of understanding about the issues at hand, through a physical reductionism. They stay on the groove because it feels good, not because they have been instructed to do so. If they try to digress from the issue, their ability to drum will reflect that avoidance.

There are two rhythm structures in the universe, two beat and three beat. Everything else is a variation from these two basic building blocks. A steady two or four beat with a downbeat elicits a relaxed trance conducive for releasing trauma when it is slowed from 80 beats per minute to as slow as the client can go. Using alternating hand technique is important. Brain hemispheres speak to each other in an equal way. Drumming is one of the few times that this happens for our brains. Most of the time people favor one lobe, which makes for a lopsided body and mind coordination. As a result, many people distrust their "weaker" side. In drumming, this can be overcome, and as a result, people's behavior changes.

In anger management, rhythmic programming might actually rewire how the system gets angry. Instead of losing control, the new commands allow the person to become calm. This seems to be a permanent modification for many people who have drummed-it-in to their own operating system.

This type of rhythmic programming seems to have an effect in the body/mind interface. It addresses physical as well as conceptual behavior. For instance, in one case of adult autism, we drummed in a phrase like, "I process correctly". This is in relation to the sensory signals that were missed in social interplay. He was elated to be able to stand quietly and listen and respond based on what he was seeing and hearing. It worked for him.

"I compete with grace" became a successful drum mantra for one high achiever. I could give many examples, but each mantra should be customized for the client. Generalized statements just approximate what the precise effect can be. A proper introduction and inclusion of subdirectories is important for the belief system to accept the drummed instructions. This means that there is an active conversation between the therapist and the client while the slow downbeat is being played. The groove becomes the subliminal soundtrack for the therapy. It is a comforting friend and an activity that imparts confidence as the patient slows down, getting "better" at drumming. Musical ability can sometimes interfere with the therapy when the player cannot get past their performance concerns. Nevertheless, the slowing of the downbeat usually clears the path for deeper insight work. The slowing of the downbeat, "laying back" of the groove, even in our everyday lives, gives us a safe space to heal within. The steady groove seems sacred, protecting us from harsh realities, past, present and future. Within this safe space, we can reprogram our belief system with simple self-generated commands. With this new belief system in place, we can move forward in our lives with confident intentions and joy.

We can also use the drum to celebrate and dance with our friends, sharing the joy that is inherent in the grooves of our lives.

TONING...
A JOURNEY TOWARD SELF-DISCOVERY

ELLE SPEED

                  Intention...
                        Breath...
                              Sound...
Start the air moving all around
It changes...it's affected by the tone
It seeks a balance...it seeks a wave to ride upon
To free the need it's found...
The limits are endless...
The opportunity overwhelming...
The possibility thrills....
The sound I tone gradually finds the fear...
The fear I clearly hide within
The tone invites me to begin a process of growth
A process of transformation....
There's no limit to the tones I hear....
So why not put a positive balancing spin on the world I'm in...
Sound your tone...
Experience the freedom...
Influence the frequency in which you reside...
Set an intention for peace of mind and sacred bliss...
With your sound, you become your own personal advocate/activist

    The vowel sounds ...A E I O U are in every language. They connect us. The dressings of varying consonants create an illusion of separateness, which sets each one of us apart from the other. The vowel sounds are the glue that binds us together in body, mind, and spirit. Toning is the conscious elongation of a vowel sound using intention, breath, and sound for the purpose of balancing the body. Sound in many different forms has been used as a healing tool for thousands of years and today has been scientifically proven to aid in the healing process. You do not need any previous musical knowledge to learn the technique of toning nor do you need to be ill to receive the benefit. Let's begin.

Jonathan Goldman in *Healing Sounds* states

"..everything in the universe is in a state of vibration. The chair you may be sitting on is in a state of vibration...Sound may be understood as being vibration." He continues, "Resonance is the frequency at which an object most naturally vibrates. Everything has resonant frequency...every organ, bone and tissue in your body has its own separate resonant frequency." (2002:20)

Toning affords us the opportunity to discover our fundamental sound and frequency, and thus engage in the healing process.

What? You are afraid of the sound of your own voice! Or maybe you've never taken the time to "feel" the sound of your own voice. Feel it resonating through you. Allowing it to caress you or express its emotions to you. Don Campbell suggests you sit comfortably in a chair, close your eyes, and spend five minutes **humming**...not a melody, but a pitch that feels comfortable. Relax your jaw and feel the energy of the hum within your body. Bring the palms of your hands to your cheeks and notice how much vibration is occurring within your jaw. This five-minute massage will release stress and help you relax. This "**Humming**" moment brings you one step closer to achieving balance and healing within yourself.

In your own time, let's continue with an **ah** sound. The **ah** immediately evokes a relaxation response. You produce it naturally when you yawn, and it can help you both wake up and go to sleep. If you feel a great deal of stress and tension, take a few minutes to relax your jaw and make a quiet **ah**. There is no need to sing. Just allow the sound to move gently through your breath. After a minute or so, you will notice that your breathing is much slower and that you feel more relaxed. In your office or at school, where toning may disturb others, you can simply close your eyes, breathe out and think the **ah**. Although this is not quite as effective, it is still useful.

Is there an all important vowel sound?

Eeeee..is said to be the most important of all vowel sounds. It can awaken the mind and the body, functioning as a kind of sonic caffeine. When you feel drowsy while driving or are sluggish in the afternoon, 3-5 minutes of a rich **eee** sound will stimulate the brain, activate the body, and keep you alert.

The sound which is considered the most powerful by toning regulars is the **oh** or **Om**. These sounds are considered the richest of all. Make the **oh/Om** sound. If you put your hand on your head, cheek, and/or chest, you notice that the **oh/Om** vibrates most of the upper parts of the body. Five minutes of the **oh/Om** can change the skin temperature, muscle tension, brain waves, breath and heart rates. It's a great tool for an instant tune-up.

Now that we have experienced some of the fundamental sounds of toning how do you attain the richness, the fullness of resonance, which you need to experience an inner healing? One of the important elements is in the breath.

"Every breath,
As word or wonder-ous sigh,
Precipitates change.
Now
Imagine our bodily waters flowing,
Breath by breath,
Covering all creation in a mist of intentioned time.
As focus goes, so will creation flow.
Breathe easily,
Releasing vaporized sighs of matter, realized through intentioned Gratitude.
Ah – oh – mmm"

The ideal position to experience the natural flow of the breath is lying down. In this position as we inhale into the nose we can watch and feel the lower abdomen fill up, followed by our stomach, then our chest area (but do not raise your shoulders.)

We then exhale through the nose feeling the movement of the air from our chest cavity with the pulling in of our lower abdomen and our stomach area. Allow yourself to feel the flow of air throughout your body and with each breath concentrate on this airflow. The movement creates a sense of well-being and serves to strengthen your sense of purpose and self-reliance. You are all you need to be. Take the time to do the sounding exercises we have previously discussed and as the tones move with the breath, allow yourself the freedom to feel their power. Allow them to reach their own frequency. Yes, at this point experiment! Improvisation coordinates reason, intuition, emotion, movement, and imagination to create a unified act. Improvisation and free play create a place where thought is muscular perception, and body is simultaneously mind.

Start at the lowest part of your voice and let it glide upward, like a very slow elevator. Make vowel sounds that are relaxing and that arise effortlessly from the jaw or throat. Allow the voice to resonate throughout the body. Explore ways in which you can massage parts of your skull, throat and chest with long vowel sounds. Let your hands trace the upper parts of your body very slowly, and you will see which vowels emit the strongest, most stress-releasing energy for YOU.

During one of these sounding sessions, you may come across your own fundamental sound. Fabian Maman, in *The Role of Music in the Twenty-First Century*, states that when you reach a note or frequency that puts you in total resonance from within to the space around you, you have found your fundamental sound. Both you and the space around you feel full, vibrating. He also writes:

> "After a few minutes of sounding this one note, you won't know whether it is you making the sound or the walls or the trees around you making the sound. You will feel completely filled with your own sound — your fundamental sound. This frequency can make your body tingle or tremble. It can momentarily clear not only your physical eyesight, but your inner vision as well, opening access to the higher realms of consciousness" (1997.)

A goal well worth pursuing.

What is the difference between these exercises and a toning practiced by a more formalized toning group? I think the answer is that within a group you have the opportunity to not only experience the resonance of a single tone but also the vibrational impact of blended tones. Western music has defined these tones as intervals. These intervals influence us with their unique resonant qualities. Some create tension (Second, C-D, Seventh, C-B), others influence our emotional and psychic life (Third, C-E, Sixth, C-A) Fabian Maman considers the Fifth interval (C–G) the most stimulating. "It frees the creative potential," and facilitates the movement of energy (1997.)

In Hindu Ayurvedic medicine, the use of the voice to balance and align chakras has been a practice for thousands of years. Contemplate the importance of "Frequency + Intention = Healing." What does it mean to experience healing? Consider this answer:

> "Healing at this spiritual level is more than alleviating symptoms. It means rearranging the energy of a person or a circumstance so that it reflects a

clear image of his or her divine nature. Healing means bringing something or someone into full alignment with the level of soul, while rooting them more deeply in the level of form. A truly healed person is fully embodied, fully present, fully available to the realm of form, and yet fully in communication with the divine. A healed being is one who experiences unity consciousness and sees the interconnectedness of all beings and all actions, awake or asleep" (Kaplan, 2002: 143.)

When a person is using their vibrational modality, the potential for achieving their healing goal is imminent. Directing their tone to an energy center with an intention to stimulate the movement of the "chi" to create the healing balance begins with knowledge of the chakras. Chakras are energy centers located along the center of the body. In summary form there are seven chakras, each located in a specific area of the body moving from the base of the spine upward.

The first Chakra is located at the base of the spine. It is called the Root Chakra. It is related to the adrenal glands and associated with issues of survival. The "I AM." The musical tone associated with this chakra is C and the common vowel "seed" tone is "UHHH."

The second Chakra is located below the navel. It is called the Creation Chakra. It is related to the sexual organs and associated with our creative abilities. The "I FEEL." The musical tone associated with this chakra is D and the common vowel "seed" tone is "OHHH."

The third Chakra is located above the navel. It is called the Power Chakra. It is related to the digestive organs and associated with our power and self-mastery. The "I WILL." The musical tone associated with this chakra is E and the common vowel "seed" tone is "EHHH."

The fourth Chakra is located at the heart cavity. It is called the Heart Chakra. It is related to the organs of the heart and respiration as well as the thymus gland and associated with our ability to love and express compassion. The "I LOVE." The musical tone associated with this chakra is F and the common vowel "seed" tone is "HAAA."

The fifth Chakra is located in the throat area. It is called the Throat Chakra. It is related to our voice box, ears, and thyroid gland and is associated with our ability to speak and hear our truth. The "I SPEAK." The musical tone associated with this chakra is G and the common vowel "seed" tone is "AAAH."

The sixth Chakra is located between the eyebrows. It is called the Third Eye Chakra. It is related to the pineal gland and associated with our imagination, psychic abilities and the seeking of the Universal Truth. The "I SEE." The musical tone associated with this chakra is A and the common vowel "seed" tone is "OOMMM."

The seventh Chakra is located at the top of the head. It is called the Crown Chakra. It is related to our brain functions and is associated with our ability to control every aspect of body and mind as well as our ability to seek full enlightenment and union with the Universal Truth. The "I KNOW." The musical tone associated with this chakra is B and the common vowel "seed' tone is "EEEE."

Again, I repeat this is only a summary of the Chakras and the possible "seed" tones used to activate them. Experiment! Experiment! Experiment! Only you and you alone, have the opportunity to discover your fundamental sounds.

Perhaps you are wondering what effect these tones have on our cellular make-up. Fabian Maman has followed through with experiments showing the effect of the human voice on actual human cells. His work has produced photographic evidence of the effect the human voice has on healthy as well as diseased cells. His findings prove that the human voice has an added element that cannot be found with any other instrument. "The voice can be considered the premier instrument because its inflection carries not only the physical aspect (vocal chords, pitch of the note) and emotional colors, but also a finer, subtle element which comes from the conscious and un-conscious will of the toner. The human voice carries its own spiritual resonance" (1997.) This difference, evident in his photographs, is what makes the voice the most powerful instrument, particularly in therapy when the person requesting the work produces the sounds with the toner.

Our toning group, Tones for Living, at Bayfront Medical Center, invites each member individually to come into the center of our circle and express an intention along with a "seed" tone or a word or, most commonly, their name that is then toned in a harmonic fashion by the group, using intervals improvisationally. The individual intention becomes a group intention. The resulting "Song of the Self" is toned and the intuitive vibrations of the intervals are sent forth to achieve their goal. The response from the person in the center is so often "I've never felt more relaxed." "Thank you for this gift of self-awareness."

And what happens in between the tones, when the desired frequency has been reached and is still resonating almost silently through the room? We are listening, and like swimming mammals, we are hearing something in the distance. We call it Silence. Within the parameters of the Silence, the energized molecules are resonating and we feel it. We know the sound is there. To move or speak would disturb the moment...would break the Silence.

> "...we are ourselves musical vibration and we live in a universe of vibration ... that is nothing less than pure music" (Maman 1997.)

This is the power of toning. By affecting the vibrational patterns within and around us, we affect change. We achieve balance. We get to know ourselves wholly. We connect.

Consider this...every sound you hear has the potential to change how you feel. Whether it is the singing of a bird, the roar of a fire truck, the melody from an instrument or the tone of the human voice, it has the potential for awakening your deepest fears...or creating a newfound peace. The choice is yours.

Note: I would like to thank the following people who are a part of Soundwave, and did the recording for toning that is included in this book:

> Kathryn Bolen
> Sally Harkness
> Robin Hill
> Kathy Luethje
> Lindsay Mainland

Soundwave is a group of peers who believe in the philosophy of toning for self-discovery and gather as able for regular group sessions, presentations, and special events to tone.

"A Journey toward Self-Discovery," our CD, includes the following text:
A journey toward self-discovery takes many pathways. Toning is but one. You will be introduced to traditional "seed tones" used through the centuries with new innovative variations which Elle Speed has embraced as significant to the experience. Soundwave responds improvisationally, i.e. with no previous rehearsal, with the intention of encouraging you to join them and to add your sound to the mix. There is no wrong sound. You are on your own journey. Dissonances are embraced as individual representations of soul-power. Finding your energetic voice is presenting yourself as being worthy to be heard by the

Universe. You become a part of the movement. Your self-worth is illuminated and the Absolute Power sees you as being responsive to a necessary transformation.

Listening with earphones may be preferable for it encourages you to go within.
Breathe deeply while listening with the intention of adding your sound to the creation.

Join in the journey.

You are co-creating a unified field of unique vibrations as you are meant to do. So it is.

(Do not participate while operating a motor vehicle)

References

Campbell, Don G. *The Mozart Effect.* New York: Harper Collins. 1997.
Goldman, Jonathan. *Healing Sounds: The Power of Harmonics.* Rochester, NY: Healing Arts Press. 2002.
Kaplan, Connie. *Dreams are Letters from the Soul.* New York: Harmony Books. 2002.
Maman, Fabien. *The Role of Music in the Twenty First Century.* Boulder, CO: Tama-Do Press. 1997.
Rojcewicz, Peter. "A View from the Conservatory: Noetic Learning through Music and the Arts." *Current Musicology.* New York: Columbia University. Fall: (1998) 65.

Websites

http://tonesforliving.com
http://www.GoGratitude.com

SING FOR YOUR SOUL

LAUREN LANE POWELL

I used to believe that everybody could sing. Now, not only do I believe everybody CAN sing...beautifully and on key... I believe that everybody NEEDS to sing! Let me tell you about my journey into these beliefs, and then I will share with you a way to get started in your own healing through singing for your soul.

My mom says I was singing before I could speak. Humming was a very natural thing for me to do. Before words came, oohs and ahs were my lyrics. Everything had a song and I knew them all by heart! Mom still almost glows when she tells people I was singing harmony at the age of three. Actually, SHE sang the harmony to our family's favorite song, *You Are My Sunshine* and that's all I heard. So at a party when she had to sing the melody to lead the song, naturally I sang what I knew-the harmony!

Before I was old enough to go to school, my mom and I sang with Captain Kangaroo on TV every weekday morning. One of my own original songs is based on a melody that was played often in that show as a closing- where a little rag doll, whose job it was to clean up, sweeps up the spotlight as she dances to this beautiful melody written by Leroy Anderson. My use of that melody is a Tribute to my mother and to the composer Leroy Anderson.

When I was three and a half, I sang to my sister when she was new to the world. Very quickly and naturally, she sang with me. Our greatest joy as kids was performing together. We created the kind of harmony you could feel inside. Our mother has a beautiful voice and would teach us songs, sing us to sleep, sing us to awaken and sing our day into being. When the three of us sang together, the density of the intensity grew and we felt as if we wound raise the roof! I remember singing songs from the musical Sound of Music: Do a Dear, Edelwiess, Climb Every Mountain and the Lonely Goatherd. From Hans Christian Anderson, a musical starring Danny Kaye, we would sing Thumbelina, Ugly Duckling and Copenhagen. Mom and I sang our favorite from the movie, the duet Inch Worm, every night before bed. Looking back on it now, as a musician, that is a very unusual song and very difficult to sing because of its two different time signatures sung at the same time. At 6 years old, I nailed the ¾ part, or "2 and 2 are 4"... All I knew is how we sounded together and most of all how it felt to sing it with my mom.

Mom played the piano for ballet classes as she was growing up and kept up with it as we grew. I remember loving to hear her practice Chopin and Rachmoninov. I took for granted having an accompanist as a mother! She could play anything. So in time we added all of Rogers and Hammerstein's works, then Jesus Christ Superstar and Hair, then all the other Andrew Lloyd Webber works as they came out. But I'm getting ahead of myself. My dad, too, had a very musical, artistic side. He had a radio show, "Larry Powell's House of Sound," that he recorded weekly in our basement. We would tip toe around the house during his sessions, trying to be as quiet as three females could possibly be. While we 3 were usually successful, inevitably one of our seven Siamese cats would break the silence with a typical *HOWL* followed by Daddy's howl of frustration, which would span more than a full octave and would be louder and longer than the cat's! When he suffered from "record-us interrupt-us" he would howl. But when Daddy played the saxophone, he would wail!

Dad played the Saxophone and some piano all by ear. He played for the sheer joy of it and would add soul and spice to our family sing-a-longs and parties. It was great fun for my sister and me to pretend to eat a lemon or drink lemon juice when he was playing. When we puckered, Dad puckered and couldn't play! I wonder now how much of that was all an act of fun for us kids. We sang in the car on every trip, long or short. Our favorite car riding song was from an old play, made for the radio called Seven Dreams. "Are We There Yet?" became our standard and it would be repeated all the way, to wherever it was we were going. Singing kept my sister and me from fighting! As long as we were in song, we were in harmony. Then the oh-too-familiar "She touched me!" started again. So we'd sing another song. Mom was a genius!

Perhaps everyone should write his or her musical autobiography. Mine is going to be a full-flown book one of these days. Through the writing of "Sing For Your Soul!" I have had confirmed and reconfirmed how important music, singing, has been in the very salvation of my life, all my life. The fact that I didn't recognize the calling until I was 25 still eludes me. My love affair with singing has always been as natural as breathing. However, I never thought about making a living at it until a friend suggested I might make a good teacher. The seed was planted, and 6 years later began to flower. I got my degree in music Education with an emphasis on Voice in 1992. I sang classically, like an opera singer, for 10 years.

When I began teaching voice lessons in 1989 I, too, was teaching classically. And I was frustrated. My own voice felt false and forced singing the way I was taught to sing. I had many recurring throat illnesses throughout the years. My students weren't serious or enjoying the lessons either. After 3-4 years of rotating students and having a few successes, one of my students also studied with a man in Chicago. She came to me with the missing piece! I saw the same teacher for a couple of hours myself and he gave me some strange and wonderful vocal exercises that gave my voice a completely new feeling of freedom.

I saw him once more 3 years later. He had more weird and wonderful exercises. He could not explain why the vocal gymnastics worked to my satisfaction, just that they did work. I had to figure out why myself. Hey, I am a Virgo! What awakened in me instantly is the inner knowing that our human voice *deserves to feel good* coming out of the body. Our voice *deserves to feel good* to those listening to us. Now it certainly did not feel good right away. I spoke with my tight angry sounding throat muscles and was misunderstood often. My singing voice was throaty and operatic. For a long time, I had the natural and I had the operatic, but 'never the twain shall meet!' However, as I slowly learned that what felt the best also sounded the best, my own human instrument shifted from being a mechanical, mind-driven force to a physical, air-lifted flow.

Now, not only is my voice more pleasing and consistent for myself and my audience, my singing range has increased in both directions, high and low. I've had 3 "colds" in 10 years and those illnesses I can attribute to lengths of time without vocalizing! You know, life gets in the way, you get busy, you forget. WHAM! I learned my lesson! What follows is the first set of exercises designed to remind the body how to breathe, then strengthen and put to use your waistline muscles, using them in a different way than they may be accustomed to being used. As basic as this is, this is the very foundation on which all natural vocalization lies.

When we don't feel comfortable with our source of expression parts of our body can and often do break down. We develop stress in our chest and shoulders. Our throats react and hold a lot of tension. Even our digestion can be affected all because we're not breathing the way we were born to, nor are we using our voice the way it was built to be used. Just think for a moment. When we are infants, we yell and scream perfectly! We express and emote from the gut muscles! We breathe perfectly! Watch a baby breathe some time and notice what part of their body moves. It's the tummy! Right? Now watch most people over the age of five and you'll probably see the chest rise and fall. Sometimes the shoulders heave as well. This is our stressed out breath! This is learned...not natural! Why do you suppose we've forgotten how to breathe, speak and sing naturally? If you guessed stress, you're partly right.

More specifically, *fea*r. Whenever we encounter our first fear, even if it's some adult saying "Hush! Don't show off!" We hold our breath. It's that fight or flight response. We learn the *untruth* about our world that it is an unsafe place to be. We learn the *untruth* about ourselves, that we are not perfect, beautiful, and magnificent! We then continue to breath shallowly to keep that artificial sense of protection around us. When we hear "Children should be seen and not heard." Or "Cut out that racket you kids." We learn that what we have to say is not valuable, another *untruth*. Think now about the very worst, child abuse.

I was in Ft Lauderdale, FL, doing a workshop and working with individuals. One woman I worked with there came to me because of her throat challenges. I could hear as she spoke that there was friction and resistance in her throat muscles and her vocal chords. Rita was a therapist and needed her voice. Her specialty was adult survivors of child abuse, in particular sexual abuse because that is the abuse she herself had endured. As a therapist, of course she had dealt with her own issues most of her life. Nevertheless, this voice thing was beyond her scope of healing.

When we met, it was early 1999. I was out to teach the world to sing! That was my only mission at the time. I had been recognizing the healing effects singing naturally had on people for the 10 years prior but working with Rita validated all my intuitions, heightened my understanding and helped evolve my workshops from Sing For Your Soul to the Harmonies of Healing. I thought I was just getting her to sing, to use her waistline muscles to vocalize. She was ok on the low notes, but there was no high range at all. All of the exercises we did would stop in that mid range, right where she spoke, and go no higher. I was stumped. Finally, in frustration I had her sigh, long, loud, and high.

She did it! A high tone came out that was strong, clear, and very surprising! All at once, she was crying. She tearfully exclaimed "Oh, my God! I never screamed!"

Since then, I have delved more deeply into healing powers of sound and music, but most importantly to me, the healing powers of the human voice, how it is produced, how it feels as well as how it sounds. As I scrutinized my own voice and listened with new ears, I discovered that what *felt* the best to me physically also *sounded* the best to me. As I released my classical education in vocal training, my internal awareness strengthened, as did my waistline. I discovered how physical vocalizing really is! That is only part of why singing is so healing.

When I got "tuned in" to my gut muscles and used them to push air out quickly, not only did those muscles start to remember, but also my throat muscles started to relax! The stronger those muscles got, the more they would work and the less and less the throat would. Vocalizing naturally causes me to breathe deeply every breath, which causes me to stay relaxed. More oxygen in the brain and all my cells! No wonder I stopped getting sick! No longer do I get sick, since I sing and speak with my natural, authentic voice, which by the way sounds and feels like velvet, as opposed to the burlap voice I used to have.

Speaking of that old burlap voice, it is the voice that sounded angry even when I wasn't. It is the voice that would get high and screechy when excited. I could cut through a noisy room by being shrill. That was my speaking voice. When I was studying Opera, my singing voice was vastly different. The 6 years I was in college, I was sick all the time. I had one throat problem after another. I was checked out for viruses and allergies and was a candidate for a tonsillectomy twice! In retrospect, I was singing with one voice and speaking with another. Not only was there no consistency, but both voices were unnatural for me and in time began to hurt me. When I relearned how to vocalize with my whole body instrument, I stopped getting sick!

The Healing Power of the Natural Voice

Does your voice feel and sound wonderful every time you sing or speak or do you feel restriction and hear tight, edgy sounds? Are you "in your body" every time you sing or speak, or are you in your head and throat? Do you always speak your truth or do you say what is expected, or perhaps, nothing at all? Do you always sing with all you've got, on key and with a beautiful, healing tone or do you hold back and hit wrong notes, or perhaps avoid trying altogether? Do you use tones that are anything but healing? We are born to sing on key and speak our truth, very physically, but most of us do not. Below are the first steps to reclaiming your authentic voice! This is also an excellent set of warm up exercises to do prior to singing, speaking and toning for health.

The BREATH

Sit tall and allow your waist to expand as you inhale and release the breath back out again. Now puff the belly out as you inhale even more, on purpose. This allows the diaphragm to drop, filling all of the lungs instead of just the top third. Notice how different it feels than the breath you're probably used to, high in the chest, heaving. And exhale. Most of us take a shallow "thoracic" breath that puts us in the state of fight-or-flight, yes, into a state of stress! By contrast, breathing with the whole body not only brings in more oxygen but you stay more relaxed more of the time because you are "in your center." Until I rediscovered my authentic voice, I didn't realize how truly physical being "in my center" really is!

The SUPPORT

So with every breath in, push the tummy out from the inside. Now HISS! Hard and Fast! Faster! Harder! Feel your whole waistline contract. Relax. Notice anything familiar? Women who have had natural childbirth recognize this push, but it's also same group of muscles that we laugh with! Remember the last time you laughed so hard you almost wet your pants? Didn't your gut ache when your sides split? These are the very muscles we're working with now. These are the muscles we were born to sing and speak with, not the muscles in the walls of the throat! HISS again, hard and fast!

Notice how many muscles around your waist are working and how low in your groin you feel the grunt! Now notice if any upper body muscles may want to help you HISS. So, last time, deep, low, belly breath in and HISS it out! This time as you HISS, roll your shoulders. Make them do something else instead of getting into the action. Can you feel even more intense contraction in your lower gut? When the body pushes the air so quickly through the vocal chords that all they can do is vibrate perfectly, the freedom of the natural voice is insured. So I recommend HISSING a lot! It only serves to strengthen those original muscles.

The TONE

Every time I am to sing or speak I HISS for a about 5 minutes then I do the fun, silly exercise that I thought I had created for kids! It's such a great exercise that I know it will keep me singing well into my hundreds! Ready? Take a deep, low, belly breath and motor boat...you heard me, raspberry with your lips. Can't buzz your lips yet? Push more air out faster, harder. Make those lips PRRRRRR! If they still don't want to do that, stick your tongue out. Yes, it's messier, but it works! Now, add a tone to it, as if you're humming but motorboating, too. PRRRRR. This is harder to describe on paper than I thought! Think of how a baby bubbles his lips as he learns to make sounds of his own.

When you do this in the car, and I know you will, please stop short of passing out. You will get a bit light headed for a while! Think of all the oxygen you're getting! I bet you've yawned a few times already, too, haven't you?

Now use that motorboat sound to sing three notes up and back. That's it; just Do, Re, Mi, Re, Do. Try to sing very short notes starting with the letter "p" to get your motor started. Keep the tones short and explosive and think only of getting your lips prrrring on every single note. Notice what muscles are working? They can't help it! You're not teaching them something they don't already know, you're just reminding them how to work in their original capacity! Where the lips stop and start is the indication of where those ordinary throat muscles still want to help. Push more air out, faster and force those lips to vibrate until you can PRRRR on every note.

I warm up this way every day to remind my waist to work and to remind my throat not to. After I do those three note passages all the way up and down my range, then I sing a song…with the motorboat, all the way through. Once you get past the giggles, you'll notice how much fun it is to sing with your whole body, why it feels so good to express from your gut and how physical vocalizing naturally really is! And very soon, you'll notice how those lower body muscles kick in when you sing or speak and how relaxed your throat is! Very soon, you'll notice how relaxed your whole body is!

If this is the most natural way we can breathe, speak and sing, why have we forgotten? Why are we a nation of chest breathers, throat talkers and head-dwellers? That answer is simple, yet profound: FEAR, as I mentioned before. We learn, at a very young age, how to hold our breath when we hear "NO!" "HUSH!" "Don't show off!" "Children should be seen and not heard." With this now very shallow breath serving as an artificial protection, we disconnect from our center, our abdominal muscles and our feelings. Consequently, the only muscles that can sing and speak for us are our throat muscles. This is why singing naturally is so emotionally therapeutic and very often singing leads to tears. With every note coming from our gut muscles, so too are all of the reasons we shut up in the first place!

So with just these little exercises, 10 minutes a day, you'll be on your way to raising your serotonin levels, releasing endorphins, oxygenating your body, staying relaxed and focused, getting healthier and happier and raising your vibration! All from vocalizing naturally! Wouldn't you say that is worth the time and effort it takes?

Over the last 2 decades, I have discovered these techniques and more that I share in my Lesson CDs and in my workshops across the country. I'm 45 years young and feel 18. I sing when I'm happy. I sing when I'm not, to help me get happy. I sing to ease pain. I sing to release toxic emotion. I sing to pray and give thanks. I sing to create peace. My mission has indeed broadened. It is my mission to remind people how to use their authentic natural voice to sing, speak and to heal their body, mind, spirit and world.

META SOUND- THE FREQUENCY OF LOVE

ROSEMARY WARBURTON

Beyond sound...where does that take us? Sound is a powerful transformative ingredient in our lives. It is so much a part of us that our awareness of it, especially in the Western world, has become dampened. The goal of a sound healer is to light the spark that reawakens our awareness of the sound that surrounds and pervades our being.

The sense of hearing is a truly amazing phenomenon. It is the first sense to develop, after only 4 months *en utero*. Our first expression when we are born into this world is a cry- the triumphant affirmation of new life. One of the wonders of the sense of hearing is that it reaches far beyond the body. We can only touch that which is "within arm's reach." We can see that which is within a given distance, but we have to actually be looking in the direction of that which we are seeing. Yet we can hear sounds that are sometimes miles away, and not only sounds that are in front of us or within some peripheral range, but also the sound can be far above us, or behind us. Direction is of little or no consequence; and not only that, we can usually tell what direction the sound is coming from. We can be in the middle of a conversation with someone two feet away and suddenly stop, in total distraction, because we hear a distinct, though very faint sound- maybe a child's cry, an unusual birdsong, perhaps a plane with an interesting overtone, wind rustling in the trees, or a distant train whistle or fog horn.

What is this magical ability that sound has to suddenly captivate our attention and totally shift our focus in the matter of an instant? It can be disorienting at times in the sudden unfamiliarity- or just the opposite. It can also reorient us, help us find our way, ground us into a familiar reality. Do you remember walking in the woods when you were a child? Maybe you weren't quite sure of where you were, so you stopped and stood very still, barely breathing, until you could hear the highway, or a busy road, or maybe a train on the tracks, or the neighbor's dog- some familiar sound to tell you that you were safe and had not lost your way. And then you continued on the path.

As we develop our "outer" hearing, our "inner" sense also develops. The human body is fantastic; it is a myriad of resonance, tones, pulses, rhythms, and frequencies. In a healthy body, all parts are in harmony, a brilliant symphonic work of art. As we begin to expand our awareness through the art of listening, our consciousness grows on every level. The stillness grows more profound and we realize "silence" doesn't exist in our world. We hear sounds we have never heard before because we couldn't get quiet enough. Listening to our inner sound is an art, and can have profound effect on our consciousness. The ancient Essenes talked about the "sound current." Hindu yogis speak of *"shabda Brahman,"* the sound of creation, and *"anahata nadam,"* the "unstruck sound," or inner music, divine music, celestial harmony. This sound is heard when we learn to listen deeply within; it is the cosmic vibration which lies within each of us and leads us to our true Self.

Many people complain of "tinnitus"- ringing (or humming, or buzzing) in the ears. This is an example of the inner "nadam." The next time you hear this sound, rather than trying to suppress it, listen to it, meditate on it. This is a powerful practice that can transform your mind and your entire being. Ride on this inner current of sound and see where it takes you.

One of the things I remind people of, as a sound therapist, is this: If you hear a sound that is uncomfortable or causes distress, don't resist it. Rather, breathe it in and make a conscious effort to allow it and to integrate it. Become one with it; allow it to become part of your being- your walking, waking meditation.

Infants are able to fall asleep no matter how loud the sound is around them, because they have not yet developed the quality of "resistance." They haven't learned that they need quiet, or pretty songs, to help them go to sleep. They're tired- they sleep. Period.

There are many different kinds of music from all around the world that may be used for healing. The Bioenergetic Psychotropic Music of the Russian composer and sound healer Boris Mourashkin is just one form that has very powerful healing properties. It is typically played with the volume quite loud and there are many strange sounds, dissonances, and juxtapositions of rhythm, melody, and timbre. Over the years, I have closely observed what happens as I listen to the music or play it for other clients through a vibroacoustic sound bed. First, the conscious mind simply cannot follow the shifts that are happening, so one quickly goes into an altered state. Many different areas of the brain are being affected at the same time and it is like having "sonic acupuncture" in the brain. It seems to recharge and even "re-educate" the brain. All of this affects the entire being in countless ways, from relief of physical pain, to emotional release, heightened creativity, expanded awareness, and much more.

Another interesting point about Mourashkin's music is that it may initially be perceived as very disturbing due to its unusual nature, combining many elements in a way that we have simply never experienced before. He has created videos that combine light, color, and sound as well. They can be just as disconcerting to some people due to the volume at which he plays, the "weird" sounds presented, and the computerized images. However, it is extremely powerful due to the impulses that are being received both aurally and visually. While watching this, I realized that if we can learn to enjoy—to love—every frequency, **every** vibration, of color and sound, then we will also learn to love each other more fully. We can actually learn unconditional love, and suddenly the possibilities extend so far beyond the healing of the body, and reach to the mind and the emotions. Suddenly the healing expands to our spirit and thereby heals the planet. Because really all we are is frequency, and we can and ultimately we must become the vibration of love. All discord, all pain, all fear, melts before the vibration of love.

Practice the art of releasing resistance. Breathe in all of that which causes the tightening, the contraction, the holding of the breath. The next time you hear a loud siren as an emergency vehicle goes whizzing by, or perhaps a voice that you find grating, don't resist it. Don't block your ears or tense up. Try to simply breathe and expand your capacity to love just a little bit more. Breathe, travel on the frequency of sound, and love. Then see where it takes you.

A TRILOGY: FROM TONE DEAFNESS TO UNIVERSAL MUSIC DAY

SUSAN PATRICIA GOLDEN

Part I—Essence of Essential

You may ask, "Why, Essence of Essential?" "Why Art and Music?" and soon you will ask, "Why Universal Music Day?" Everybody knows we have music, right? Everybody knew we had an Earth thirty-eight years ago. Gaylord Nelson and John McConnell wanted to safeguard the earth for us and for the generations to come so they created Earth Day. Now, we are taking better care of the Earth. Those associated with Universal Music Day want to call attention to the importance of Music, Musicians, Music Teachers and Music-Making. These people and activities are essential to our health, healing, stress relief, LOVE and FUN. Music and Art are too important to leave only to the professionals.

According to Webster's Unabridged Dictionary:

ESSENCE: is that which makes something what it is. That which constitutes the inward nature of anything; true substance.

ESSENTIAL of/or constituting the intrinsic fundamental nature of something; necessary to make a thing what it is, indispensable.

I believe Art and Music are Essential. I want to tell you why and I invite you to make your Art and Music on a daily basis. Our Essence is Art and Music! The creative expressions of our Art and our Music send out messages from our soul that then reflect back to us who we are. In addition, the "Art and Music" around us resonates with us in ways that inform us. This soul information is Essential to our well-being because it allows us to follow the dictum, "to thine own self be true." How can we be true to ourselves, if we don't know who we are?

It all starts with the Breath. So, I invite you take a few deep breaths. Listen to your reaction to what you have just read. Listen to the relative silence and most importantly breathe—breathe deeply. Listen to your breath. YOUR BREATH is ESSENTIAL TO YOUR LIFE. We all know that, however, few of us give our breath the attention it deserves. The breath as taught by the sages for centuries is not only *essential* to our lives; the breath also opens pathways to listening deeply to that which is within us. That which is our *essence*. When we listen deeply to that which is within, we gain a better understanding of who we are. We learn about our gifts, and sometimes we even learn why we are on this planet! We learn about our own ESSENCE and knowing our Essence is Essential to living a satisfying life.

Notice I did not say "happy life." Not all of our lives are happy, and certainly not all the time. We all have challenges and none of us will get out this life alive, or so I have been told. However, no matter what is going on—illness, injuries, worries about the recessions, lost loves and even elections, we can learn to LISTEN, we can learn to be true to ourselves at any given moment. We can be true to our *essence* and thereby make choices consistent with who we are. We will then live in a way that we know we are doing our best. Even when doing our best falls short of the mark of getting us what we want or what we think we want. Even then, we can still feel a sense of satisfaction and that satisfaction fills our souls. Making Art and Music offers us that satisfaction. The experiences are rich even when dissonant!

On the other hand, when we ignore ourselves, pretend, mask our essence with our drugs of choice: nicotine, alcohol, TV, shopping, sex, computers, or food we stay unconscious. When unconscious, we have little control over ourselves and our lives because we are on "automatic," and usually reactive rather than thoughtful or soulful. We then often act on decisions that we made as children and continue to live our lives from the perspective of that 2, 3 or 6 year old. We may have decided way back then that: "life isn't fair," "I've gotta win," "I don't want to and you can't make me," "I want what I want when I want it," "I don't deserve it," "I am not loved," "I am not lovable," "I can't," or even "I am not worthy." Some parents and authority figures teach those toxins to children. Whether or not they are explicitly taught, those childish ideas often come from not living up to the hopes, expectations, or abilities of the adults around them.

From those childish perspectives, we often hurt ourselves. We often knowingly and unknowingly hurt others. We undermine our place in our communities and even undermine those communities. We seem to have versions of that in Technicolor right now [September 2008] on Wall Street and all around us in smaller ways. From my knowledge and experience both personally and professionally, as a successful psychotherapist for many years, there is nothing like making Art and Music, especially music improvisation, because the spontaneity teaches us about ourselves from the inside out—in other words, we get to know our Essence.

So much of education these days is outside-in and upside-down. The true self gets lost as children grasp for something outside to tell them who they are, who they should be, and how to live. Upside-down because learning and growing are constantly evolving explorations, not things for which there is a "right answer." Rather than living life as a creative adventure, our children are often spoon fed someone else's ideas, answers, and goals. Children are learning narrow parameters through which we define success in school and in life. They often work hard to take tests in order to live up to those outside expectations, only to get to their middle years and realize that they don't even how they ended up where they are, because they have been sleepwalking through their lives.

Let us look at this from a different angle. The scientists teach us that EVERYTHING in our universe is particle and/or wave. When they test for particles, the current technology "proves" that everything is particle. When they test for waves, they "prove" that everything is a wave. Deepak Chopra says, "Quantum Physics is not only stranger than we think it is, Quantum Physics is stranger than we can think!" So, the Quantum Mechanics experts and Physicists are telling us that the chairs, the ceiling, the piano, your body and mine all made of the same things—waves and particles, but mostly empty space. Well the next steps up from particles are Light, Color, Space and Shapes—in other words—Art! The next steps up from waves are Sounds, Silence and Vibration—in other words—Music!

Art and Music are all around us and also within us. We are made of waves, particles, and empty space. All that empty space needs the vibrations and the resonances of Music. The Music connects our heads with our hearts, with other hearts and with the Universal Energy. Just as when the "G" string on a cello is played, the "G" string on the violin, viola and base all vibrate. So also do the waves within us vibrate as the different pitches are played. We have all that music within us. Music not only resonates within us, but also gently massages all parts of our bodies and souls. Those vibrations move through the empty spaces within us and fill our bodies and souls.

Vibrations also come from within and send information back out past families, friends and neighbors into the Universe. Whether we are listening to our own vibrations or not, we affect others with our vibrations and those who are listening learn a lot about who we are, even without words. We resonate out from within us as well as getting vibrations from the outside in. This constant dialogue can inform our choices and our lives, if we are listening. Even if you disagree, I invite you to just play with these ideas for a bit and see where they take you!

If we are waves and particles; then we are Art and Music. Therefore, Art and Music-making are our Essence. If Art and Music making are our Essence, then they are ESSENTIAL TO OUR LIVES. They are not the extra fluff that many budgets would have us believe. What if we would only teach Art, Music, Dance, Drama, Reading and Writing from Kindergarten to 5th grade? Those subjects will teach what being human is all about. Our children would enter middle school with a strong sense of who they are, they would know what their gifts are, they would have had many experiences of taking safe risks so they could develop their courage, and they would be less likely to be negatively influenced by peer pressure.

A Call to Action

When the following text is spoken, a musical interlude of about 15 seconds between each section gives space for digestion. As you read the following, I invite you to breathe a few deep breaths between each thought.

*We gasp for breath as we first enter this world and as our last act leaving this world. Let us commit to honoring each breath and thereby honor our lives.

Musical interlude of about 15 seconds or a few deep breathes.

Breath is the Essence of Life and Breath is the Essence of Music. Therefore, it is safe to say that MUSIC is LIFE and if we allow it to be, LIFE IS MUSIC.

Musical interlude of about 15 seconds or a few deep breathes.

Let us commit to honoring our own Music from our heart song, even if only humming or playing a kazoo. Allow you heart to sing and play your heart song often.

Musical interlude of about 15 seconds or a few deep breathes.

Let us commit to making Art and living Artfully, taking care with ourselves and our surroundings.

Musical interlude of about 15 seconds or a few deep breathes.

We mark the most important rites of passage of our lives with music: weddings, birthdays, bar & bat mitzvahs, church services, national holidays and funeral ceremonies. You may remember that just after 9/11 when our political leaders could do nothing else and were speechless, they stood on the Capitol Steps and SANG.

Musical interlude of about 15 seconds or a few deep breathes.

Just as we take our breath for granted, most of us take Music for

granted, even if we love music. Certainly most people don't think of making their own Music and Art on a daily basis. Being a reformed non-singer and non-musician, I know the difference Music and Art make in our lives. For this reason, for the reasons stated above and because our Gifts of Music and Art from our hearts are important for the world, I invite you to spread the word. Many of us believe that Music is a ladder to God. Let us make our Art and Music daily.
Musical interlude of about 15 seconds or a few deep breathes.
Let us build a strong FOUNDATION on which EVERY THING else can rest. A foundation based on our ESSENCE.
Musical interlude of about 15 seconds or a few deep breathes.
Ancient people in all parts of the world began, and many still begin, their days with Music, Chanting, Drumming, and Dance. They sweat their prayers. Let us make every day a Music day and then come together in a World Wide Sound Wave on Universal Music Day the second Saturday of October each year.
Musical interlude of about 15 seconds or a few deep breathes.
Music and the arts help us to live life on life's own terms, which brings us back to the Essence of Essential and the prescription for a satisfied life.
Musical interlude of about 15 seconds or a few deep breathes.
From that place of deep feeling and deep listening we can then do for the "actively living" what hospices are doing for the "active dying." We can enhance the beauty, love, joy, compassion, comfort and support in the human experience so that we all live with dignity.
Musical interlude of about 15 seconds or a few deep breathes.
By now, you know the WHY of Universal Music Day. It has been established so we may safeguard making Music and Art for ourselves and for the generations to come. We will connect our heads with our hearts, our hearts with other hearts, and we will work together so we may all live in peace, bringing our gifts to the world.

Part II: My Personal Journey Begins: From Tone Deafness to Healing the Voice and the Spirit

February 1989, Susan Osborne's April "Seeds of Singing" Workshop Flyer attached itself to me as if by some gooey sap. The flyer wouldn't let go. For two months every time I opened my purse, it sang mysteriously like *Bali Ha'i*, "Come to me…"Come to me." I tried to throw it away. It just wouldn't let go. "Come to me."…Come to me."

For two months, I resisted. "No thanks, I don't sing—not if anyone can hear. I am tone deaf. I will spare people the torture. I sound terrible." Someone had even said to me, "Please don't sing Happy Birthday." My nephew was only three years old.

It seemed just a tad strange to have a running dialogue with a sheet of paper. But you should have heard that flyer! Gently at first, then building to a mighty crescendo… "Come to me…COME TO ME….. COME TO ME." Two months of that flyer beckoning, nagging, bullying got on my last nerve. "I am not going to that stupid workshop. Period! Besides it's probably too late."

To let myself off the hook I called John's Hopkins University, certain that the workshop was filled. Sweet, bubbly Sophia said, "No, you can register right now."

"No, no I can't register yet; I'm not sure about tomorrow. I think I have to work. I'm… I'm not sure… I have to…. I have to… I have to do my taxes."

In her best bubbly tone Sophia said, "No problem, if you can, just come and register at the door." She hung up. I slammed the phone down. "How could they? They should be full. I'm not going to that workshop." As I opened my purse the flyer sang again, "Come to me…COME TO ME….. COME TO ME." I made a deal, as if with a relentless child. If I wake up early, without an alarm, I'll go. Surely, I won't wake up!

Saturday morning's spring sunshine tapped my shoulder at 6:30 AM. The sun seemed to bubble like Sophia. I lashed out. "I am not going!" Then I bargained. "OK, I'll get dressed BUT I don't have to go. OK I'll go but I don't have to go in. The whole time, I continued to reassure myself, "I can always turn around." Instead….

I arrived early. Sitting in the Hopkins parking lot, I said, "OK, I'll go in BUT I don't have to stay." I mentally shadowboxed with myself up the steps and through the door. Wouldn't you know: Ms. Bubbly herself sat right inside at registration! We recognized each other's voices. "You came; terrific!" In my mind I was saying, OK, I'm here but I don't have to stay. She took my check, directed me and said, "You'll have a great time. Susan Osborn is amazing!" I half smiled and walked away thinking, OK, I'll stay for a little bit. But I'll be the exception to her no-one-is-tone-deaf, anyone-can-sing rule.

I looked around, barely making eye contact with anyone. I got a drink of water, admired the rotunda's high glass dome, went to the bathroom, got another drink of water, and commiserated with a scared soul at the water fountain who said, "Why are we wasting time inside on such a beautiful day?" I then noticed Susan's collection of CD's. Impressive! I took my seat.

When Susan entered, her long, green flowing dress highlighted her beautiful complexion, and short reddish brown hair. Susan gave a few guidelines, and then said, "Tell us your name and why you're here." Some also responded, "I am tone deaf," or "people say I can't carry a tune." Others sang in a choir, chorus or with friends. Some were professional singers. Some sang jazz, rock, and even opera. What an impressive range of people and styles. One woman, a professional Jazz singer, said, "Every time I come to your workshop, I improve. It's worth the effort and three hour drive. I wish you lived on the East Coast." That got my attention.

Then Susan began singing. Her voice reflected the sun beaming through the dome; her bright eyes and shimmering spirit lit up and filled that rotunda. Her-clear-as-glass sounds cut right through the ceiling and opened a pathway to the Universe. Amazing, Susan Osborn became one of the most beautiful women I have ever seen. Her glow radiated to the sun and back, melting my glacier of anxiety. She then began to speak.

"It is all about the breath!" We are just going to breathe. Take deep breaths and release the breath with a sound. Just let whatever sounds you make come to the surface. The uglier the sound—the better. "Basically that was what we did for most of the workshop. Breathe with sounds and feelings. In just eight to twelve hours Susan Osborne transformed a painfully tone deaf person into a singer.

She invited me back to my voice and I gratefully accepted the invitation. That was not something that at forty-five years old, I believed was ever going to happen. I finally began to let myself know how important Music is to me. I finally began to face my fears, my discomfort of allowing others to ridicule me about my voice. I forgave myself for joining in with others to ridicule my voice and lack of ability to match pitch. I finally acknowledged that sitting on the edge of my seat to look up at the choir as I listened to and felt the sounds and vibration rock my heart and soul meant something. It meant that my denial and fear deprived me of nourishment for my spirit for forty-five years and now I would have that feast of sound and vibration for the rest of my life. I went home and joined our summer choir. That talking flyer started a life-transforming journey. That sustains me and continues to take me to my musical Bali Ha'i. In my heart I still hear it call, "Come to me…COME TO ME….. COME TO ME." I am so glad I listened.

Part III: Come Alive and Thrive: Road to a Livable Bottom Line

Ravel's "Pavane for a Dead Princess" bathes my body in luscious sound waves from the Bose speakers in my living room. Nature bathes my eyes with another majestic sunset of bright orange waltzing over Jerry Lake in Dunedin, Florida. My mind drifts north to another ending — a Music for People (MFP) weekend workshop in Pennsylvania. I wonder:

   Who and what have I missed?
   What sound waves would have massaged my spirit?
   What miracles large and small might I have witnessed?
   What gems of wisdom would my Music Mentor, David Darling, have generously tossed to participants?

Then waves of gratitude wash over me for all the MFP workshops I have enjoyed since 1989. I shudder to think what my life would be like, had I not bolstered my courage to reclaim my voice and Music just before and just after the most challenging crisis of my adult life. Life happens to all of us! One day we're in charge, we're creating a life we love. We believe we're invincible. We have arrived!

The next day we begin sweeping up the life we knew, like the shards of a crystal goblet dropped on a brick patio. Shattered illusion invites us to, once again, recreate ourselves. And so it is!

Susan Osborn of *Seeds of Singing* took me to the top of the world in April 1989 at Johns Hopkins University in Baltimore where she masterfully helped me reclaim my lost voice, at age 45, in just two days. Two months later a car collision shattered hopes and dreams and crumbled my physically strong, active, sportswoman's body (like week old bread) and turned me into a human shaped glob of pudding. Needless to say, I wasn't laughing. Instead, I allowed my fear and disbelief to turn to anger. When the trusted systems pulled away the promised safety net and discredited me for the next seven years, that anger turned to rage. The insurance industry and legal system took me to hell; in some ways, I colluded. It was not a fun place to spend eight to ten years of my life. But perhaps it was the alchemy I needed for my life's mission.

I sometimes wonder how different my experience would have been had I continued laughing? The way I see it now, had I kept laughing, singing, or humming almost constantly, I would have more quickly reduced the constant pain and stress that made me incoherent and less effective. I would have fared much better. The healing power of sound would have done its magic. I want others to get this message and learn of the Power of Sound and Vibration—Music for their challenging times.

Lucky for me, a sense of adventure and good support systems could take me back to heaven on earth; I found it in friends, family, work, church (an Uncommon Denomination, which invites us to "Nourish Our Spirits and Heal the World,") Seeds of Singing, Music For People, the Omega and Esalen Institutes, and Living Tao. All offered that security, which I so desperately needed. They gave me a respite unlike the promised safety nets from before.

These supportive organizations balance self-interest with participants' needs and community interests. They supported, nurtured, nourished and sent me on my way to recreate myself. They gave me life. They provided caring and compassion during difficult times. Their minds and hearts work together, creating a "livable bottom line." Love is their mantra and healing their business.

Before the collision, Susan Osborn invited me to reclaim my voice. Post-collision, David Darling and Bonnie Insul, co-founders of Music for People, helped me find my "Lost Musician." Kaye Gardiner and Jonathan Goldman introduced me to Music for Healing. Ysaye Barnwell built Vocal Communities. I recreated, re-created and re-learned the healing power of laughter and play. I remembered that life is too important to be taken seriously. David Darling's last words to me that momentous August 1989 were, "You will never LISTEN in the same way again; your life will never be the same." That listening adventure has taken me to many amazing places. Finally, in 2007, after eighteen years, I discovered how I wanted to "pay it forward." I have known all along that I need to do something for the 80% of people who believe they are not musical but wish they were. I want to pass on what these amazing teachers and organizations offered me. But how?

In addition, to not knowing how to accomplish that noble task, the harder I tried to rebuild my business, the worse I did. It was like trying to piece together that shattered crystal goblet. The pieces just didn't fit together. I now had the nuts and bolts of many more tools but not the training or experiences to pull it all together. I am still working on this. In 1994, I started writing. I spewed venom back at the industries that hurt me. Then in 1998, I wrote a poem, "The Listening Game." That poem helped me to realize that there was enough venom in the world. I wanted to focus on the heaven that I experienced and put that out in the world. So I wrote a few children's books. Then I realized that first, children should know about instruments, see and hear the ones that everyone can play. I created the *ABZ's of Musical Instruments Book 1* with pictures of rhythm instruments and a glossary to teach something about the instruments. The sounds are on our website "FamilyMusicNetwork.net". I encourage everyone to make music at least 10 minutes a day. Book 2 will be the more traditional instruments that everyone knows. The time and financial investment to learn all that I needed to publish my own book was significant. The other books wait in the wings!

Doing the books required that same courage and determination that drove me, at age 45, to break through personal barriers and limitations to become a singer, a musician, an artist, and a writer. Those creative experiences drove me forward. The process offered me a deeper connection between my mind, heart and spirit. I was able to listen in new ways to myself, to others, to the world within and all around me, an exciting journey.

But there was still something missing, something more that I needed to do with all the gifts I received from these compassionate, loving people. How could I translate what I have learned and am still learning into something that will enrich the lives of others? I needed something that would continue to enliven everyone, not only during good times, but also when life shatters one's illusions. But what?

Just after Earth Day 2007, as if struck by lightning, this bolt of energy zapped me with the awareness that I need to do for Musicians, Music Teachers, Music Making and all of Humanity what Earth Day is doing for the Earth, Environmentalists and Humanity. I want to help create a world where we bring the kind of caring and compassion to the "actively living" that Hospice offers the "actively dying." I FINALLY knew what this journey is about.

Therefore, I invited friends to join me and we declared that the second Saturday of October would be Universal Music Day from now on. Some might say, "Why? Everybody knows Music!" The answer is, for similar reasons that Earth Day is important, because too many take the Earth and Music for granted. Thirty-eight years ago, most of us knew we lived on planet Earth. It was just always here so we paid little attention. We somehow missed the lessons of our Native American ancestors and didn't think about our responsibilities for caring for the Earth or making sure it would be a healthy place for future generations. Now many more view supporting the Earth as a right, a responsibility and a privilege. Making Music to support us is also a right, a responsibility and a privilege. While we have a long way to go, many people now ask and explore the important questions about the Earth and Music.

Since Musicians talk of "playing" Music, some people diminish the importance of Music. After all, these people would rather be "playing" than "working at a *real job*!"

Universal Music Day teaches others about the importance of adding Music to their lives because:

Music enriches our lives just for the sake of Music.
Music heals.
Music and Music-making parallel other experiences and challenges in our lives.
Music-making energizes many parts of the brain and strengthens lines of communication.
Music-making teaches about modulation: fast-slow, loud-soft, hard-easy.
Music-making conveys emotions through tone and intonation.
Music-making exposes our own style, as we do with Music so we also do in our lives.
Music-making with a chorus, often in parts, requires that we hold our part even when others around us are doing something totally different.
Music-making teaches cooperation as we sing or play in unison. We keep up with the Music and accompanying Musicians or we fall behind and miss out.
Music-making demonstrates that when each of us takes responsibility for our own parts, the whole ensemble works beautifully.
Music-making demonstrates the importance of starting on time and finishing right on cue.
Music exposes us to poetry, history, rhythm, pitch, volume, tone, expression and melody, all at the same time—the quintessential multi-tasking!
Music-making gives our lungs and body a physical workout as we breathe deeper.
Music-making massages every cell of our bodies.

Making music, we learn all the above, usually while performing someone else's Music.

Music Improvisation, a major focus of Music for People, puts one's heart and smart guts in charge. While doing many of the tasks above, we strive to come from that truth inside, see what is there, share our heart song and play in a way that enhances everyone's experience.

The learning includes wonderful:

Give and take
Offer and receive
Having our say and listening to others
Creating from nothing minute to minute
Just like life; we never know what is coming next. We are right in the moment.
The louder instruments sometimes play pianissimo to make room for the softer instruments.
At times, they blast a statement of exactly who they are and what they can do.
We solo, form spontaneous duos, trios, quartets, small groups or even a whole symphony of world instruments.
We offer our silence and actively listen to see when and where we can make a useful contribution.
Sometimes our best contribution is harmonious.
Sometimes it is dissonant.
We reach out with Love in our hearts and a commitment to truth, usually resolving the dissonance.
We laugh.
We cry.
We stir often forgotten thoughts and feelings.
We can experience a microcosm of life and the world in as little as one 'improv' or workshop.
We are fulfilled and satisfied.

David Darling and Music for Peoples' genius is in creating Democracy in Action through Music. We learn about listening, integrity, sharing, acceptance, respect, living fully, taking risk, being kind, and keeping a positive, loving attitude even when we make mistakes or react to the mistakes of others. Just as we learn to make room for the more quiet instruments, we learn to encourage the shy or less-practiced musicians to participate. As they become stronger, the group and community becomes stronger and more musical. We learn about the worth and dignity of every human, and we learn about citizenship!

The experiences and research from the Sound Healing Disciplines suggest physical, mental and emotional benefits of music. For instance, The Music for Healing and Transition Program (MHTP) reports that Music:

> Reduces blood pressure
> Accelerates physical healing
> Stimulates memories
> Relieves anxiety
> Induces mental imaging
> Provides a way to release emotions
> Reduces stress
> Facilitates the transition process for birth and death
> Provides a way to express feelings
> Augments pain management
> Provides an opening for verbal communication
> Aids mental focus
> Supports the grieving process
> Relieves mental tension
> Provides distractions
> Relieves body tension
> Provides companionship
> Provides time for contemplation—see website www.mhtp.org

Rich experiences with Sound Healing Groups, Susan Osborn, Seeds of Singing, David Darling, Bonnie Insul, and Music for People have inspired my life and planted the seeds for UMD going back to 1989. Now we are building on what these wonderful people offered in ways that help us heal from our challenges and find greater joy in the richness of our lives. Those of us involved with Universal Music Day, join many others around the world, who are committed to bringing love, caring, compassion, integrity, and an intelligent, sane way of living to the World Community so everyone can find ways to deal with the dissonance of life and create peace and harmony in our hearts.

When we do that around the world for at least one day every year, people will begin to understand that we can create peace and harmony in our world. We can learn that we are enough and we have enough. There is plenty in this beautiful, wonderful world for all to share.

Bibliography

Campbell, Don. *The Mozart Effect: Tapping the Power of Music to Heal the Body, Strengthen the Mind and Unlock the Creative Spirit.* New York: Avon Books, 1997.

Custer, Gerald. *The Open Door: Three Elementary Talks About Music.* Ann Arbor, MI: Stockton-Taylor Music, 2003.

Golden, Susan Patricia (Aunt Susie). *ABZ's of Musical Instruments Book 1.* Silver Spring, MD: FamilyMusicNetwork, 2001.

Green, Barry and W. Timothy Gallwey. *The Inner Game of Music.* New York: Doubleday, 1986.

Green, Barry. *The Mastery of Music: Ten Pathways to True Artistry.* New York: Broadway Books, a division of Random House, Inc., 2003.

Hull, Arthur. *Drum Circle Spirit: Facilitating Human Potential Through Rhythm.* Tempe, AZ: White Cliffs Media, 1998.

Knysh, Mary and Betsy Bevan. *Boom Do PA: the Creative Music Classroom, Rhythmic Connections.* Litchfield, CT: Music for People, 2002.

Mathieu, W. A. *The Listening Book.* Boston: Shambhala Publications, Inc., 1991.

Oshinski, Jim, et. al. *Return to Child.* Litchfield, CT: Music For People, 2008.

Suzuki, Shinichi. *Nurtured by Love.* Athens, OH: Shinichi A Publications, 1969.

Shawna, Carol. *The Way of Song: a Guide to Freeing the Voice and Sounding the Spirit,* New York: St Martin's Press. 2003.

Werner, Kenny, and Jamey Aebersold. *Effortless Mastery: Liberating The Master Musician Within.* New Albany, IN: Jazz, Inc.

Other Resources

Chopra, Deepak, speech at Omega Institute, Rhinebeck, NY. 1996.

David Darling, www.daviddarling.com

Music for people, www.musicforpeople.org, 860-491-3763

House of musical traditions, www.hmtrad.com, 301-270-9090

Susan Osborne, www.rockisland.com/~songhaus, 360-376-5180

Sweet honey in the rock, www.sweethoney.com, 202-829-4899

Suzuki Musical Instruments, 1-800-854-1594 or 858-566-9710

The Gift of Music, Music Educators National Conference, 1806 Robert Fulton Drive, Reston, VA 22091, 1986

Yamaha music (USA): email: infostation@yamaha.com, 714-522-9011

SING AND SWING:
A PERSONAL APPROACH
TO AN INDIVIDUAL VOICE

ANNETTE TEWES

There once was a king, who reigned with joy and wisdom. One day a visitor came to his country, full of admiration for this honourable ruler. However, at night, he suddenly found the king throwing dice.

"Your Majesty, allow me to ask you this: You are highly respected as a great king, and yet I find you gambling at night!"

"Well," answered the king, "I tell you a secret: If you wish to do a good job, you first have to bend like a bow, but to reach the goal, you then must let the arrow fly."

"There will come a time when a diseased condition of the soul life will not be described as it is by psychologists, but it will be spoken of in musical terms, as one would speak, for instance, of a piano that was out of tune."

—Rudolf Steiner

Our individual voice can become one of the most basic expressions of ourselves, when we are open and able to "let go," when we allow ourselves to enter the space of self-forgetting during our highest concentration. Singing always has been part of my life, but only now, at the age of 48, I am beginning to get a glimpse, a very first idea, of its power and healing energy. Sharing my experiences and visions, written down during the process of healing after a disastrous personal crisis, might serve as examples to the interested reader and encourage his/her own approach to learning about the powerful tool called music.

Modern physiologists like Eckart Altenmueller, of Hannover, Germany, have proven that melody and sound reception for non-musicians take place in the right half of the brain, but these move to the left part of the brain during the process of music practicing. The brain has no specific "music area" like the speech or visual centers that have been identified. Music, according to Oliver Sacks, is "at home all over the brain." Music appeals to brain and spirit, intelligence and wits, to creativity and emotions—to the entire person.

Sir Yehudi Menuhin, the famous violinist and conductor, believed that singing is the native language of humankind. Through music, we come into contact with our center; through the breathing, the giving and taking, we know the inside and the outside. But there have been severe changes to the way we approach singing over the years, mainly caused by the development of the mass media and modern communications. "The most beautiful, the most elementary human ability of singing has withered throughout the last decades or has even vanished. 'Noise' comes out of sound recording media all around, but the people themselves fall silent, they unlearn, they forget how to sing" (Jacobs, 1988:16.)

But little children have not forgotten how to sing naturally. They can show us the differences between the measure, the beat and rhythm. There is a natural musical wisdom in children. We cannot help to admire how young children tweet and chirp, and naturally sing in the highest pitches.

My own journey with music began with my "little-girls-world" behind our home. Lying in the green grass of the old enchanted garden with roses around the house and all kinds of beautiful flowers in the back yard, I looked into the clouds or counted numberless little bugs while humming. Sometimes I sat beneath the old black currant bush nibbling berries and sang to myself. Yet my first true childhood memory of song belongs to my mother, and to listening to her beautiful voice. She met my father in a church choir, and together they had found soothing comfort in choral music, something they greatly needed after the many years of war and destruction our homeland of Germany had seen. Some of my own dearest memories are the family gatherings, listening to the piano-duets of my grandmother or singing together all kinds of tunes, depending on the season: Christmas carols, Easter songs, tunes of summer frolic, or some of our own compositions.

Visits at my father's workplace, Oldenburg University, especially the orchestra concerts he led, but also his viola playing, impressed me deeply. It was for the first time there that I began to realize music could be a subject of scientific studies. Music was an important, self-understood and connecting part of our family life, and without pressure to perform, it meant natural fulfillment and joy. I was wrapped in a world where music was naturally present. Using my voice felt natural as well. My voice opened freely without intention, with no reason but being; it unfolded without my thinking about it. Singing was like playing – it had no end but itself.

During a stay in Connersville, Indiana, as an exchange student, aged 16, I joined the Senior High School Choir, not even knowing the German translation of this 'funny sounding' word, "choir." I found myself in the middle of a group of teens who enjoyed singing just as much as I did. Choir class included serious practice, and for the first time, there were goals to achieve: participation in a choir contest throughout the whole state of Indiana, producing a Christmas recording, and two big concerts in the school's auditorium—true events in that small town.

The fun we had, the mutual effort and the joy we brought to the audience, but especially the work of our gifted choir teacher, Shirley Henson, all combined to create some sort of a melted musical grounding for me. At this time, my voice began to relate to my self-assessment. A Solo, required in the senior class, and done in front of several hundred people in the audience, was most challenging and very frightening—and one of the most valuable experiences in my life.

Back in Germany, I found no equivalent to "my choir" at all. It took another five years until I came across the method of "Uncovering the Voice," and I was surprised to find that it proved to be an advantage that I had had no formal singing training. This method was the basis of a school, invented by a Swedish opera singer, Valborg Werbeck-Svaerdstroem (1879–1972.) She and her musician husband Louis Werbeck of Hamburg, developed a new understanding of the human voice. Between 1912 and 1924 in collaboration with Rudolf Steiner (1861-1925,) the founder of Anthroposophy, she designed her singing school for artistic, educational and therapeutic reasons. Steiner's spiritual science encouraged people to look at the original and natural, sensual parts of life, not only the materialistic. Her school was based on this kind of understanding. She did not, however, see herself mainly as a founder of a school, but more as a mediator of universal knowledge.

Valborg Werbeck-Svaerdstroem's biography can be divided into three parts that seem to have had different musical tasks in each: the performing singer, the founder of the singing school with educational value, and the therapeutic assignment.

A naturally born singer, Valborg Svaerdstroem grew up in northern Sweden. In her biography, she describes intimate contact with the beautiful nature of her homeland; she was a wild child with loads of energy who had understanding parents who did not interfere to 'tame' her. Singing was her life elixir, and as a young girl, she never experienced hoarseness. At the age of 15, she joined the Royal Music Academy of

Stockholm and aimed for an opera career. So far, singing had been an unconscious procedure for her. But during voice lessons, she felt a slight unease; her focus changed, causing her to notice as she sang. Trying to help her achieve a "great voice" led her teachers to forcing and pressuring her.

Very successful concerts all over Europe could not gild over her increasing voice problems; Valborg had to face them. She finally suffered a complete paralysis of her vocal cords. In that desperate moment, she remembered the hint given to her by a colleague who told her about nasal singing at an earlier engagement at the Munich Opera. She tried the new tactic. "I spoke nasal, and tried to cling to the sound, to broaden it, until it became a halfway sung note. On this, I concentrated with all my power of listening. Suddenly, in an outrageous way, the memory of my childhood voice appeared out of this listening! The foremost silvery sound came to my mind and made me search for the tone, the sound that expressed this best....Thus I found the syllable—NG!" (W. Verbeck-Svaerdstroem, 1975: 11.)

Practicing nasal speech, and later nasal sounds, she gained back her voice step-by-step. Between concerts, she practiced her newly invented exercises: "It was a constant compromising between the new and the old way to sing. The old way, of course, tried to dominate, while the new way was so tender, so different, that I found myself as if I was in between two hostile worlds" (W. Verbeck-Svaerdstroem, 1975:12.) At the pinnacle of her career, she resigned, with only one wish. Since she had observed her own healing process closely, she wanted to assemble a new Anthroposophical Singing Education, combining an anthropological and a spiritual approach with the natural children's voice as her main guideline. It occurred to her that something which is hidden inside the individual is allowed to come out into daylight through her process, so the name "Schule der Stimmenthuellung—School of the Uncovering the Voice" was chosen.

After decades of research using the pedagogic and therapeutic secrets of her inventions, she passed the essence of her knowledge on to her pupils. From her 88th to her 93rd year, she laid the groundwork for them to continue her teachings. After V. Werbeck-Svaerdstroem´s death her work has been continued in the artistic, pedagogical and therapeutic spheres under their leadership, and has been distributed all over Europe and into the other continents as well.

This school works beyond prejudices, without conditions concerning any talent or lack of talent in its pupils, referring to the standpoint of the individual, and only to some extent to anatomical circumstances. Of course, there are some singers that are apt to become professionals, but the first consideration is the fact that everybody has a voice to be unveiled! "Great artistic achievements will not exceed the adventure of the most tender beginning in the creation of tone...it is actually nothing more than removing hindrances and barriers...the human 'Voice' is ...there, complete, perfect, and waits to be freed" (Ibid., 18.)

Looking at the exercises taught through the Werbeck method, one finds a strictly technical-methodical part, but even that part is always based on the statutes for human voice and its spiritual origin. Vocal exercises might reveal an emotional flow, but remain an active work on consonants. They feel like a sculpturing with lips, tongue, jaw, and cheeks. The sound is a means to unblock energy and vitality, and all this is based on the breath and imagination working together. Pupils balance being active and passive in the work. It can be a rich and fulfilling experience.

The central pathway for the method is in finding and achieving one's own musical quest. Every individual shows a unique voice, and everybody has a different starting point. It is not the operation, the activity of the pressing and pushing force of gravity in the body mechanism, that counts; the goal is to find a sphere of effortlessness, easiness in singing. Students must find it and recognize it within themselves.

I found the "Uncovering the Voice" method to be comfortable partly because it fits with my own philosophical sensibilities. My personal approach to Anthroposophy included artistic as well as educational experiences, especially through contact with one of the Waldorf Schools in the town where I lived. However, the most impressive experiences have been my singing lessons. They opened the door to a new world, and a day without practice felt like I was in a black-and-white, not Technicolor, world ever since. I need Technicolor.

Within a few years of making these discoveries, I had signed up for the study of landscape architecture at the University of Hannover. Looking back on those years, I seem to have lived in two parallel worlds—singing, creativity, on one hand, and my scientific studies of ecology and nature on the other. Soon, family life, establishing a small family business, and working as an expert of ecology and landscape planning provided many tasks and demands. My singing diminished, almost fading away entirely. And my voice changed again: The experience of motherhood especially changed me; the basic life energy moving through birth deepened my relationship with the arts and religion, as well as my spiritual connections. A ripening of my voice was obvious. At the same time, I felt exhausted because children need their mother's living energy, the same well of energy, perhaps, from which creativity draws. Renewing my pursuit of singing exercises helped alleviate this situation.

Through various coincidences in my life, the "Uncovering the Voice" method pushed its way back into my personal focus. Twenty years later, I have now come to the point of re-defining myself. With (almost) grown-up children, and after separation from my husband and losing my job in the family business, a well-known phenomenon to many women my age, I am discovering my very own talents again. As Julia Onken, a famous Swiss Psychologist, puts it: "We often carry hidden abilities, which we could not develop throughout daily family life, and now they lie somewhere narcoticized in the attic...Then we ask ourselves, which preferences, which affections we used to have as a child, and suddenly the old long lost favorite activities show up again..." (2002:166.) During this period of my biography, after 7x7 years, it is time for me to unveil qualities and aims that could not previously be a part of my life on earth.

Giving birth to and raising my children taught me to let go, and know that through the detachment I might be rewarded with the most precious gift! Witnessing the wonder of a newborn child and watching it grow up taught me about the divine origin of life. Taking care of the children's needs helped me to realize that my own desires are not that important. But a time comes when it is my own turn to focus on my potential as a human being beyond the role of motherhood. I have practiced the art of letting go, which I need for my singing, and learned partly within that role.

"Letting go" while singing rewards me with very special moments of realizing the strength and beauty of my own voice. The sound and the music take the lead, and it feels like 'something is singing' through my voice as if it was an instrument. My emotional crisis and the breakdown of my accustomed life already included the seed of a new beginning. It seems to me that the deepening of my feelings goes along with a widening of the range in my voice. Witnessing, watching the floating energy, becomes a process of self-recognition I can experience while singing, especially when I express emotions like anger or rage. My high notes suddenly begin to sound clear, not when I use a certain technique, but when I am feeling my courage.

Mystics and scientists of ancient cultures knew about sound, as audible vibration, and its use in harmonizing, healing and expanding consciousness. "All of life is sound...[Spiritual] silence contains all sounds of the universe, just like colorless light contains all colors" (Sharamon, Baginski, 1988:237.) Standing near a huge Tibetan singing bowl almost immediately sets free my tears. For me, the experience of creating sound through my voice takes me to a sphere of inspiration, just as the creative self-expression of singing did for me as a child so many years ago. It opens the door of self-reflection, it connects to something greater than me that I can only receive, but not force. It brings back my own tune:

> "As long as we try to balance, we are moving forward, as long as we are moving, we are alive."

Editor's note: All translations into English of text, titles, and quotations were done from original German texts by the author.

References

Albohm, Paer. Die Sonnentrommel und andere Lieder (original title: „Soltrumman"). Jaerna, Sweden: Choroi-Foerlaget,1968.
Altenmueller, E. In: Held, W. Die Organe des Denkens 8. Das musikalische Gehirn. A tempo 11 (2008): 17.
Jacobs, Rita. Musik fuer kleine Kinder. Stuttgart: Verlag Urachhaus, 1988.
Knigge, Klaus. Kanons. Stuttgart: Edition Bingenheim im Verlag Freies Geistesleben, 1993.
Onken, Julia. Altweibersommer. München: Beck'sche Reihe, 2002.
Sachs, Oliver. Musicophilia. Tales of Music and the Brain. Vintage books, 2007.
Sharamon, S. und Baginski, B.J. Das Chakra-Handbuch.- Aitrang: Windpferd Verlagsgesellschaft, 1988.
Werbeck-Swaerdstroem, Valborg. Die Schule der Stimmenthuellung. Ein Weg zur Katharsis in der Kunst des Singens. Dornach, Schweiz: Philosophisch-Anthroposophischer Verlag am Goetheanum, 1975.

(Translation by the author)
Albohm, Paer. *The Drum of the Sun and other Songs*. Jaerna, Sweden: Choroi-Foerlaget, 1968.
Altenmueller, E. in: Held, W. "The Organs of Thinking 8. The Musical Brain." *A tempo* 11 (2008): 17.
Jacobs, Rita. *Music for little Children*. Stuttgart: Urachhausverlag, 1988.
Knigge, Klaus. *Canons*. Stuttgart: Edition Bingenheim im Verlag Freies Geistesleben, 1993.
Onken, Julia. *Indian Summer in Female Life*. München: Beck'sche Reihe, 2002.
Sharamon, S. and B. J. Baginski. *The Chakra-Manual*. Aitrang: Windpferd Verlagsgesellschaft, 1988.
Werbeck-Swaerdstroem, Valborg. *Uncovering the Voice. The Cleansing Power of Song*. Dornach, Switzerland: Philosophisch-Anthroposophischer Verlag am Goetheanum, 1975.

YOU MUST SING TO BE FOUND...

SUSAN GREGORY

Morning sun pours through the studio windows, lighting up a singer as she stands with arms raised, feet planted, chest expanded, mouth open, eyes shining, sustaining the full last note of a song. She remains a moment with arms uplifted when the music stops, then bursts into a grin and declares, "I'm back! I feel alive!" Lowering her arms and gaze, she quietly adds, "I never thought I'd want to sing again." This 72-year-old professional woman had been depressed since September 11, 2001. She came to me in 2002 hoping to use singing to regain her love of life.

We worked with a modality that mixes singing study with therapeutic movement and conversation, using singing as a catalyst for self-discovery and growth. Songs that she chose, at first those that had been part of her history and later new ones, provided a context that engaged her interest. She expressed feeling a sense of safety in the structure of our work. Within that safety, we began our vocal experiments, first with pure sound-making, which fostered her attending to somatic experience, including grounding and breath, then with short rhythmic atextural patterns that allowed us to widen the inquiry. We then moved to aesthetic experiences of melody, timing, pitch, vowel color, and dynamics, and finally, to singing with words.

Through attention to these stimuli, emotions began to flow that we accepted without interpretation, held by the field of our therapeutic relationship. This led to her revisiting unfinished business in her life, which became expressible not only in therapeutic conversation but also through song texts and sound itself. Her choices of songs became more adventurous and far-reaching as our work progressed; and our processing conversations after the singing included attention to the inter-subjective field of our work together. Our therapeutic relationship provided an environment for experimenting with voice, and from that, the possibility for personal growth emerged (Amendt-Lyon, 2003).

Singing and listening to songs involves deepening breathing, mobilized body movement, heightened sensing (Desjarlais, 1996,) intensified emotional flow, and sustained aural contact with the environment, the whole of which has been shown to promote health (Rousseau, 2000.)

Singing is an integrating experience in which musical structure and composed text makes it possible for people to manage strong feelings. Therapeutically oriented singing lessons provide a rich relational field between therapist and singer, who co-create ways to encounter both the satisfaction of skill mastery and the changes that occur through uncovering heretofore-unexamined patterns of learning, expressing and interacting.

As a Gestalt therapist and a singing teacher, I have drawn the case examples in this essay from my seventeen-year practice of weaving these areas of expertise together into an action therapy (Cook & Wolfert, 1999) called GestaltSing. Vocal growth cannot be separated from personal growth. Emotions are quickened through the aesthetics of music. Awareness is heightened through the poignancy of lyrics. The body is mobilized through breathing and supporting vocal tone. All of this provides an enlivened functioning for therapeutic exploration. Moreover, it is grounded in the neurobiological and developmental underpinnings described below.

Neurobiological Considerations

Dr. Steven Porges (2002/2008) has established experimental programs in which he uses enhanced recordings of human singing to treat both adult depression and childhood autism. The work is based on laboratory studies he pioneered regarding neuronal connections from brain to ear, face, mouth, larynx, pharynx and diaphragm. Those connections are a branch of the vagus nerve that innervates what he calls the muscles of social engagement. This neural plexus is so important for an infant's survival that it is the second nerve to mylenate in gestation. With good functioning of this nerve complex and its associated muscles the infant is able to call or cry for help and then to hold the attention of caregivers by use of appealing facial expressions and prosodic sound making. Porges points to the strong connection between ability to vocalize and success in social interaction.

If the neural regulation of muscles of vocalization and facial expression is dysfunctional, a flat affect is observed, typical of depression and autism. Porges has found that listening to enhanced human singing activates the vagus nerve complex and its associated neuronal controls. Through a program of regulated activation, Porges has shown that facial and vocal expressiveness can be aroused, and that a range of social affects appears, improving social contact and life quality. It has been suggested that Porges's ongoing work provides the scientific explanation for the success Tomatis (1969) achieved in his program of therapeutic listening.

Voice scientist Alison Behrman (2004) is also interested in the relationship of brain functioning and voice use. She speaks of an area deep within the midbrain called periaquaductal grey matter or PAG. When that area is stimulated, the subject emits wordless, affect-laden sounds. Behrman notes, too, that nerve endings involved in stimulating movement of skeletal muscles closely approximate, and in some cases penetrate, the PAG.

From this, she posits that overt body movement and expressive sound-making are intrinsically connected. As a phenomenon, we may observe the connection in all cultures where people dance, stamp, clap, or sway as they sing. Anthropologically, in many cultures, the words for "sing" and "dance" are the same word. Based on this, I have found it productive to have my GestaltSing clients engage in movement while singing. This often heightens their self-awareness.

Infant Development and Voice

The intrinsic connections between movement and vocalizing are most observable in infancy. Infant researchers M. and H. Papousek (1989) have shown that singing begins in the first months of life with prosodic exchanges between infant and caregiver. In those wordless duets, relationship grows in a co-created field of sound, gesture, touch and gaze through which attachment occurs and the self is elaborated (Shore, 2002.) In order to have their needs met, infants vocalize. While attending to those needs, caregivers may respond by making a variety of sounds that soothe or stimulate their charges.

Caregivers' sounding is essential to infants' well-being. This was proven pragmatically as early as the 12th Century when Frederick the Great had an experiment performed in which 30 infants taken from households around his empire were cared for in his palace with every need assiduously attended to, save one; the caregivers were forbidden to talk with or sing to the babies. Within a year, every otherwise-healthy infant died!

Sound exchanges develop between infants and mothers as part of development. These dialogues, a form of play, are musical in nature. Papousek and Papousek (1984:142) state, "It is not just the empathic mother who adapts flexibly to her infant, but the infant too is alert, sensitive and responsive to the mother's own variations of communications." Thus, self is a relational self, forming in interaction with other (Fogel, 1993), and prosodic exchanges—earliest singing—are important components of those interactions.

Trevarthen (1999) studies how babies teach good-enough mothers to sing with them, often taking the initiative. On research tapes of mothers and their babies of five and six months of age, intricate songs are sung with obvious delight. At about nine months, complex cross-modal action begins in which they combine singing, movement and facial expression. Infants and mothers reinforce attunement between themselves with gaze, gesture and vocal toning. Stern (1985) stated that mothers constantly introduce modifying imitations or else themes and variations. Vocal duets between mother and baby are one of the ways that babies develop their sense of self in relation to an important other.

The ability to hear begins in the fourth month of gestation. A baby is already familiar with its mother's voice before birth and is thus primed to communicate with her vocally and to be receptive to her vocalizing. The aural/oral field that babies and caregivers co-create supports the infant's developing awareness of self/environment. These prosodic exchanges may be seen to be the infant's first experiences of group singing. These earliest experiences create the patterns with which we listen, speak, and sing throughout our lives. In the therapist-client singing relationship, those established patterns are revealed.

This example reveals the presence of early patterns of interaction in a singer's contemporary functioning:

In her first few lessons, Joan chose to stand to the side of the piano and slightly behind me. That way, we made no eye contact. After a few weeks, I asked her to experiment with a different position in the room. She tried, and reported feeling frightened. Her voice became much quieter. Yet, in moving back to her original position, she became aware of being disappointed. When she said this, her voice was fuller. We experimented with changing positions regularly. We devised some eye-contact experiments for her to try outside the session. Over time, Joan reported feeling more present in life. We kept up this work using songs Joan loved to sing as a supportive resource while she continued to enlarge her contact with the world.

Approaching Trauma with Singing Activities

There are many examples of the power of singing in sociopolitical contexts. Here is one I find very moving.

In 1997, Ugandan musician Samite Malundo visited a refugee camp in Rwanda where the child occupants were survivors of horrific massacres.

One day Malundo sat down next to a silent young boy and sang him a song. The boy quietly sang another back to him. Soon, a group of orphaned children gathered around them. They exchanged songs for several hours; and slowly, their trauma-related flat affect began to change, the heightened breathing and movement helping them undo a frozenness that had set in as a survival strategy.

While they had lost everything—homes, families, villages—they began, through singing, to experience their pre-traumatic memories, feelings and group identifications. In slowly reclaiming these, they began to lay ground for possible recovery. After having been mute and in shock for weeks, many of the children began to cry and to tell their personal stories to Malundo, with the support of the music and the group. By the end of his one-week visit, the children had begun to talk about a future: "When I leave here...When I am big...I want to introduce you to my new best friend." Through singing, these shocked and uprooted children had begun to reorganize their life field, self-mobilizing and forming new social connections.

Peter A. Levine (2002), the founder of trauma amelioration work called Somatic Experiencing, has reported how utilizing singing and dancing with mixed groups of Bosnian and Serbian mothers and babies enhanced communication among all members of the community and promoted a general relaxation of tension in a town whose inhabitants were traumatized by war. He believes that changes of brain states were promoted by their singing and dancing together.

Bessel van der Kolk (1996,) a clinician specializing in trauma work, has spoken of working with spontaneous singing in both groups and individual sessions with sufferers of PTSD. Observing the efficacy of singing in helping persons revisit their traumatizing experiences without their then becoming retraumatized, he has put out a call for formal research to backup the results he is seeing in his practice (2003.)

Working with Individuals

Singing and speaking are important ways of connecting. Our vocalizing transforms the aural/oral field of which we are a part. The activity of singing, in which breath and movement are mobilized to support sound, activates all parts of the field. Therapist Bud Feder (2005) sometimes asks clients, "Were you to sing any song right now, what would it be?" And Laura Perls often asked clients who were verbalizing uncontactfully, "Can you sing that?" (Goodman, 1951)

Here is a student describing the therapeutic effects of her singing lessons, even without psychotherapy *per se* having been practiced:

> I was involved in developing a true body instrument, requiring a mind-body unity from the inside out. It also meant overcoming an area of previous failure and disability in my life. I experienced a combination of trust in my teacher's diagnostic ear and prescriptive methodology and trust in my own neuromuscular capacities. It took more faith and perseverance to overcome the obstacles of my past vocal history than anything I ever did in my life. I had an awareness of owning a voice that could command attention. My speaking voice had more nuances and was expressly connected to my thoughts. My body seemed to be standing behind my voice. I found I could use more of my voice in the world.

Almost everyone has a song that has been important in his or her life, important because of the context in which it was sung or listened to. Songs can be markers of one's personal history. Drawn from my practice, here are examples of songs as personal narratives:

A professional singer chose Kurt Weill's *Trouble Man* to perform. Working on it led to an outpouring of emotion about her father having brutalized her, something she had kept hidden for twenty years.

A teenage baritone selected *What I Did for Love* from *A Chorus Line*. Through exploring the lyric's meanings, plus facing his feelings around having chosen a song sung by a female character in the show, this young man was able to find support to become clear about his sexual orientation, first with me and then with his family.

A European film actor brought Brahms's *O, wüsst ich doch den Weg zurück* (Could I but find the way back.) The poet speaks of longing to return to childhood. Through singing this song, she mourned a lost childhood in her war-torn homeland.

A bass-baritone struggled to sing Papa Germont's aria from *La Traviata*, which he had chosen for a concert. Finally, he broke down in tears, "I wish I were a tenor. I'm frightened by my low sound. I sound like my father. This character and my father are so unbending. I don't want to be that kind of man."

In each of these cases, the singers and I combined singing study with therapeutic conversation, adding a variety of voice and movement experiments to engage with concerns that came foreground through singing the song.

Group Singing

In his book *The Singing Neanderthals*, Mithen (2006) shows that singing is an activity whose roots are evolutionarily deep within us. Singing is an ancient way that groups prepare to carry out mutual activity and soothe themselves when activity is done (Berger & Del Negro, 2004.) Soccer fans, field hands, army squads, birthday celebrants, church congregations all demonstrate this. There is a sense of group support and group identity that develops when people sing together (Wade, 2004.) Singing has been an aspect of group organization throughout human history (May, 1980.) It provides opportunity for participants to experience strength and solace by "simultaneously coordinating the emotions of a group of people" (Storr, 1992:114.)

Campbell (1997) reported that group members singing together have been measured to have similar pulse rates, blood pressure, and pupil dilation; and a study of people singing has shown their brain wave patterns to be synchronized (Rider, 1997.) Human beings are neurologically primed for this somatic entrainment by the vocalizing exchanges they first participated in during infancy. They are thus neurologically available for a kind of light trance induction (Rossi, 1993) which group singing may facilitate. In group settings, these understandings can help therapists use singing to create either soothing or stimulating therapeutic experiences, which aide in bringing about brain wave changes (Taylor, 1997,) evince phenomenological qualities of arousal, expansion, and the blurring of boundaries between self and other which some have called spiritual.

Since in infancy most of us have engaged in vocal exchanges with caregivers, we are primed in our neurons to be moved in various ways when we participate in group singing. Under differing circumstances, singing in groups may encourage heightened individual awareness facilitated by the experience of group aural support, or dulled individual awareness facilitated by an experience of group domination.

Daniel Stern (1985) describes a process called "automatic induction" whereby heightened auditory experience, spoken or sung, may move people to respond on a preverbal level to the prosodic elements of oratory, including timbre and melodic line, pitch patterns, pace, volume, and relationship of phrasing to breath pauses. Based on early developmental patterns of sound exchange, humans are deeply susceptible to qualities of vocalization, and may be moved toward an orator's or singer's ends as much by the sounds of voice as by the meaning of words.

Anthropologist David Attenborough (2002) investigated the uses of singing in preliterate societies and in group activities of several other species. He found songs to be important coordinators of group effort, signifiers of readiness to mate, and a means to denote group boundaries or territory. The singing of structured vocal activities was once thought to be exclusively a human activity. Research at the Department of Biomusicology at the Massachusetts Institute of Technology now shows that singing structured songs antedates human evolution. Articles in *Science* (Angier, 2001) compare the structures of songs by birds, whales and humans. Biomusicologists describe what they call a *music instinct* identifiable in vertebrates brain functioning. They show many inter-species parallels in range of pitches, variety of rhythms, harmonic relationships, melody patterns and song forms. Based on this research as well as his own, Attenborough (2002) proposed that singing, rather than being exclusively cultural, might have biological roots. Some MIT researchers proposed that human beings may be "hard wired to sing" (Angier, 2001.) This evolutionarily deep connection of human beings to singing may point to one of the reasons that working with singing therapeutically has such potentially powerful effects.

Conclusion

"...you must sing to be found; when found you must sing..."

These words were written by contemporary poet Li-Young Lee (1990). A therapy client, a visitor to New York from Ireland, brought them to me. She told me of wanting to sing and having been forced to fall silent. We were able to hear how her mellifluous speech and skillful storytelling have become her singing. We spoke of the rich oral tradition of her culture. We noticed together how, in times of social emergency, group singing comes to the fore.

We saw that in New York City on the nights following September 11, 2001, when neighbors spontaneously gathered in the streets to light candles and sing songs of solace. On the streets, we heard people say that singing allowed them to express the intensity and complexity of their experiences, something for which conversing alone was not enough.

Singing facilitates manageable discharge of held-back energy. Moreover, when we can do that in tandem with others, the community holds our expression and, through its aliveness of functioning, points toward the future. In singing, we engage body, emotion and thought simultaneously. In that sense, it is an integrative undertaking, and thus therapeutic. Singing in a group, in addition, allows us to experience both the individual and social aspects of self. Singing is a mode of lively contacting through which we can experience self-in-community.

Singing connects people with their histories, remembered and hidden, and with each other, and helps people renew their energy for life's challenges. Grounded in neurobiological and infant developmental experiences, singing connects us to our present relational field and to our evolutionary and anthropological past. Expanding Li-Young Lee's thought, we may say:

> "...we must sing to be found; when found, we must sing... "

References

Amendt-Lyon, N. and M. Spagnuolo-Lobb,"Toward a Gestalt Therapeutic Concept of Pro-Moting Creative Process." *Creative License.* Vienna: Springer. 2003.

Angier, N. "Sonata for Humans, Birds and Humpback Whales.", *The New York Times,* (2001) Sept. 9:C5.

Attenborough, D. "Song of the Earth." New York: *Nature*, WNET. 2002.

Behrman, A. Speech delivered at the New York Singing Teachers' Association". New York: Dept. of Otolaryngology, Beth Israel Hospital. 2004.

Berger, H., and G. Del Negro, *Identity and Everyday Life.* Middletown: Wesleyen University Press. 2004.

Bloom, D. "Aesthetic Values as Clinical Values in Gestalt Therapy." *Creative License*, Vienna: Springer. 2003.

Campbell, D. *The Mozart Effect.* New York: Avon. 1997.

Cook, C. and R. Wolfert, "Beyond Talk Therapy: Using Movement and Expressive Techniques in Clinical Practice." *Gestalt Therapy in Action,* Washington, D.C.: American Psychological Association. 1999.

Dejarlais, R. "The Performance of Healing." *Presence*, London: Routledge. 1996.

Fogel, A. *Development Through Relationships: Origins of Communication, Self and Culture.* Chicago: University of Chicago Press.1993..

Gregory, S. "A Gestalt Therapist Teaches Singing." *Australian Gestalt Journal,* 10 (2),(2001) 114-117.

—. "The Song Is You," *British Gestalt Journal,* 13(1).(2004) 24-29.

Lee, L. "You Must Sing." *The City In Which I Love You.* Rochester: BOA Editions. 1990.

Levine, P.A. "Trauma, Rhythm, Contact, and Flow," *Caring for the*

Caregiver, Silver Spring, MD: American Music Therapy Association. 2002.

May, E. *Musics of Many Cultures*. Berkeley: University of California Press. 1980.

Mithen, S. *The Singing Neanderthals,* Cambridge, MA: Harvard University Press. 2006.

Perls, L. *Living at the Boundary*. Highland, NY: Gestalt Journal Press. 1992.

Papousek, H. and M. Papousek, "Forms And Functions In Vocal Matching In Interactions Between Mothers And Their Precononical Infants," *First Language*, 9(1),(1998) 137-158.

Porges, S. Speech delivered at meeting of the United States Body Therapy Association. Baltimore: Johns Hopkins University. 2002.

—.Speech delivered at the Music Therapy Association. New York: Louis Armstrong Foundation, Beth Israel Hospital. 2008.

Rider, M. *The Rhythmic Language Of Health And Disease*. St. Louis: MMB Music. 1997.

Rossi, E.L. *The Psychology Of Mind-Body Healing*. NY: W.W. Norton. 1993.

Rousseau, G. "The Inflected Voice: Attraction And Curative Properties." In P. Gouk (Ed.), *Musical Healing in Cultural Contexts*. Aldershot, Hampshire: Ashgate. 2000.

Shore, A.N. *Affect Regulation and the Repair of the Self.* New York: W.W. Norton. 2002.

Stern, D. *The Interpersonal World of the Infant*. New York: Basic Books. 1985

Storr, A. *Music and the Mind*. New York: Ballantine. 1992.

Taylor, D.B. *Biomedical Foundations of Music as Therapy*. St. Louis: MMB Music. 1997.

Tomatis, A. *Dyslexia*. Ottowa: University of Ontario Press. 1969.

Trevarthen, C. *An Emotional Symphony*. London: BBC Radio. 1999.

—. *Music Therapy in Context: Music, Meaning and Relationship*. London: Jessica Kingsley Publishers. 1997.

van der Kolk, B. *Traumatic Stress: The Effects of Overwhelming Experiences on Mind, Body and Society*. New York: Guilford. 1996.

Wade, B. *Thinking Musically: Experiencing Music, Expressing Culture*. Oxford: Oxford University Press. 2004.

III: ENGAGING BODY

META-PHYSICAL:
FROM MOVEMENT TO MAGIC

ROGER N. MILLEN

Have you ever wanted to feel happy, but could not see yourself that way? Have you ever wished that you had a reference experience for empowerment, but just could not imagine what that would be like for you? What if you could access (or create) powerful reference experiences ... feeling energy surge through your body, bringing with it the ability to see yourself in action, hear yourself speaking confidently, tasting victory, and smelling the sweet smell of success. The interrelationships between our feelings and physiology are well established and form the basis for the work described below. Our physical condition is a somatic display of the psychological life that we have been living to the present moment in time. Deepak Chopra, M.D., author of *Quantum Healing*, says that our physical bodies are the metabolic end product of all our experience. That our bodies are, indeed, ourselves has been known and a part of various cultural practices and disciplines since pre-history. Ritual dances, various yogic practices, fire walking, the whirling of the Dervishes, Qi Gong (Ch'I Kung), and Tai Ji Quan (T'ai Chi Ch'uan) are but a few examples of man's attempts to transcend the physical plane of existence using the physical body as the vehicle of transcendence. Meta-Physical is based on these principles and is designed to more fully involve the kinesthetic aspect of processing in both the accessing and creation of subjective experience.

As practitioners and healers, we often ask others, and are frequently ourselves asked, to re-experience some past episodic event or to create a powerful experience to be integrated into the actually-experienced past ("change history") or to be inserted into the yet-to-be-experienced future ("future pacing.") Typically, during this process, the subject is seated and in a light-to-medium trance state. The entire process is cerebral in nature, the "experiences" being created by mentation alone: imagination and visualization. The physical body, save by conjecture, is not involved. Any somatic responses are reactive, not proactive. These experiences occur in the body (i.e. in the brain/mind), but not with (i.e. using) the body.

For those subjects who would be classified as processing primarily through the visual, auditory, or cerebral channels, the above procedures can, and often do, produce dramatic results. But what of the remaining category: the kinesthetic? Common sense dictates that body-oriented approaches would be more than appropriate. Virginia Satir utilized family and other group "sculpture" as a means by which relationships could be expressed kinesthetically as well as visually, with very powerful results. M.H. Erickson observed that, "all of us have a tremendous number of these generally unrecognized psychological and somatic learnings and conditionings, and it is the intelligent use of these that constitutes an effectual use..." One's relationships with oneself, as well as with others, is often dramatically felt when it is expressed kinesthetically. While in some situations it may be useful to allow the subject to express himself completely freely and spontaneously, or to impose inferred structure, based on learned or intuitive understanding, it is often very useful to have the subject express himself in archetypical postures and movements based upon a current situation, presenting problem, or relationship to the change process.

One of the great treatises on change is the *I Ching*, which means literally "Annals of Change," originally part of one of the great contributions to philosophy and world literature, the *Wu Ching* (the Five Classics) of ancient China: *Shi Ching* (the Book of Songs), *Shu Ching* (the Book of History), *Li Ji* (the Book of Rites), *Chun Ch'iu* (the Spring and Autumn Annals), and *I Ching* (the Book of Changes.) Ordered destroyed by an early Emperor in his bid to control knowledge, only the *I Ching* survived intact. Embodying the essence of the Taoist philosophy of the universality of change, the *I Ching* remains to this day one of the deepest philosophical insights of history. Its wisdom is universally applicable for insight and self-reflection, as well as an inexhaustible source of clarity and inspiration.

While a complete explanation of the structure of the *I Ching* is far beyond the scope of this article, a brief introduction to the basics follows. The underlying basic concept is that of Yin and Yang, the two complimentary and opposing forces in the universe that continually die and give birth, each to the other, following life's only certain rule: change. While more commonly represented by the familiar black and white "double fish" diagram, Yin and Yang are also depicted by a broken and a solid horizontal line respectively. These are arranged into all possible three-line configurations to form eight trigrams, the Ba Gua (Pa Kua). The eight trigrams represent the members of various relationships, e.g. familial, natural, organizational, heavenly, etc. The eight trigrams are, in turn, combined into all possible six-line configurations yielding the sixty-four hexagrams which comprise the *I Ching*. Each hexagram represents a state or situation occurring in the world and the complete cycle of sixty-four is said to represent all possible situations and changes that exist in the world of experience.

Less well known is that the hexagrams also represent postures from T'ai Chi Ch'uan, literally: supreme ultimate boxing. The upper and lower trigrams of each hexagram representing the upper body position and lower body stance of the various postures in the T'ai Chi Ch'uan form. These lower body stances and upper body positions are also used in another Chinese discipline, Ch'I Kung, literally: energy development. These various postures and movements are kinesthetically and energetically congruent. There is evidence to suggest that they may be emotionally congruent as well.

A frequently encountered presenting problem is the issue of "grounding" or "centering". With an ever-increasing number of professionals spending more and more of their lives, both on and off the job, planning and conceptualizing, as opposed to doing, their connection to the earth becomes ever more tenuous. In response to the simple question, "Where are your feet?" I have observed a large variety of responses including the ever popular "going into down time," various types of search procedures, and the all-time-favorite "I don't know." Re-grounding, i.e. reconnecting, begins with re-experiencing the feeling of being on the earth and the pull of gravity. A posture called Wu Ch'I (no energy,) which is based on the *I Ching* hexagram Hsu (waiting, nourishment, meditation,) is employed to create this experience. The posture is one of preparation, of being in equilibrium; from this position one can either give or take, advance or retreat, but, for the present moment, one just is. Once the body is correctly structurally aligned and proper breathing is established, an awareness of internal energy circulation can begin. Little by little, one level at a time, the awareness comes to center—to stillpoint—and the reconnecting process, the re-grounding experience, can be felt. Subsequent sessions explore balance and centering, movement off and from the center, and direction of energy with intention.

Another often-heard complaint is that of feeling or being "stuck." The cognitive understanding that something needs to be done, that some action (long overdue) must be taken, and even understanding what it is that needs must be done, is often insufficient to "move" someone to action. In cases like these, a direct kinesthetic experience of initiating action can be the difference that makes the difference. Using the t'ai chi movement Ch'I Shi (raise energy), based on the *I Ching* hexagram Chin (progress), potential energy is transformed into kinetic energy and the body is moved from static equilibrium to dynamic equilibrium. Thus, while remaining grounded and centered, movement toward some goal, objective, or outcome can be felt in one's direct experience.

Correct use of the postures and movements of both Ch'I Kung and T'ai Chi Ch'uan can provide experiences and releases of both an energetic and emotional nature. Deep, basic, and archetypical experiences can be both recalled and created by proper use of these systems. Typically, the desired state is accessed or created using Ch'I Kung and any changes accessed or created with the movements of T'ai Chi Ch'uan. While Chi Kung practice is limited to the individual, T'ai Chi Ch'uan can be practiced as a martial art and offers opportunity for the exploration of interactions and relationships.

Using the system of Tui Shou (push hands,) the adversarial relationship is transformed from one of "struggling against" to one of encounter, or "struggling with" one's opponent. An opportunity is created to explore balance and harmony in the relationship. By means of a directly experienced kinesthetic metaphor, struggle is transformed into a mutual endeavor accompanied by respect and challenge. The normally combative encounter with one's adversary is transformed into an opportunity to discover and explore balance and harmony using movements based on the concepts of Yin and Yang as they are manifested as continuous and cyclical advance and retreat, push and parry, and directing and receiving energy. While there exists a plethora of books on Ch'I Kung and T'ai Chi Ch'uan, the majority describe the outward physical postures and movements with little to no attention to the aspects of breath, energy, and internal experience.

Here are the beginnings of an exploration of these topics as they apply to postures and movements particularly effective in the accessing and creation of internal reference experiences.

> I begin by centering and grounding the client and bringing their awareness of experience into the internal here and now. I first have them assume the Chi Kung position called Wu Chi-Empty Energy. This position is based on the *I Ching* hexagram 5, Hsu—Calculated Waiting. In T'ai Chi Ch'uan, this position is referred to as Preparation. Have the client stand (with no shoes) with feet directly under the hip sockets, equally weighted on both feet and between the ball and heel of each foot, knees unlocked, pelvis is rotated down (tucked under) to allow the lower spine to relax and flatten. A sense of "opening up" in the spine should be experienced. The spine is extended vertically to encourage more opening, the head is held high and light above the spine, aligning the head so that it is directly over the center point between the feet. The shoulders, elbows, wrists, and hands are

relaxed and opened, the opening between the thumbs and index fingers, referred to as the "tiger's mouth", is allowed to rest against the outer thigh muscles, palms to the rear. I have the client ever so slightly shift the weight off-center: side to side, and then forward to rear, to allow the experience of being slightly off-center to determine when s/he is "centered".

I instruct the client, clear nasal passages permitting, to place the tongue at the roof of the mouth, with the tip behind the upper incisors, and breathe through the nose. Drawing the attention to the breath, I have the client "slow down" and deepen the breathing, then instruct him/her to imagine the body as a large, empty vessel and the air that surrounds it as liquid. Allowing the lower abdomen to relax and expand, as the air is allowed to pour down into the body, will fill it from the bottom up. Then, as the center of the abdomen begins to fill, we allow the ribcage to expand outwards to the sides (NOT up and forward) and sense the skin as it tightens over the ribs.

Next, as the upward filling continues, we allow the upper back to expand to convex. This permits the tops of the lungs, which are above and behind the collarbones, to fill with air (a rare occurrence for most.) The chest is relaxed and allowed to become a little concave. The breath is held, consciously, for a moment or two. Then, emptying the lungs from the top down, as if pouring out the liquid, we slowly release it.

Coaching the client through several breathing cycles, we are concentrating on the submodalities of the internal experience associated with the external experience. I verbally pace, and lead the client to a centered, grounded, rooted, relaxed state and a sense of "being ready without being poised." I have the client "feel" energy rising in the body during inhalation and sinking during exhalation.

The third step is to prepare the client to move into empowerment. With the client's arms completely relaxed, I have him/her allow the shoulders to sink down and slightly back during an inhalation. If the client is truly relaxed, the hands will begin to rise slightly. The sensation is similar to hypnotic arm levitation. As inhalation continues, I instruct the client to lower the body gently down, at the same rate that that the air is filling up the body, by bending the knees. It is important to coach the client to have the rate of body descent and air/energy ascent synchronously equal and opposite. As the arms reach the level of the lower ribcage, the client is instructed to gently begin to raise the body at the same rate that the air is filling up the body by straightening the knees. The legs should be straight, with knees unlocked, and the arms at shoulder height at the peak of the inhalation. The air is held for a moment and, then as exhalation begins, the upper chest collapses a little, the elbows first and then the wrists are "sunk," allowing the hands and arms to begin to lower. At mid-exhalation, the arms are at low chest height.

As the exhalation continues, we allow the arms to return to the starting position and then I coach the client through several repetitions of this process, until it becomes smooth. Once the process is learned, I will have the client remain in the position as preparation for what follows. The arms are at low chest height, as in mid-exhalation. This position is based on the *I Ching* hexagram 35, Chin—Progress. In T'ai Chi Ch'uan, this movement is referred to as The Beginning. It is the position from which all movement of energy originates.

Thus, the client is now kinesthetically grounded. This is the reference point of our empowerment; our energy is ready for whatever may come. Thus empowered, we feel magically able to handle the stresses and strains in our life with ease and balance.

"CIRCLE OF DANCE" – MEDITATION, MOVEMENT, AND MINDFULNESS

KAY PLUMB

"A person's ability to move is probably more important to his/her self image than anything else."
—Moshe Feldenkrais – Awareness through Movement

"Circle of dance" calls upon each person to reconnect with his or her inner spiritual landscape, with the primalness arising from the body. As a result, this kind of movement contributes to healing and quality of life for each participant. The dance process lets us take a second look at our breath, our bodies and our spiritual selves. It becomes our emotional choreography.

Expressive Art experiences utilize *process* rather than product. The concept of *process* and its therapeutic value, through actual experience, is one of the major components in empowering individuals to facilitate their own healing. It is the body in movement that helps the body to remember the breath, to find the heartbeat, to calm its rhythm, to change its image in the mind, to shift, and to slow the body down. *Process* diminishes stress and restores a sense of well being.

Dance, Yoga, ShiBaShi, Feldenkrais, awareness through movement, TaiChi and Qi Gong are some of the forms that aid us in understanding this internal process and the wisdom of the body's cellular memory. Many people using dance for healing feel that the body, including its organs, bones and flesh, hold responses to emotional, mental and external events. This idea is also reflected in what is known as network chiropractic. Even our reactions to life are held in the physical body, according to Daria Halprin in "Living Artfully," found in *Foundations of Expressive Arts Therapies* (2000:136 – 137.)

Body movement is one of the tools used for communicating, calming, centering and connecting. It is inherently an expression of non-verbal communication. When we move, we are experimenting with boundaries, limitations, space, wholeness and oneness. Many sources of writing remind us that life itself is movement. Linda Hartley discusses in *Wisdom of the Body Moving* (1995,) that "even by contemplating the actual form of a movement before we try it allows us to have an idea of the 'mind' it evokes." The following are examples of this process that I have witnessed in my participation in an arts in medicine program at a local hospital. Each plays an important part in translating the immediacy of the meaning:

- Communicating can be exemplified through spontaneous non-verbal theater.

- Calming and graceful forms of movement in Yoga, Tai Chi or ShiBaShi can help to de-stress the body. Gentle participation, even watching such patterns of movement, can move people to feel relaxed, slow down breathing, and take time to stop and allow the body to experience less stress.

- Centering becomes apparent when people gather to watch, listen and participate with song, drumming, toning and swaying movement.

Connecting comes naturally when participants are encouraged to hold the edge of a hand painted 54" x 54" silk scarf. Individuals in groups, painting their favorite colors and designs, created these scarves. None of the people may have known each other at the start. The group of people holding the edge of the scarf simultaneously moves the scarf in a circle to the right then to the left, and as they lift the scarf up over their heads, they watch the scarf's mesmerizing floating qualities. The painted silk scarf provides a metaphor of both the strength of the silk fabric and its lustrous, seemingly fragile, beauty. Voila! People, who have not moved or danced, have just experienced connection, simply by holding on to the edge of the scarf. From the edge of tension, each one's consciousness may have been transformed. They may have experienced a feeling of floating, or the colors of the silk may have lifted their spirits through beauty.

There is no right or wrong in this kind of movement journey. All of these experiential tools, communicating, calming, centering and connecting help us to be physically, emotionally and spiritually in the moment. The movement toward healing, or becoming whole, is in the give and take of the conversation, the give and take of being the listener and the listened-to. There is a sense of connectedness, which takes root with us in this process of mindfulness through the body.

Movement exists within the molecules of our body and between the neurotransmitters. Molecules are literally working through the mind and the physical body systems, such as the nervous system. Research has shown that awareness of this interaction can serve to give a sense of well being. In a recent article in the St Petersburg Times (St. Petersburg, FL, Oct.12, 2008) the Nobel Prize winning Brainbow project at Harvard was detailed with pictures of neurons lit with fluorescent colors, to reveal the movements that occur during synaptic connections along the trail of sensory input to muscle and brain. Sensory input is essential, but consciousness plays a part in well-being in other ways. It is imagination brought into the expression, with elements of surprise and mystery, which allow people to make mental shifts and dive into the moment. And it is within their present moment that people experience themselves as whole.

Anna Halprin's book, *Dance as a Healing Art*, alludes to the healing power of dance.

> "Our body houses our feelings, our emotions and our spirit. It holds memories of our ancestors, our past, our present and our future...It has wisdom, wonder and magic in it to perform the great dance of life... it is crucial if we have become ill, and may feel let down by our body, that we return to our bodies, return home, reawaken the senses, and the natural healer within can renew its strength and power" (Halprin, 2000: 21).

The following story offers an illustration. At a recent open studio, a woman, the wife of a patient, had had a long and taxing day. She and her husband had received some news that delayed her husband's discharge. Although things were progressing medically, the patient was not ready yet to return home. The caregiver heard the song and music "The Kentucky Waltz" being shared by musicians playing for patients down the hall. The acoustic instruments of auto harp and hammered dulcimer, as well as the singing, created an atmosphere of reminiscing and hopefulness. The alchemy of instruments and voice transfixed the caregiver "in the moment" and swirled around her. Her eyes lit up, even though her body was lagging behind. The strains of the waltz tempo and the song lyrics were pulling at her shoulders.

Our open studios are prepared with "props" such as items of clothing for dress up: hats, purses, boas, and scarves. Putting a green boa around her shoulders got her ready to sway to the waltz. I joined her. The music filled in, allowing us to slow down and listen to our bodies. As she glided back and forth, I could see that her spirit really needed to dance. She needed some uplifting, and the shift in the dance tempo gave a shift to her body as well. She began to hold an image of hope. By the end of the dance, the caregiver's shoulders had straightened, her head was lifted, and a smile was back on her face.

No matter where people are in their life journey, as a patient, caregiver, family, or friend, what matters is that each person is still a part of the dance. Sometimes I dance with a scarf so that people can watch the swirl of color. It occurs to me that each time I move, or ask another person to move, with the chosen colored scarves, we are really standing for each person no matter where they are in their life. I call this Life Dance. I want Life Dance to let people experience the beauty they have inside, no matter where their life takes them. The open studio concept focuses on holding the space. The "space," which includes the actual physical space, is designed with the intention to hold expression, surprise and creativity born truly in the moment. People may say that they are not an artist or a dancer. The expressive artist or facilitator helps to hold the space for play, for experimentation; actually, there is a kind of stopping of time. Gary Izzo points this out in the *Art of Play* (1997.) He reminds us that this space is a sacred space, partially because it is a space for bringing people together, for gathering in like spirit and like mind. Participants may feel a sense of connectedness as a result of merely trying or playing together. A kind of *temenos* or a sacred circle may be created. When entering such a *temenos*, we all hold this space with a certain respect and protection (Izzo, 1997: 9.)

Why is play so powerful? As children, we learn though play, through exploration and discovery of our movements. We learn how to be people in the world. Louise Steinman reminds us that storytelling, improvisational movement, or miming call on a sense of play and discovery that is an integral part of us (1995:99-100.) The term *Improvisio* means "to not know before," hence improvisation in mime or storytelling is an act of discovery. We must discover through experience. Through "storying" a memory by using movement as the language, one heart can speak to another. Often one can add an element of hope or a healing metaphor by improvising in the moment. This requires full presence.

I once experimented with this very thing in a warm-up exercise during an expressive arts class. We were asked to pick a picture out of fifteen nature scenes. There were also some simple props laid out for us from which to choose, including things like hats and belts. The picture I chose had a red barn on a backcountry road with trees and rolling hills. It reminded me of a bicycle trip I had taken in the Vermont countryside. I picked a red cap, which I wore backwards for my bike helmet. For a time during this imaginary scene, I felt like I was back on that bike. I threw my leg over the "pretend" bike; I made peddling movements, lifting up one knee and pushing down, and then the other. I took the position: arms down, head down, rear up, to give the group watching an image of my idea. This action piece became the vocabulary of art. The essentials of metaphor were expressed through the body position...I was thinking to myself, "Bicycling through life...up strenuous hills...I may be the last one up, but I will make it, and I may have a glorious ride down."

Movement calls on our whole body to participate, not merely engaging our mind. The cells of the body do the talking whether we are moving or not. As we have seen, cells are a part of a magnificent system of messengers that allow our body to celebrate good news, but also to hold onto bad news, like trauma. Traumas get caught-up in the synapses, those pathways of neural talk going up and down as discussed in the Brainbow project; and the nerve axons and dendrites can become frozen. This can block communication in our nervous system. Working with all of the senses and especially the kinesthetic can help release these blocks and tension bundles. Movement and dance help get the story out. Sometimes words are the last to come. Sometimes to get to the words we must first use metaphor, find our heartbeat, be quiet in meditation, or participate in toning, all forms of language that can by-pass the mind and ego. Other media can contribute to releasing the verbal story, such as painting and then dancing the painted image. It is essential to our wellbeing that our story be told and "heard." Movement and meditation are powerful tools to facilitate this sense of wellbeing, work to reduce stress, and create the necessary shift needed to find words or images for our story.

I am hopeful that looking at the concept of movement will call up awareness of the senses overall, and the kinesthetic in particular, as healing tools. Through the use of movement, we can re-pattern some disabling life patterns. Movement can move the pent up patterns into awareness and move them into freedom. It is an agent of change in the physical body, but also an agent for change in mood; movement can channel emotional responses and can shape the way we think. We are made of body mind (In our field, some now say "bodymind") and spirit, as our parts on both micro and macro levels work and move together in harmony or disease.

When we practice being in the moment, as in movement used in mime for instance, the movement of the extemporaneous storying, we hone in on what a certain emotion feels like. Strong non-verbal expression feeds back to us this powerful communication. Our non-verbal expression is difficult to disguise, and we cannot see ourselves, or be seen, as integrated and authentic unless our non-verbal expressions match our verbalizations. Everyday examples of non-verbal expression are not hard to find. Think of this...you are in a line with 15 other people, seated at the post office or driver's license bureau. You would probably shift in your chair, tug on your keys, tap your fingers, or run hands through your hair. There is a lot of expression just in shifting your weight from one hip to another, not to mention your facial expressions. Facial expressions are very powerful. Sometimes we are not even aware of our own, and they inform the emotional context of our day. Now, you might try putting a sad expression on your face. Really feel it. Are any emotions ("e-motions") accompanying this look? While holding that expression, try writing a cheery note to someone to tell them "thanks" for something nice they have done for you. Keeping that sad look and at the same time saying something cheerful is a very difficult thing to accomplish!

Movement, meditation and mindfulness are all forms of expression, which lead to personal growth and healing. We work with the senses and do experiential activities in order that, over time, a person will feel a sense of the body as home. Each time we participate and experiment, we expand our awareness, our mindfulness, and our worldview. We have a sense that we are not feeling things alone, and frequently learn that we are not too different from people around the world. What happens to us can happen to others and vice versa. A simple exercise for changing perspective through body shift in Yoga asks you to take a deep breath, lift the rib cage, and extend your arms out to the side. Simple gestures like this one expand how you feel in the moment, and how you look at the day. They increase your mindfulness.

We are all artists at heart; we have imaginations and the capacity to play and improvise. We all have a repertoire of behavior patterns. Our bodies already move. Being alive means we are in motion, participating in movement. If we enter the expressive process, through movement, we can calm our body and our mind to a restful, healing pace. Our inner dancer can help us find our inner healer. Working from the cellular level out, we involve our bodymind and our spirit.

Recently, in a workshop I co-facilitated for Latin women cancer survivors, a colleague brought the huge painted scarves. The group was large, so we used two of them. To bring the attendees together, we invited everyone to hold on to the scarves, and we played some cultural music in the background. We had an interpreter to help us, but the movement spoke its own language. The mindfulness of the moment together with the movement of the group united us, extended hope, and suspended the "moment in time." The image of it is forever imprinted in my mind and heart. This exercise was a rallying point and allowed each woman's body to do the talking, coloring in turn each woman's experience and making space for each one to share her story in words when she felt it right to do so. Such experiences bring to mind a saying from a card I found at a book store by Brush Designs. "I may fall down and I may fall short, but I am the dancer of my own dance." So, when your spirit wants to, dance!

References

Benson, Herbert. *Timeless Healing: The Power and Biology of Belief.* New York: Scribner, 1996.

Chodorow, Joan. *Dance Therapy & Depth Psychology*. London and New York: Routledge, 1991.

Halprin, Anna. *Dance as a Healing Art.* Boston: Shambala Press, 2000.

Hartley, Linda. *Wisdom of the Body Moving.* Berkeley, CA: North Atlantic Books, 2000.

Izzo, Gary. *The Art of Play: The New Genre of Interactive Theater.* Portsmouth, NH: Heinemann Trade, 1997.

Levine, Robert and Ellen Levine. *Foundations of Expressive Arts Therapy.* London: Jessica Kingsley Publishers, 1999.

Oriah. *The Dance.* San Francisco: Harper, 2001.

Steinman, Louise. *The Knowing Body.* Berkley, CA: North Atlantic Books, 1995.

HEALING, CREATIVITY, AND TRANSFORMATION: A PATH TO THE DIVINE

ELIJAH GARY WOHLMAN

I have been developing my Wohlman Method of deep tissue healing for over 30 years after investigating, comparing and contrasting many other systems of healing. This highly interactive session engages participants in a revolutionary modality to facilitate swift, long-lasting breakthroughs for the clients. What makes this approach to healing unique is the multi-sensory integration of deep tissue body therapy with affirmations and guided visualizations in a choreographed, creative ritual. Each phrase is whispered, spoken, rhymed or sung—to match every stroke—in concert with breath and sound. As a result, there is a synergistic effect of integrating the deep muscular stretching with breath, visualization, sound and affirmations spoken in rhyme. I have uncovered a streamlined pathway to healing that frees blocked physical and psychic energies. Results are often immediate and life changing, in transforming outmoded physical patterns to vital ones, as well as in awakening pathways for clear communication with the self and others, unparalleled emotional freedom, and renewed full self-expression.

From what I have consistently experienced and witnessed hundreds of times, I see that I have come across a pathway to healing that frees blocked physical energies that have accumulated over time and become bound in the body, in the neuro-muscular systems. This method can offer far swifter and longer-lasting healing and restoration of vitality and creative energy than many other methods. This innovative hands-on session is an exciting opportunity for holistic practitioners of all kinds to enhance their skills and effectiveness with clients by adding this multi-dimensional approach of healing to their own. It is my wish that those learning the method will take this work even further than I have. I can only imagine the potential impact this work can have in making this world a more harmonious and fulfilling place to live for all of us. This is my living legacy to the world.

The following is a description of selected strokes, affirmations and guided visualizations. They are used with a participant lying face down on a massage table. Lighting and music have set the tone of the environment. You will need some knowledge of anatomy and physiology to make the placement of your hands and arms for the strokes.

When directions below use the word "say" that can mean whisper or sing as well. Use theatrical voice to create your own emphasis where you feel it is needed. Your own sense of presence with the person on the table is part of what makes the method work. In addition, remember to set the pace according to what you feel is needed; timing may not be everything, but it is important...

The following series of photos and descriptions contains selected excerpts from my *'Wohlman Method for the Whole Person'* training manual. Since a full session comprises of approximately 101 strokes, the following selected strokes (edited from the totality, with numbers removed yet taken in sequence) will serve as a preview as to what typically takes place within a complete healing treatment:

Description of Strokes and Selection of Photos of Strokes along with Affirmations & Guided Visualizations

With client facing down, you at their head: Slide thumbs from top down alongside spine, applying pressure on client's exhalations—lengthening the back along its vertical axis. Then use pads of thumbs and your own body weight to move upwards. Say:

> "Picture and feel waters falling as you take long exhales, sunrise lifting as you inhale...Breathing out long, picture and feel what you are ready to release at this time. Breathing in strong, what you are ready to receive..."

Continuing to face client from above their head, now apply pressure with the length of your left forearm—sliding up alongside the belly of the para-spinal muscles on the left side of the spine. Shift angle of pressure to your elbow through thoracic area. Say:

> "Breathe back, release holding in your back. Breathe back, release holding back—in any way you are ready. Breathing back, releasing having to hold back—in your body, in your life."

Placing flat the heels of hands on either side of the sacrum, apply pressure while rotating in both clockwise and counterclockwise directions

—increasing the flexibility and range of movement throughout the sacral joint. Say:

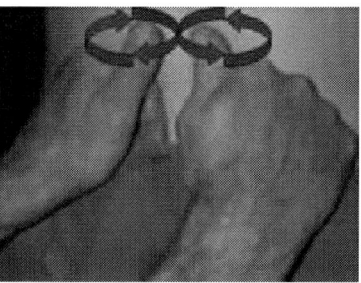

"I shift old patterns of rigidity to flexibility. I let go of holding stiffness, stubbornness, stuck-ness and tightness—no longer needed and wanted. I now allow greater range of movement and choice of positions to express myself through..."

Standing on right side of client, press knuckles of soft fist along the gluteus maximus muscles—moving from top to bottom, along the inside, medial and lateral vertical lines. Say:

"I release my "yes, buts"—once holding me back from moving forward in my life direction. I mobilize what I've been sitting on to fuel my most passionate purpose here."

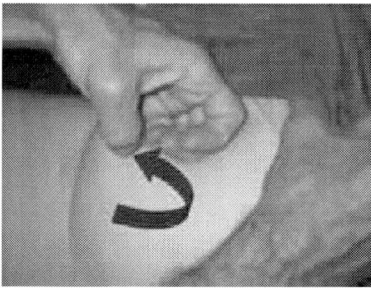

Slide flat of forearm up along hamstring muscles. In three parallel strokes—on the inside, up the centre and laterally along outside, both sides. Say:

"My vulnerability is my strength, and my hamstrings stretch. Sharing my humanity is my strength, and these muscles become more flexible, fluid and flowing. Sharing my caring is my strength, and my hamstrings become elastic."

The participant turns to rest on their right side, slide elbow down gluteus muscles in 3 in three parallel strokes—along inner vertical axis/sitz bone. Say:

"I turn my "yes, buts" into "yes, ands" "I release patterns of unconscious sabotage holding me back from moving forward in my life direction."

With client lying on right side, pull down their left shoulder with your left hand—applying pressure during each exhale. With a soft fist of your right hand down their trapezius, towards the sternocleidomastoid muscle, then tapering off pressure as you approach bones of their skull. Say:

"As you exhale, feel your shoulder dropping away from your ear… Giving you more room to speak your truth…more room for you to clearly hear."

There is an application of pressure via fingertips at the beginning of this stroke. Concentrate on creating a counter-stretch, pulling the arm down in one direction while stretching trapezius muscles the other direction. Say:

"I let go of carrying the weight of the world on my shoulders — shifting feeling burdened and heavy with allowing flexibility, fluidity and freedom."

With client laying on the right side, place your left hand over their left shoulder…pulling it back toward you so area under scapula lifts out. Place the pad of your right thumb under the bottom of the wing tip, sliding up toward traps on exhales –"freeing the wing." Say:

"I release holding back my heart—more room for me to embrace my part."
(Lengthy pause)

"I let go of blocking myself from receiving what I most strongly desire, deserve and decree—more room for me…And the band around my chest and heart expands."

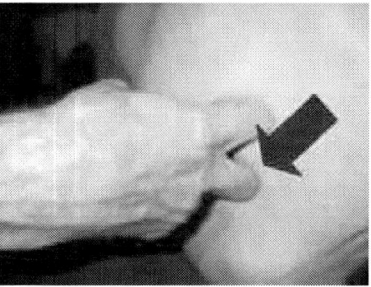

At top of spine, place the flat area between the 1st and 2nd joints of your index plus middle fingers. With these fingers splayed, each finger on either side of spine, slowly move down spine—increasing pressure on exhales. Say:

> "Breathing back, release holding back. Breathing back, release having to hold back—in any way you're ready. Breathe back, release holding in your back. Longer than before, taking longer exhales—all the way down to the floor."

Sliding flat of forearm along inside of inner thighs while client is on the side, apply pressure along inside/center/medial vertical axis to lengthen tissue with exhalations. Say:

> "Feel your inner core—all the way down the inside of spine, down your thighs—lengthen and widen to the floor... Giving you more room to stand your ground, trust what you stand on, and have faith in a flexible foundation."

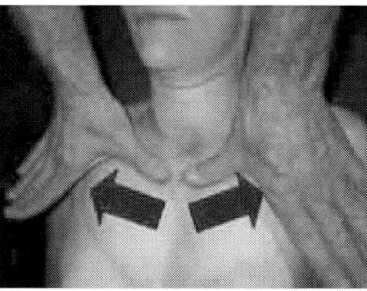

Press thumb pads along inside crest of clavicle, tracing a line inside out, as you apply pressure on exhales to stretch and expand the horizontal band around the chest and heart. Encourage strong inhales, to embody the following affirmation:

"I fully receive what I most strongly desire."

Slide length of forearms along vertical axis of hamstring muscles, increasing pressure on exhales—apply pressure along the inner, central and medial vertical axis. Say:

"My vulnerability is my strength, and my hamstrings stretch.... My humanity is my strength, and my hamstrings become elastic.... Sharing my caring is my strength, and my hamstrings become flexible, fluid and flowing."

With right hand holding fingers together in firm "C" shape under occipital ridge, and palm of left hand resting firmly on forehead, lean back on exhales while lengthening neck from base of the spine. Further each exhale (Repeat 3 times,) saying:

"My spine lengthens, and I stand tall and free on a firm and flexible foundation. I stretch further than I thought I could—in my body, in my life."

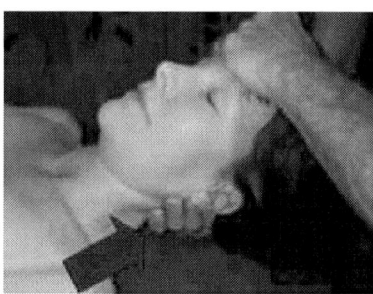

Standing at head of client, place your body mid-way between shoulders and head so you can use heels of both hands to stretch shoulder away from ear on their exhales—each exhale stretching further than the one before (Repeat 3 times,) saying:

"More room for me, between my shoulder and my ear...More room for me to speak my truth, more room for me to clearly hear."

Standing behind client, press thumb pads along length of trapezius muscles on exhalations, leaning your body weight towards client's toes to increase pressure and elongate traps. More on each of three exhales, saying:

> "Feel your shoulders drop away from your ears—giving you more room to speak your truth, more room to clearly hear.... Feel yourself letting go of carrying whatever "weight-of-the-world" on your shoulders that no longer serves you"

Facing upwards towards client's head, place right shoulder underneath left knee—on exhales, lean body weight so their knee approaches the ground just to the side of their shoulder—relax on inhales, increase pressure on exhales, saying:

> "Mobilizing what you've been sitting on, feel yourself freeing stored energy—to fuel your most passionate purpose here…More room to put your foot down, take your stand, be in command!"

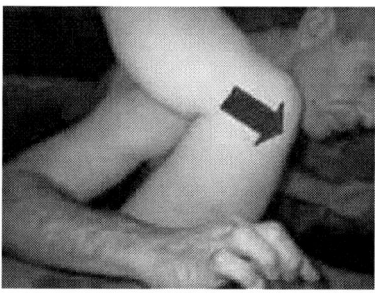

With client sitting and spine tall, apply pressure with left elbow along length of left trapezius muscle. Create counter-stretch with your right hand pushing head [with nose facing forwards] to tilt to the right. As right ear approaches right shoulder, press left shoulder towards left hip. Say:

> "I feel my shoulder drop away from my ear—giving me more room to speak my truth, more room to clearly hear…I am heard! And I trust my inner Guidance, my internal eternal word… The more my shoulder drops away, the more I trust what I have to say ~ the more I am free to play. Hip! Hip! Hooray!"

With client sitting, stretch head to one direction laterally with hand—pressing soft fist of other hand onto trapezius and levator scapulae muscles. Move shoulder away from the ear, increasing the distance between them on the client's exhales. Say:

"I let go of carrying the weight of the world on my shoulders & burden of responsibility for other people's pain...I let go of guarding what I have to say, freeing more room for lightness and play."

Use length of forearms to move all the way down along long muscles on either side of spine. Pause on inhales, stretch closer towards ground on exhales. Say:

"I release holding back, I move forward with ease."

Continuing to move both elbows and forearms along length of muscles on both sides of the spine, place hands together in prayer position as you set specific intention for healing with your client. Say:

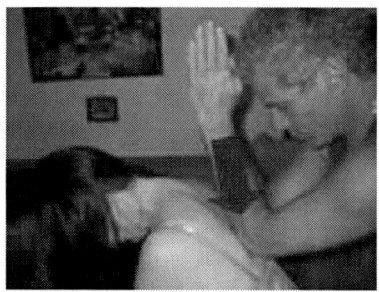

"I breathe in the new, pushing out the old—further than I thought I could, longer than I knew."

With client sitting, have them place their left hand in center of chest, right hand at base of spine. Have them breathe between these places. Place your hands on theirs, while suggesting they take long, letting-go breaths towards base of spine. Say:

"Sunrise lifting. Waters falling"

Picture and feel all you've received during this time, taking strong inhales...Each inhale a sunrise—"Behold, with each breath, I make all anew!"

"With each long exhale, picture and feel waters falling long, imagining dark and heavy colors falling down the spine—getting a sense of all you are releasing at this time..."

"Out with de-dark, in with de-light!"

"More room for you, more than you once allowed and knew—all the way in, all the way through…"

"More room for me to be fluid, flexible and free! Just as I've always wanted to be!"

The whole sequence can then be repeated.

LAUGHTER: NATURE'S HEALING REFRAIN

SUSAN M. STEWART

Have you ever caught your breath after a particularly good laugh and exclaimed, "I needed that —I feel better!" If so, you have experienced the wonder of a potent form of natural medicine: the healing power of laughter.

Someone sagely observed, "Life is the dash between two dates on a tombstone." As we make that dash through life, it is hard to miss the connection between laughter and feeling good. We laugh, we feel better— hey, it's not rocket science—this simple formula has worked for humans since the beginning of time. The act of laughter is a built-in, mind-body core defense system designed by nature to keep us well and give us joy.

Ancient folk wisdom in virtually every culture recognized—indeed revered—the power of laughter. The familiar phrase "laughter is the best medicine" originates from the book of Proverbs in the Old Testament which proclaims "For a merry heart doeth good like a medicine." There are numerous historical examples of traditional Chinese, Tibetan and yogic practitioners who incorporated laughter meditations and other rituals that contained laughter as a part of their daily health practices.

Most readers of this essay won't require much convincing that laughter is beneficial to the body, mind and spirit; and there is now abundant scientific evidence that laughter is absolutely essential for optimal well-being. So, do we need fancy-schmancy scientific studies that tell us what has been known anecdotally for thousands of years? Well, yes. These scientific studies are exciting and important because they validate the role of complementary and integrative mind body medicine. I am grateful for every white-coated scientist who has wielded test tubes and measured such things as blood levels of stress hormones before, during and after laughter, to determine if laughter helps reduce stress. This data lends me credibility when I teach a class about the benefits of laughter and tell participants that laughter is a natural antidote for stress.

I must confess, though, that I agree with my friend and mentor, Steve Wilson, founder of the World Laughter Tour, Inc, who states simply "To me, the bottom line is clear: laughter is its own reward. Even if there were not a single shred of evidence that it affected my biology or health, I would opt for a life filled with laughter because a life absent of laughter is too dreadful to contemplate."

This essay starts with a brief review of the benefits of regular chuckling. Later, I'm going to offer some practical ideas for getting more laughter into daily life, and suggest that laughter can be used effectively to engage the body in a health practice that many people neglect: movement. Movement? (Yes, gasp—I am euphemistically referring to the dreaded E word: exercise!)

But first....

Drum Roll Please... The Benefits of Laughter

Norman Cousins stimulated the contemporary laughter movement and the scientific study of laughter with his best selling autobiographical book *Anatomy of an Illness as Perceived by the Patient*, which was published in 1979. Hospitalized with a painful, progressive illness, he practiced daily bouts of laughter to test his theory that positive emotions promote healing. In his book, he documents (among other findings) the "joyous discovery" that ten minutes of genuine belly laughter gave him two hours of pain free sleep

Laughter is a whole brain experience. The act of laughter engages both the mind and body. Some scientists, including Dr. Candace Pert assert that the distinction between the mind, body and spirit is artificial, these entities cannot be separated. Psychoneuroimmunologist Dr. Lee Berk of Loma Linda School of Medicine has documented that during laughter, brain chemistry changes and orchestrates the way virtually every system of the body is affected, in a healthful way.

We know for sure that laughter: relaxes muscles, reduces stress/anxiety, decreases pain, stimulates the cardiovascular system, strengthens immune function, promotes healing, lifts our spirits, shifts perspective, increases creativity and helps us get along better with the members of our tribe. Research shows that laughter relaxes blood vessels and increases blood flow—it has been used effectively as adjunct therapy in cardiac rehabilitation; and used therapeutically to improve mood in patients with mild depression. Laughter and a sense of humor help us cope with and rebound from life's adversities.

The human brain is hard wired for laughter and infants are born with the capacity to laugh—providing survival advantages for our young because laughter enhances immune functioning and increases bonding with caregivers. The sound of genuine, mirthful laughter is recognized between cultures and has a contagious effect. Laughter connects us with other people, aptly described by Victor Borge who observed, "Laughter is the shortest distance between people." In the symphony of life, laughter is nature's healing refrain.

Vitamin L – Make Time for Your Daily Dose of Laughter

Today's lifestyles are fast-paced and "I don't have time" is a common complaint. Have you ever stood in front of a microwave oven that is cooking your food and found yourself urging it to "hurry?" Hmmmm – if so, you may be sinking under the heavy malady "over-scheduled-it-is." Laughter to the rescue! Grab onto a laugh line and take an honest appraisal of the things that now fill up your time.

Much has been written about living mindfully, savoring the present moment. Laughter is an excellent tool to enhance living mindfully because we laugh in the present tense. During mirthful laughter, conscious thinking is seemingly suspended as our brain is caught up in the physiological response to laughter. This provides, if only momentarily, a brief respite for our brain, but it is often enough time to shift perspective and allow us to see problems and challenges from different angles. Laughter restores our energy, rejuvenates our spirit and grounds us in the present.

I became a Certified Laughter Leader (CLL) in 2000 through the World Laughter Tour, and although I valued laughter prior to that, the training heightened my awareness for the need of daily bouts of laughter. The World Laughter Tour method is based on the theory that jokes are not a requirement for laughter—we don't need jokes to laugh. One of the texts recommended for the course is *Laughter: A Scientific Method* by Dr. Robert Provine. This informative book gives an historical overview of the role of laughter throughout civilization. It also deconstructs the mechanics of laughter. I was surprised to read that the majority of laughter (90%) is the result of everyday human interactions and experiences.

Since we only get about 10% of our laughs from jokes, we can explore many other options for getting our daily requirement of giggles. It has been my privilege to teach laughter classes around the country and I often share the following ideas with my participants:

- Begin each day with **gratitude** for waking up on the green side of the grass. Yahoo!

- **SMILE** before getting out of bed each morning and many times throughout the day. I'm talking about a big, tooth-exposing grin—not just some little lift-the-corners-of-your-mouth-while-your-lips-are-pressed-tightly-together sort of smile. Let's practice right now—smile broadly for a few seconds. That's right, keep smiling....smile big, smile from the heart, put that smile out there…....terrific! Smiling changes the blood flow to the brain and this simple act can jump-start a positive effect on our mood.
- Start each morning with a **LAUGH**. Practice laughing in a mirror. You don't even need to *feel* like laughing—just start chuckling, giggling and wiggling or guffawing and make the person in the mirror crack up!
- **Choose to lighten-up**. Be open to laughter opportunities throughout the day. Look for the unintended funny side of life and learn to laugh at life's incongruities. The drama of life's parade can be just ridiculous at times. When you observe something funny, write it down, share it (these are the stories that inevitably begin with "You're never going to believe what happened...." Or "I swear I'm not making this up …") and refer back to it when you need a laugh.
- **Read, listen to or watch something** that you find humorous *every day*. Develop your own laughter library. Collect cartoons or jokes that tickle your funny bone; books, short stories, and comedy videos, DVDs or CDs, or your own funny anecdotes about life's incongruities (see above.) Borrow items from the library for an ever changing and fresh supply of materials that *you* find humorous and inspiring.
- **Have a laughter buddy**. Be around people who laugh. Find a designated laughter friend(s) and share laughs over the telephone, Internet, or in person. Join a community group like the Red Hat Society or a professional organization such as the Association of Applied and Therapeutic Humor (AATH) to find kindred spirits who value laughing.
- **Go after laughter**, seek it out, schedule it, put in on your "to do" list. You will look forward to it – and this actually provides positive benefits. Studies by Dr. Berk found that even the *anticipation* of a laughter event decreased the amount of stress hormones in the blood.

An Epidemic of Inactivity –What's a Body to Do?

Rock 'n roller Jerry Lee Lewis swiveled his hips and sang in the 1950s that "there's a whole lotta shakin' going on!" Sadly, fifty years later, a more apt description for the activity level of the general population is "there's a whole lotta sittin' going on!" Computer and commuter lifestyles, laborsaving devices, dependence on television for entertainment and a dizzying abundance of food certainly contribute to inactivity and the growing obesity epidemic in the United States.

Public health officials wring their hands and make dire predictions about the increase of "lifestyle-related" health problems, including diabetes and cardiovascular disease. An alarming number of children and adolescents are being diagnosed, with type 2 diabetes—the type of diabetes that used to be referred to as "adult onset" because most people who developed it were older adults. Times have changed and our bodies reflect the change.

Incorporating laughter into our daily routine is just one aspect of making healthy choices for leading a vibrant life that is filled with joy. Our bodies are designed for movement, our muscles crave it. This book contains other chapters about engaging the body in movement. I hope you read these thought-provoking sections for specific techniques on incorporating more movement into your life. I respectfully suggest taking a slow, deep, breath and reading the ideas with an open mind and eagerness—who knows what pleasurable moves and experiences await?!

Please honor your body's capabilities and limitations and do the amount of movement that is appropriate for *you*. Movement and exercise can be done while seated, as well as standing; gently, as well as robustly. Check with your physician before starting any exercise regimen. Actually, you should probably check with your physician if all your parts work and you choose not to exercise—because inactivity is surely hazardous to your health and well-being!

I teach laughter classes around the country. Part of the laughter class consists of gentle deep breathing and stretching, followed by several minutes of laughter exercise movements. Frequently I hear comments from participants such as "Usually, I don't like to exercise, but doing the laughter exercises was fun!" or "I feel energized after doing the laughter exercises!"

I have observed, repeatedly, in my laughter classes that many participants enjoy exercising and moving when they are having *fun*. EUREKA!!! Exercise can be fun when you are having fun! Laughing and smiling during exercise appear to stimulate a positive response to the experience and makes the time pass quickly. I began to see a connection between the need for daily movement and daily laughter and how the two are closely related.

My observations are based on experience with adults who have attended my laughter sessions. D. Hutchins, a second grade teacher in Florida, sought my recommendations for ways to increase exercise in her classroom. Ms. Hutchins, like many elementary teachers today, is faced with the challenge of incorporating thirty minutes of exercise for her students during the school day. I introduced her to CDs that have musical exercise songs that are geared for children. The songs encourage children to stretch, move, count numbers, recite alphabet letters, make funny faces, laugh, etc. After using one of the CDs with her class, Ms Hutchins wrote a note to me that exclaimed, "My class got so tickled when I played the exercise songs. Laughter and fitness are very complementary!"

EUREKA!!!

Her observation paired with my own, made me wonder if other forms of exercise could be perceived as being more fun if participants—of virtually any age—smiled and or laughed during at least part of the exercise. I began an "unscientific study," using myself and friends as subjects.

First a disclosure: I *like* to exercise and move—it makes me feel bliss. The term "runner's high" was first used to describe the euphoria that runners experience during and after a run (due to the release of endorphins, the body's natural opiate and feel-good chemical.) Laughter and exercise/movement affect mood—think of these activities as delectable and satisfying mood-food! I look forward to getting into what I call my "feel-good groove" by either laughing or moving.

Like everyone else, though, I can think of lots of excuses for not moving. Over the years, I've developed strategies that work for me to regain a positive focus during times when my enthusiasm to move waivers. If exercise has not been savory to you in the past, perhaps one or more of the following ideas will have you going after a heaping helping of this natural mood-food:

- Reframe a negative perception of exercise by simply eliminating the E word. Refer to it in a positive, upbeat manner such as scheduling thirty minutes to "get into my feel-good groove—I'm gonna move!"
- Set your *intention* to move more. Start out easy, but *start*—even a few minutes of natural movement every day is beneficial. Norman Cousins noted that humans move in the direction of their intentions and expectations. Expectations provide energy. Repeat an affirmation such as "Movement feels good."

- If you are able to move, begin with gratitude that movement is a choice you can make. Be aware that there are many folks who would like nothing more than to have the ability to move, but due to poor health or other limitations, do not have that option.
- Listen to music—lively music energizes movement and engages the mind and body.
- Vary movement activities throughout the week: purposeful walking one day, biking the next, swimming, T'ai Chi, Chi Kung—the options are limitless; listen to a lively CD and free-form move to your own beat (make the movements relaxed and flowing;) borrow DVDs from the library and learn new dances—you don't have to do the dances *well,* just have *fun,* and be playful. Keep a big smile on your face while you do these activities. If you find your enthusiasm sagging, start chuckling and think or do something funny. Do the "chicken dance" with gusto or imagine someone else (perhaps someone who *annoys* you) doing the "chicken dance!") What a satisfying image—you may find your energy level soaring!
- Take advantage of everyday opportunities: deliberately pass by that close parking spot and park further away from your destination—what a great and easy way to get in some extra walking; use the stairs whenever possible; avoid "saving steps" (i.e., make several trips when unloading groceries, don't carry one "huge" load.)

In her provocative book, *Sweat Your Prayers: Movement as Spiritual Practice,* Gabrielle Roth attempts to persuade the reader that movement is an antidote for inertia and each of us has a life dance inside, indeed "we are the dance." She contends that movement is a powerful connection with the divine—that movement is a spiritual practice. Her perspective is compelling and you may find inspiration to leap from your chair and move that body. This book underscores the concept that movement and exercise are gifts from nature to be experienced and celebrated.

Get in *Your* Feel-Good Groove –
Ya Gotta Laugh, Ya Gotta Move

Come on everybody—let's get a whole lotta laughin' going on!
Come on everybody—let's get a whole lotta movin' going on!
Let out a hearty laugh right now—ahhhh, what beautiful music. Laughter is nature's healing refrain, it is the sweet melody of life—let its beat move you.

Laugh. Move. Live. Enjoy!

References and Suggested Reading

Cousins, N. *Anatomy of an Illness As Perceived by the Patient.* New York: W. W. Norton & Co., 1979.
Pert, C., and N. Marriott. *Everything You Need to Feel Go(o)d: The Science and Spirit of Bliss.* Carlsbad, CA: Hay House, Inc., 2006.
Provine, R. *Laughter: A Scientific Investigation.* New York: Penguin Books, 2000.
Roth, G. *Sweat Your Prayers: Movement as Spiritual Practice.* New York: Putnam, 1997.

Websites

Association of Applied and Therapeutic Humor: www.AATH.org
Hop To It Music: www.jackhartman.com
Wilson, Steve and The World Laughter Tour: www.WorldLaughterTour.com

DARING TO RIDE OUR IMAGES: THE MAGIC OF MASK, STORY AND MOVEMENT

FAY WILKINSON

There is a story of a young Pigmy boy who goes through the forest searching for the bird that has the most beautiful song. He searched for many days and nights until eventually, his ears were full of the sweetest sound he had ever heard. The boy caught the bird and brought it home to his father. He asked his father to make sure that the bird had something to eat every day. The father agreed, but eventually decided that caring for the bird took up too much of his time, so he killed the bird. And in so doing, he killed the most exquisite song the forest had to offer. Soon after, the father died. In killing the bird, he killed the song, and in turn, he was himself destroyed. Our story is the song; to paraphrase Badger, in "Crow and Weasel" written by Barry Lopez: if stories come to you, care for them and tell them. Sometimes we need a story more than food to stay alive. For our very survival, we need to tell stories. They help us make sense of things and remind us of what is truly important.

Imagine daring to ride some of images in that story and expanding it using masks. For example telling it from the perspective of the bird or the boy, or in a mask representing the father or a tree in the forest, observing. Now imagine that story being narrated while another creates a dance in mask with live music. The story can be told without words through gesture, sound and movement. The slightest tilt of the head from a masked performer can speak volumes. These are just some of the ways we could amplify and play with this short story. The impact on the teller and the listeners/witnesses can be profound. The combination of the spoken word with the visual impact of mask and movement touches us in an ancient and mysterious way. Rumi wrote, "A tale, however slight, illuminates truth." Each of us, teller and listeners, will take from a story what we are ready to hear and understand, our truth from where we are at this moment. Working with story and mask takes us into an imaginary world—a chance to step out of the literal and ride along with images, symbols and metaphors into the unknown. Yet it is only unknown to our conscious minds; our inner knowing and the collective wisdom of all those who have gone before runs deep within us, flowing like a gentle river, waiting for us to dip in.

I created stories from a very early age. As I look back, I now recognize that was my way of surviving. Stories served me as both a distraction and as a way of making sense of what was going on around me. I became a wee expert of putting on and performing in whatever metaphorical mask was required of me. Some fifty years later, here I am continuing to explore the power of transforming images into stories, creating masks and movement pieces for myself and to share with others. These mediums are as old as humankind and have been used to heal for millennia.

The application of these combined modalities spans the continuum of how expressive arts can be used for ourselves and in our communities— from recreational workshops, to self-exploration, through deep therapy. Our training and levels of experience need to correspond to that continuum; this is especially important when working with mask. All expressive arts making carries a risk. We take chances when we step into the unknown. Even at the recreational level what we might think of as a simple, light activity can on occasion take a person to an unexpectedly deep place fast. We need to know what to do if that happens. I have found mask work to be one of the most powerful modalities in the expressive arts toolbox. This awareness reminds me of the importance of continually refining my skills and seeking out teachers who can help me push out my growing edge as a person and as a guide of expressive arts experiences that incorporate mask and story.

Finding the way in – my process

How do I find my way into mask and story? What exactly am I finding my way into? I am looking for a path that will take me into an imaginary world where there is no judgment and anything goes. I use the full complement of the expressive arts palette as tools to help me play with and rediscover who I am; to explore mysteries like what was my original face before I was born; to understand why I am the way I am today; to inhabit who I am becoming; and to greet and befriend my shadow. Mask and story allow me to explore archetypes, manifest dream images, personify emotions, and delve into paradox. The very act of masking is a paradox for it both conceals and reveals. Joseph Campbell inspires me when he talks about looking for a meaning for our lives. He suggests that what we are actually looking for are experiences that make us feel fully alive; that there is a resonance between what is happening deep inside ourselves and reality. Being aware and willing are the first steps. Hafiz, a poet from the 14th Century, says in "The Gift:" First, the fish has to say, "There's something wrong with this camel ride, and I'm feeling so damned thirsty."

I am often asked if the mask comes first or the story. How do I begin? Movement—spontaneous, improvisational dance, either in silence or to music. I experience a sense of freedom by moving just the way I feel from moment to moment. I really do not care if anyone is watching! This gives my brain a chance to rest, tells my inner critic to take a break and makes room for whatever might drop in as a result of shaking it all up and being totally present. I have already prepared the image making tools — a large piece of paper on the wall and soft/oil pastels, or paint so when my movement is finished I can go directly to 2D art making. As I cannot draw to save my life, I begin with mark making, continuing to engage my whole body. Lines, short, long, thick, thin, shapes—from a distance it would look like I was continuing to dance in front of a wall. I may think I know where I am going, or what questions I am trying to answer, but there are times when something else, seemingly unrelated makes an appearance.

In this way, it is not unlike a dream. When I take a breather and step back, I see images and symbols emerging in and through the marks. Almost always, there is the essence of a face or faces. I am learning to stay open to the images and resist the temptation to analyze or interpret them but rather feel comfortable in the place of not knowing and investing time to get acquainted. As Shaun McNiff says, the images are like guests knocking at our door—when we open the door the first thing we ask is not "what do you mean?"!

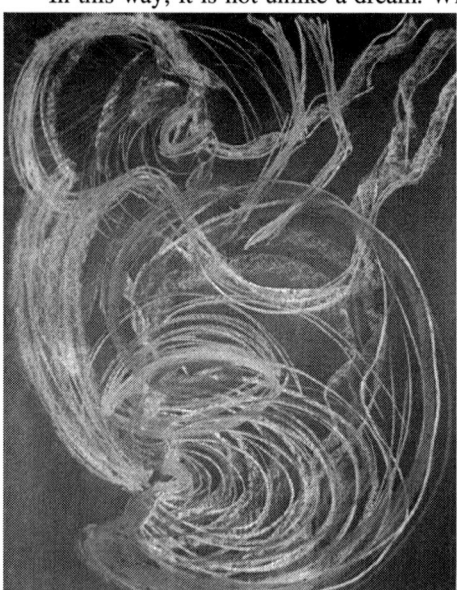

When I am ready to

dare to ride the image and see where it takes me, how do I do that? I may leave it for a while, keeping it in a place where I can see it easily. I may sit with it, writing free form, or move with it, keeping my eyes on the image, being moved from the inside—my body knows. From there I most often go to clay or felt making to see what materializes. My aim is not to impose what I think the character should look like but to allow whatever comes without editing. This preparatory work is not absolutely necessary. I do take mask forms (from Maskworx in New Zealand) and work directly with them, either building up features with a modeling medium, or using them as a blank canvas.

Before I put the mask on, I dialogue with the newly created being at times, recording the answers with my non-dominant hand. The results are the basis for the story or poem, which does not always come right away. I work in the mask with movement and sound. This part of the process is vital because it helps me find where in my body this persona resides. Which parts of me tense up or relax; where does my body want to lead from, for example, my hips or my shoulders. I vocalize the sounds that want to be heard. I am looking to love the character in me, not me in the character. The key is to get acquainted, to align and connect my head, my heart, my soul and my body—often referred to as bodymind.

In some mask cultures, the mask is an intermediary or a messenger from the gods, a means of communicating from the heavens to humans. I can become the other through mask like an ancient shapeshifter. The memories and wisdom I carry in the cells of my body, not just my mind, have an opportunity to be heard through mask. The mask can speak of things that I cannot, sees things that I do not, knows things that I am unaware of, asks questions I had not thought of, and has the power to liberate me from self-imposed chains. I see the masks I create as being envoys from my soul to my conscious mind. Storytelling has been described as the 'soul's speech.' The combination of the two with the addition of movement is transformational magic—I bring the inside out and the outside in. Rachel Naomi Remen said healing might not be so much about getting better, but letting go of all the things that are not you. The creative processes that I engage in are tools to help me figure out what that means to me. Researchers have found that the source of creativity and imagination resides in the same place in the brain where healing is activated—further confirmation of the link between expressive arts, health and wellbeing.

Working with Others

I am always in awe of the power of mask when I work with people. Linda (not her real name) attended a weekend workshop with me. She had never worked with mask, and described herself as not having a creative bone in her body. She had come to the workshop to keep a friend company. Our process was similar to the one I have described earlier, with the addition of a guided meditation and some voice and breath work. Participants were given half masks that I had prepared. They could add features, embellishments and paint. (Traditionally a full mask does not speak but a half mask can.)

When the masks were complete, we engaged in the process of mask maker and mask getting acquainted. I invited people to dialogue with the mask and record the responses. Linda asked the mask: "Who are you?" This is what came to her:

Blue of the ocean, blue of the sea,
leave the land, swim with me

deep within the silence there
find your truth, sleep without care

in the realms of the silent sea
do you dream a dream of me?

In this vast and quiet place
you shall find your state of grace
pearls of wisdom, treasure rare
if you seek, you'll find them there
amongst silver fishes and seaweed green
a crystal palace
never seen
by human eye
and clouds of fishes
flowing by
and in that place
where once, you've been
remember again that lovely scene
and
all unfolds with such great ease
all the mysteries of the seas

remember
and
remember well
your place with us beneath the
swell
and rolling thunder of the waves
and sleep, and dream of ocean days.

Linda was surprised by what she had obviously tapped into. The dance piece she created to accompany this writing captivated and touched us. We all caught a glimpse of a universal truth.

Each workshop is different. I often throw away my plan to meet the needs of the group. However, after the getting acquainted with the mask stage usually the group breaks out in pairs. One holds their partner's mask and moves with the mask intuitively—bringing it alive, also known as one of the steps in "charging" the mask. The mask maker watches. Still in pairs, the mask maker dons the mask, begins to find gestures, movements, and sounds while their partner mirrors them. This is a time of exploration and experimentation. The mask wearer may take the mask off at any time. Everyone is clear that if I say stop, remove the mask, each will do so immediately. Masks are powerful. It is possible for someone to start to lose his or her 'self' while in mask. This work is not for everyone.

In some workshops, I spend time with neutral mask. Jacques Le Coq incorporated it into actor training to develop authenticity. It is based on Japanese Noh Theatre. This is an example of how we can draw from other disciplines and adapt them to expressive arts. The neutral mask is genderless and expressionless. It can be both freeing and frustrating, particularly for those of us who rely on facial expressions and gestures to communicate. To be without attitude in our bodies is challenging, however it can help us feel what it is like to be fully present, with no past to influence our responses to what we see or hear, and no future to project. Neutral mask also teaches us about simplicity and finding the essence, a useful lead into creating masks that capture the essence of that part of us with which we are engaging.

If time permits people break out into small groups and they each tell their story in mask. It can be improvised, or given in response to questions asked by the witnesses. The story can be previously prepared or told in movement and gesture alone. I suggest there is a scribe who notes down the story. Often we cannot remember what we said while in mask and this record can be helpful. The groups then change round and retell their story with another scribe. I have found repetition to be valuable for a number of reasons, not the least of which is that it allows us to play and explore rather than trying to get it right the first time, it also builds confidence. When we come back together, the invitation is extended to anyone who would like to tell their story to the whole group. Having witnesses to our stories can deepen the healing experience for both the teller and the listeners.

Options

Not everyone is comfortable with having something on his or her face. A mask on a stick offers control, as does a simple rod puppet. Another option is to suggest that the story be told by a body part, for example a hand. The aim is not to impose the modality, but to metaphorically open up the palette so that an individual can mix their own colors, choose the tools they need to amplify their images, and tell their stories. I have also offered a blank mask that becomes a story canvas. Pictures from magazines and journals are glued to both the inside and the outside of the mask, and a story or poetry comes from that.

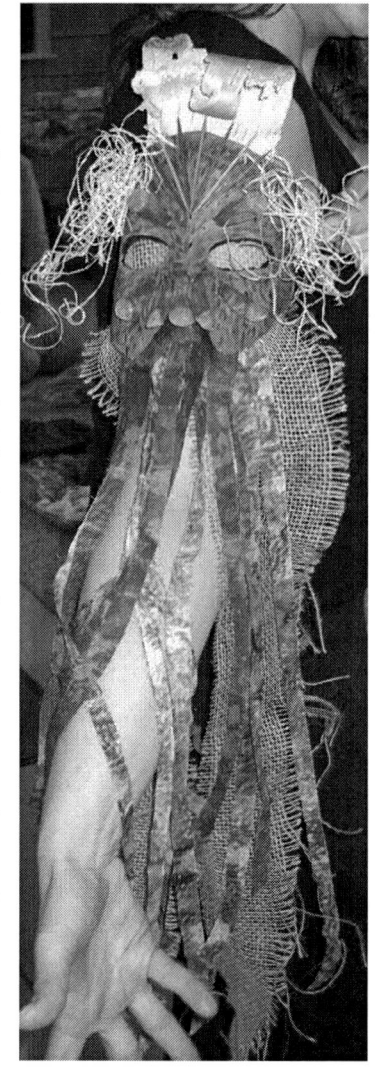

Original or Existing Stories?

Both offer possibility. It is not an either or. An existing story can be personalized and transformed. At our disposal is a world rich with myths and folktales. One of my favorites is Vasalisa and Baba Yaga. Versions of this story are found in Europe and Scandinavia as well as horse-goddess cults in ancient Greek culture. We can learn about ourselves from such stories for they speak of universal truths about what it means to be human.

The Hero's Journey can be used as a framework to create our own myths. The structures and symbols of fairytales can help tell difficult stories. Stories can be co-created by a group. I have successfully used the Saga cards and Mythos cards, part of the OH Card series, as well as games, to ignite imaginations and kick start the creative process. Spontaneous and improvisational storytelling can be exciting, fun and revealing.

Mask Logistics

When I do not want people to think too much, or worry about their skill level, I use plain or colored paper and crayons and put a strict time frame on the mask creation. The results have been astonishing, and a reminder to me that this rudimentary form of mask making can be as powerful as a highly crafted mask that has taken hours to do. The simplicity and the act of masking linked with moving, sounding, and telling a story is where the gold lies.

For workshops with limited time, I prepare half masks made from Model Magic®, a Crayola product. It is an air drying modeling medium that is light, comfortable against the skin and can take paint, glue and embellishments well. I supply additional Model Magic® for participants to build up features on this blank form and strongly encourage them to depict the essence of the character.

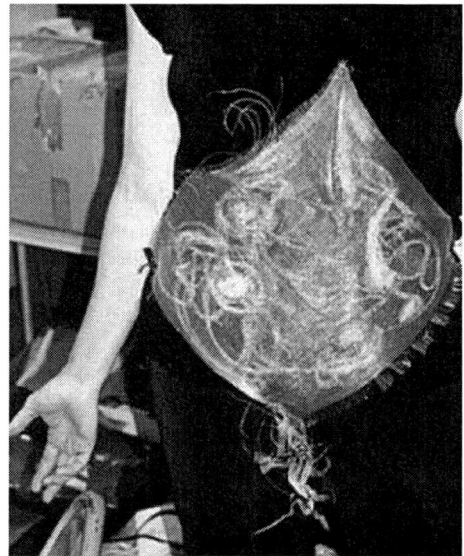

Apart from the old standbys of plaster bandage and papier mache, I have been experimenting with fly screen material that can be bent, formed and embellished with paints, oil pastels and stitching. This is intriguing to work with because it is still possible to see the wearer's face beneath the mask; a mask upon a mask. Buckram, a fabric used by milliners, can be dipped in water then draped and formed over clay or plastic masks as can simple muslin or cheesecloth that is dipped into white glue. The fabrics dry hard to the touch.

Expanding the notion of mask

As stated earlier, traditionally full face masks do not speak, but half masks can, unless the half mask has the lower part of the face covered, including the mouth. But, does a mask always have to cover the face? What happens if we make masks or maskettes as I call them that speak for or through parts of our body? In a series of recent workshops shoulder, knee, belly, and breast masks were created—all had powerful and touching stories to tell. As witnesses, we were spellbound by the movement of the personified body part and I do not believe any of us looked at the participant's face when the story was told.

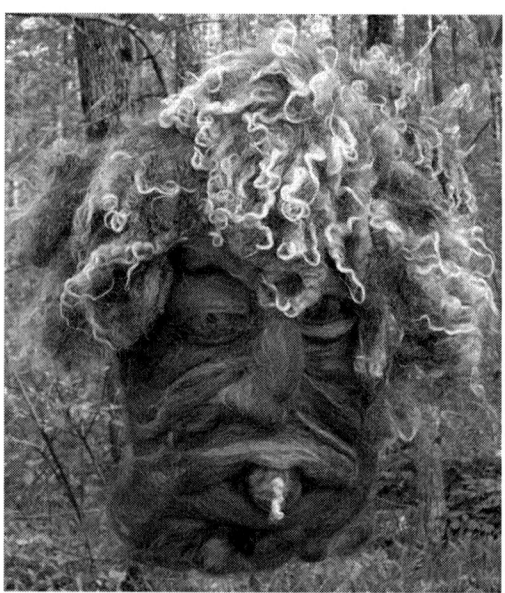

How about putting one mask on our face and one on the back of our head—then telling the story from two perspectives. I created this felt helmet style mask from handcrafted felt.

Working with expressive arts as a tool for self discovery and healing means constantly looking for paths into our inner knowing—and that means doing the unexpected, working with unusual materials, doing the opposite of what we are thinking of, and knocking ourselves off balance into unchartered waters. There lies the gold!

Full circle

I have talked about the importance of telling our stories, my process, how I work with others and some practical information on mask and story work within the expressive arts. I come full circle now to the symbols from the story I began with of the young boy who found the bird who sang exquisitely .All I know about the future is that I will continue to learn to sing my own magnificent song through the healing magic of story, mask and movement. I will hang on to the wings of my imagination that fly me into inner treasure hunts, and I will offer to help others with their own adventures.

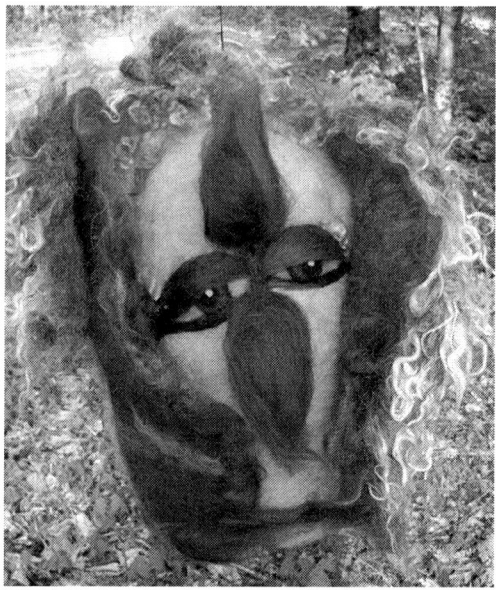

Resources

Campbell, Joseph. *The Power of Myth*. New York: Doubleday, 1988.
Ching, Elise Dirlam and Ching, Kaleo. *Faces Of Your Soul*. Berkeley: North Atlantic Books, 2006.
Coldiron, Margaret. *Trance and Transformation of the Actor in Japanese Noh and Balinese Masked Dance-Drama*. Lewiston, NY: The Edwin Mellen Press, 2004.

Eldredge, Sears A. *Mask Improvisation*. Evanston, IL: Northwestern University Press, 1996.
Lopez, Barry. *Crow and Weasel*. Bel Air, CA: North Point Press, 1990.

McNiff, Shaun. *Art as Medicine*. Boston: Shambhala, 1992.
Mellon, Nancy. *Body Eloquence*. Santa Rosa, CA: Energy Psychology Press, 2008.
—. *Storytelling and the Art of Imagination*. Cambridge, MA: Yellow Moon Press, 1992.
Pinkola Estes, Clarissa. *Women Who Run With The Wolves*. New York: Random House/Rider, 1992.

Eco-friendly blank masks Maskworx, Auckland, New Zealand.

IV: Engaging Image

PHOTO MEDITATION/INTROSPECTION

NANCY CAPPO

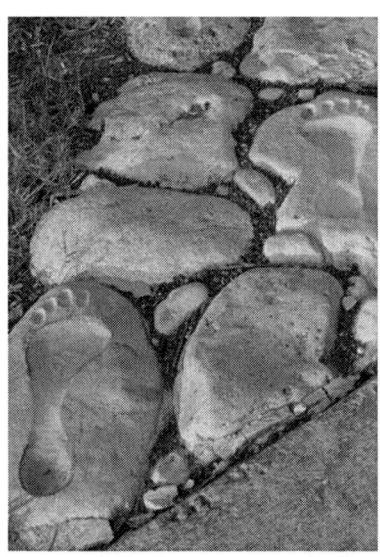

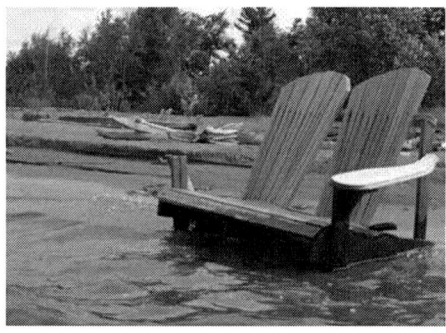

Footprints without feet, chairs without people, roots without the trees...Can these partial photographs jog the mind into deeper thought?

Certain photos can evoke emotional healing when combined with meditative words. We have all heard that one picture is worth a thousand words. For instance, a dog-eared snapshot can give a dying or grieving person a few moments of peace as a past memory is related to an active listener. Anger and fear may lessen as the "good part" of one's life is remembered. Sometimes searching into the past may be comforting and safer than living in the present. A life imbedded in confusion and memory loss may become spontaneous and alive as one thumbs through an old box of memories. Positive thoughts might offer comfort as they become an important bridge to one's own mortality.

Photographs, combined with words, are what I call "Photo Meditation/Introspection." The combination of these two disciplines gives the observer a chance to expand on the meaning behind, or beyond, the photograph of an object, person, or scene. What may normally be seen as "just a beautiful picture" opens up an opportunity for self-expression. An array of photos, from magazine pictures to personal snapshots, gives the viewer an option to go deeper if wanting to travel beyond the visual. Writing what one experiences through observation may expand this process even further. Meditation exercises require "being mindfully still." Stillness can occur as the shutter is snapped or as one examines the meaning of another's creative expression. Combining forms of visual art opens up possibilities for self-discovery by recalling life from a different angle. Adding significant words offers another pathway for introspection.

Pictures can initiate conversation or can be used as a tool for silent contemplation. Stories and emotions prompted by photographs are invaluable for both the storyteller and the listener. The ability to listen and to validate a patient's feelings, regardless of whether or not there is agreement, is an important component. A healing presence is the creation of a sacred space where one is able to be heard, be respected, and communicate freely. For an instant, life is improved, despite all the surrounding chaos and fears.

For example, listening to a 91-year-old gentleman relive an encounter with John Dillinger makes history come alive. Knowing someone who actually lived during that same era changes the perspective of a gangster on the movie screen to the reality of his humanness. Reliving these memories is an escape from the here and now. Not only does the storyteller receive validation, credibility, and undivided attention, but also this reenactment allows us to understand more about the person who willingly shares a piece of his or her past. It is a gift for both parties. Photos often allow the intricate puzzle pieces of one's own life to be put into some sort of order. Within the 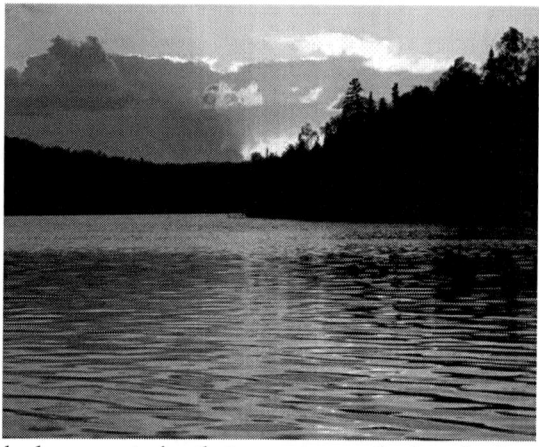 tattered and torn fluted edges are stories that may stagger the imagination and teach valuable lessons to anyone who will actively listen.

Realizing that pictures stimulate emotions, I began using them as a tool for communication. As I take snapshots, I consciously look for different angles and perspectives that can be interpreted from different lifetime experiences. I've created a method of adding text to promote an avenue for introspection. As a title on a piece of artwork gives clarity to an artist's interpretation, my phrases lead the viewer to a different dimension of thought. My intent is to present a safe place where personal experiences can be freely examined and shared. Phrases can be powerful when attached to a visual cue. The power of suggestion often works for accessing a visualization, as in guided imagery, as long as the listener has a frame of reference. Be aware of the frustration of someone experiencing dementia or whose memory is vague.

As I introduce a picture of a storm brewing on the horizon of a calm lake, the participant begins to relate a prior experience, either real or imagined. Taking enough time to allow contemplation, while providing a healing presence for her story to evolve, is essential before the next step. I would then ask her to close her eyes and listen to my words, "The calm before the storm prepares one internally." This thought allows the listener to travel to an entirely different place or emotion where introspection can begin.

Selected personal photos provide a segue for the viewer to retrieve thoughts and feelings from one's own past. Sometimes an individual may enjoy the picture from a fresh outlook without reminiscing, yet a discussion will elicit important emotions. When words are introduced, the photograph opens up possibilities to go a bit deeper or to shift one's thoughts in a different direction. A picture of a familiar scene may trigger emotions that provide a venue for discussion that will enable healing on some level.

Richard Stone writes in *The Healing Art of Storytelling*:

> "Without stories, life becomes a book cover without the pages — nice to look at, but not very fulfilling. Each time we journey inward and trace the path of a memory to its origins, we seem to discover nuances and connections that previously went unnoticed. While experience is encoded by all the senses, the primary fuel that ignites our senses is pictorial."

Jean Hunter, shares a similar technique with pictures. She has been in the professional field of photography for over 50 years.

> "As a life-long photographer, I have always found ways to use photography to connect with people. I enthusiastically share other peoples' personal pictures, knowing it provides a glimpse into their life story...and feel strongly about the joys of capturing a record of the things in my own life that have stirred or delighted me. When my husband was in his last difficult years of Alzheimer's, having lost the memory of most of his life, it was a desperate struggle to find conversational material to fill the hours I spent with him daily in a care facility. Talk of home and family further confused him, so photographs of our life together proved difficult to share. Recalling his former enjoyment of the fine photographs in *National Geographic*, I started working my way through a friend's collection of years of the publication. We spent time on each photo illustration talking about animals, people, and places, encouraging his comments and participation. It passed our hours together pleasantly, constructively, and even therapeutically, as we shared the diverse fascination of that fine magazine. As a photographer himself, something in him still responded to the visual impact of a fine photograph, giving him pleasure not to be found in talking of things no longer recalled. As a support-group facilitator for the Alzheimer's Society, I have passed this suggestion on to other family members and friends, who have also found that it lessened the anxiety and frustration of visits with their spouse or parent in similar circumstances. Interaction with loved-ones at this stage of their disease can be painfully difficult, but the photographs of *National Geographic* helped me through to the very end of our time together."

As with Jean's experience, I have also found the value in unique photographs of familiar subjects. Personally, I use a camera to capture candid moments as they unfold. Snapping the shutter to preserve the feeling or thought of a precious moment is my criteria for picture taking. Looking at life from different angles allows me to create a deeper meaning from an ordinary scene or object. For example, when kayaking the St. Croix River along the Minnesota/Wisconsin border, I noticed a steep cliff overhead where numerous trees jutted out from the protruding rock shelf. Dangling in front of me were roots partially covered with dirt. As my eyes absorbed what may have been a pile of dirt to most, I began to process the significance of roots in my own life. The deep blue sky provided a backdrop for the silhouette of the trunk and branches as they reached upward. Quickly aiming the viewfinder, I captured the image as we paddled by. In my first Photo Meditation book, *Captured*, I enhanced this picture by adding these thoughts under the snapshot. "Our roots ground us, even as the dirt erodes away." When questioning my closest friend about what she saw in this picture, I was disappointed when she limited her brief description to the physical characteristics of the object. Encouraging her to read my words and interpret them according to her own life, she was able to delve deeper. Jacky Saeger expressed these thoughts, as she looked inward.

> "Roots are the core of my values which come from the deepest part of me. Some have been established as a child, others as an adult. Many are formed as I get the final 'Ah-Ha' or understanding. The dirt that falls off is that which is not needed anymore, both good and bad. Much of my root system is buried until the dirt falls away and exposes that which is important to me. I need roots for my existence—to survive. They are my staying power and wisdom."

My intent is to take the observer to a more meaningful place in his or her life. Although personal captions define my thoughts, I encourage those who read them to tap into their own personal life stories. My photos are chosen to encourage introspection with the hope of encouraging a deeper understanding of self and communication with others.

While attending a photographic workshop in Paris, France, I learned different lighting techniques at the entrance of the famous Sacre-Coeur. A group of empty wine bottles had been carefully arranged on the church steps. Thirty photographers in our class carefully avoided shooting them as part of their pictures' composition, but my thoughts catapulted to another opportunity for life's symbolism. As I placed this picture in the format of my first book, I wrote these words. "Some obstacles are part of the bigger picture...embrace them." The viewer can interpret these words from his or her own perspective, again giving permission to think past the picture itself.

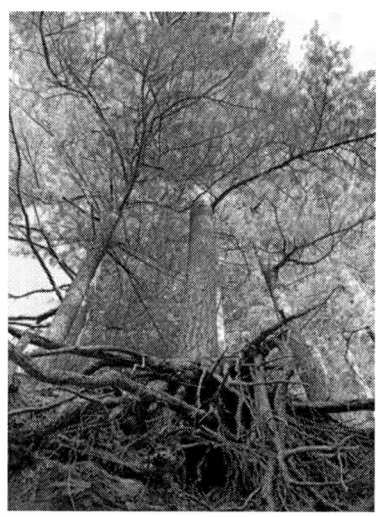

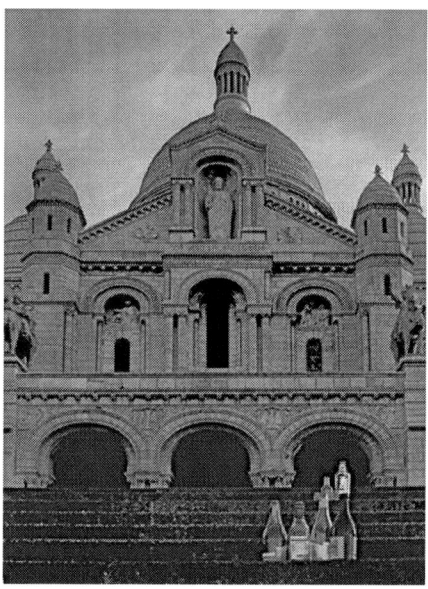

Photo Meditation /Introspection

During a recent trip to Israel, Lori Beese had the opportunity to review my second book, *Being Still*. During a museum tour, she related an awareness that emerged after reading the phrase written under a photograph of a loon stretching his wings. The sequence of words gave her insight into a personal experience with her son.

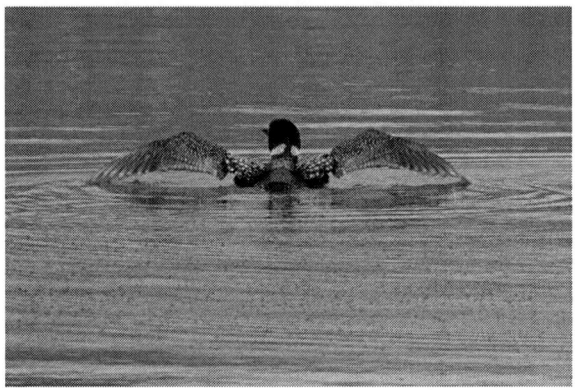

Spread your wings before choosing a direction.

"Mark, our self-supporting 25-year old son, was still undecided about a career path. After graduating from college, he moved back home and got a job, but not a career. Most of his friends were settling down, getting married, and moving up the career and economic ladder. Mark's lack of career choice had been causing him some angst and self-doubt. An old college roommate called one night, inviting him to join some friends moving out west for a snowboarding season. Moving out west to snowboard for a year, although tempting, seemed to Mark to be downright immature and irresponsible. He felt he should be buckling down and getting serious about being an adult. We encouraged Mark to go, knowing that this was the right thing for him, for so many reasons. He did go, and it has been a great experience for him, with an enormous amount of personal growth. When I saw the photo in Nancy's book, I instantly thought of Mark. It spoke perfectly to his situation. I will send it to him, because it affirms, not only his decision to move away and try something outside the norm, but also verifies our faith in him that he will find his path. Although it is the less traveled path, some people do need to spread their wings before choosing a direction."

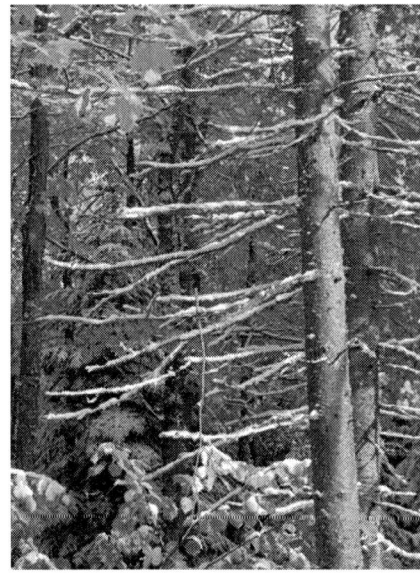

The light snowfall, like friendship, insulates bare branches.

Friendship is an important part of my life so often my snapshots represent this symbolism. Along an isolated driveway in Northern Minnesota, I spotted a maple tree laden with fresh snow clinging to its bare branches. As I zoomed in on the shot, I thought beyond the natural scene in front of me. These words may launch the reader to another direction. *"The light snowfall, like friendship, insulates bare branches."* This phrase changes the picture's perspective while giving the observer yet another thought to ponder. In discussing this photograph, another friend interpreted the snow as hope for tomorrow and the loss of leaves as crucial to the change of seasons, as friendship is to human survival.

A Hospice patient struggling with cancer shared thoughts of her favorite selections from my publication. She referred to the feelings that surfaced from the words written next to the picture. With a quiver in her voice, she expressed that she didn't know if she could have made it this far without having significant relationships in her life. She continued to explain how essential friendships had been while coping with this disease.

Reflect-Love-Laugh-Trust-Share-Grow
Discover the value of true friendship

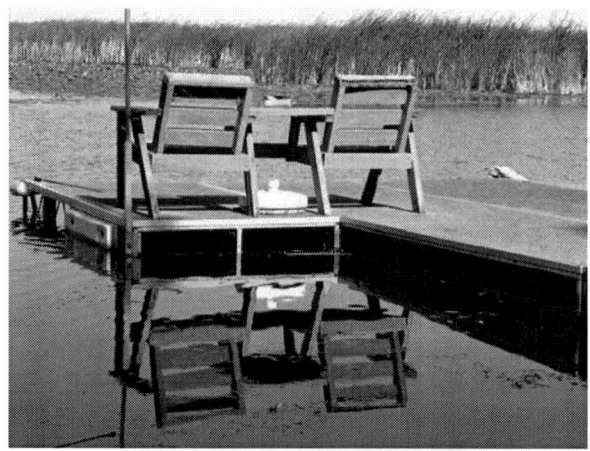

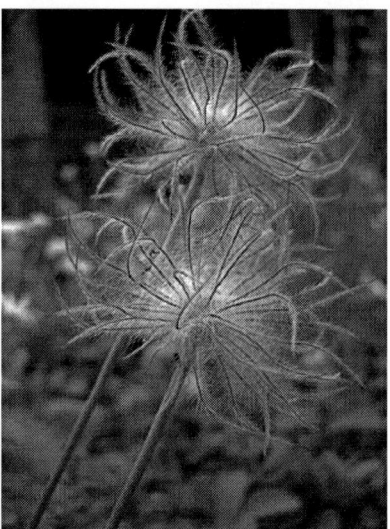

As you can see, neither of these photographs required the presence of a person to symbolize the concept of friendship, but the text took the viewer to that perspective.

Some may not want to express their thoughts or feelings verbally, but would prefer to jot them down. In a recent journaling workshop, I was asked to select three photos from a table strewn with magazine cutouts. I was not given any specific directions about the reason for selection other than to choose three which "spoke to me" in some way. Returning to my workspace, I was asked to mount one of the three on the front cover of my journal to represent my life as a whole. Without much forethought, I immediately selected the most complicated photo and began to write.

I watched everyone else in the room do the same thing without hesitation. Words seemed to flow from all different directions. We were then asked to choose one of the two pictures left to represent the reason that each of us had chosen to be a part of the Hospice organization. Again, words jumped on to the paper, as the photo selection was obvious. Listening to each participant share intimate feelings created a cohesive atmosphere within the group, even though few of us knew each other previously. The random magazine cutouts were individually selected because something resonated beyond the aesthetic value of the picture. Again, visual representations were used to promote feelings, conversation and self-introspection.

When warm fuzzies appear, relish them.
Accept, as the receiver —Send as the giver.

During my elementary teaching career, I found the teaching of "heart mapping" to be quite successful in helping fourth graders express emotions. Modeled from Georgia Heard's book, *Awakening the Heart*, we began a journey inward to learn how to access personal feelings. Creating a photo collage of the important people, places, things, and emotions in their lives spring-boarded into a writing exercise. Working in this pictorial mode helped students determine experiences that made a difference their lives. By establishing a safe atmosphere, the results of this emotional exercise were encouraged to be shared. I watched as one of the biggest bullies in the classroom shed tears as he related a story about his dying parakeet. Another classmate shared an abusive situation at home and explained how it contributed to her aggressive behavior at school. The sharing of such personal feelings, preempted by pictures, led to a different set of classroom dynamics and understanding. Again, choosing relevant magazine pictures combined with personal snapshots began a healing process.

As indicated by these examples, I have found photo meditation to be a useful tool in promoting communication and expression of personal feelings. Don't be afraid to analyze the meditative words under one of my pictures to define your own emotions. Each of us has a story to tell and individual experiences encourage each other's journey.

There is a challenge to look past the obvious and find symbolism in life's snapshots. Tilt your head, get down on the floor, look through an obstacle, squint, and bring life into focus from a different angle consciously formulating your thoughts and feelings. Just notice. Be still, if even for a moment, as you contemplate that which you have noticed. Understand that personal expression evolves from your own interpretation of what you really see. The more often you "let go" and avoid self-made rules, the more comfortable you will become with the process. Share with another, if the time is right, or treasure your own discoveries as you open your heart. Cherish each moment you create. The photographic journey can take you to the depths of your soul, capturing the moment, seeking your own truth, learning to express your feelings, and sharing with others what you have learned along the way. "Photo Meditation/Introspection" is a unique way to understand oneself and help others through the expression of their own feelings. It can promote conversation well beyond what you can imagine and begin a healing process within those who embrace it.

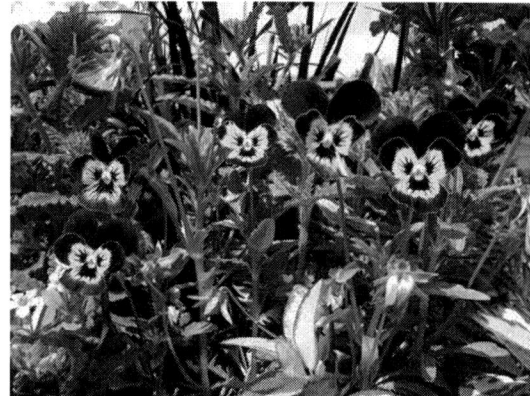

Even if one chooses to remain silent or is unable to speak, healing can occur as one enjoys the significance of a beautiful photograph. Watch for body language or facial expression that may reveal an inner shift.

Providing an array of pictures, in order to express one's emotions, encourages further communication of feelings and experiences. My method of Photo Meditation/ Introspection offers a visual representation of the familiar along with carefully selected verbiage to promote deeper thought and conversation.

Smiles can be found, if one looks below the surface.

Whether a partial photograph of an object, a symbolic representation of an emotion, or a personal snapshot, a photograph can elicit an important story. Each experience has the potential to unlock pieces of the heart or mind that may have been dormant for quite some time. Pictures, enhanced by a personal thought, may launch the viewer into a different realm of introspection. However one interprets, or simply enjoys, a photograph can be a source of healing.

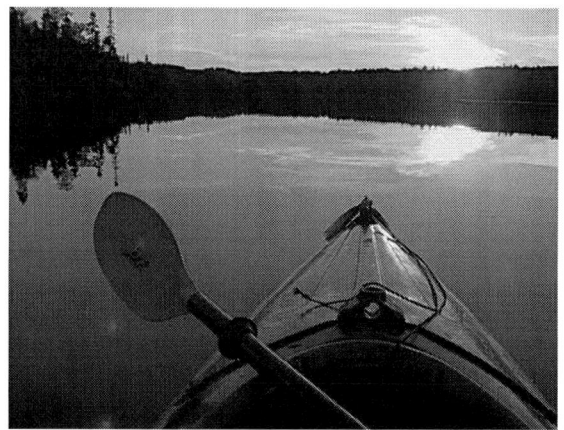

Paddle with intent, yet take time to drift.

References

Cappo, Nancy. *Captured: Photo Meditation.* Ibook by Apple, Inc.: December 2007.
—. *Be Still...Photo Meditation.* Ibook by Apple, Inc.: February 2008.
Heard, Georgia. *Awakening the Heart.* Portsmouth, NH: Heinemann: November 1998.
Stone, Richard D. *The Healing Art of Storytelling.* USA: Iuniverse.com: 2005.

AS WITHIN SO WITHOUT: AN ANCIENT SOUL MAP TO HEALING

CHRISTINE MCCULLOUGH

The labyrinth is an ancient and sacred path which has been walked through many turbulent times. A labyrinth is a path of peace, offering sublime centering, deep introspection and powerful healing. It is a unicursal path, winding in and out again, which balances both heart and soul. Simple yet complex, beautiful to experience, whether you are a walker of the path or take part as an observer. Once you experience its power, your world may never be the same.

Walking the labyrinth, we're tracing a path that winds back thousands of years, back through the history of Christianity, back through the Neolithic period and beyond, back through Old Europe when the Goddess reigned supreme, back through time out of mind, 6,000; 10,000; even 20,000 years ago.

We begin with the Goddess. The excavation in this century of thousands of Paleolithic and Neolithic Goddess figures is synchronistic with the inner journey many people are making now. The unearthing of buried images of female power is a metaphor for the way in which women, and men, are contacting the deepest layers of the collective sacred Feminine. These Goddess figures have what archeologist Maria Gimbutas calls a "Pictorial script" carved into them. The symbols reveal that the worldview of our ancestors revolved around the worship of the Goddess in all her myriad forms: animal, bird, fish, and all her archetypal manifestations, including; the self generating Goddess, Giver of Life, Fertility Goddess, Earth Mother, Death Wielder and Regenatrix.

She embodied the unity of all life in nature, and presided over a culture that was peaceful, egalitarian, creative and life-reverencing. One frequent form the Goddess figurines took was as a Bird, and one of the most recurrent symbols these bird goddess figurines display is the MEANDER, a water symbol. The Meander grows into the Labyrinth.

The oldest Bird Goddess figure with this pattern was found in the Western Ukraine and is dated somewhere between 18,000 to 15,000 B.C.

The bird Goddess frequently appeared as a Crane, a water bird who migrated over all of Old Europe, and whose mysteries are intimately connected to the Labyrinth.

Another frequent image—the oldest of the old—is the spiral. It is the pattern we carry in our cells, in our DNA. The spiral is the oldest form of labyrinth. It is the single path that winds in to the center and then out again. Spirals, single, double and triple, appeared all over the Paleolithic and Neolithic world, and they remind us of a time when the cosmos was experienced as whole rather than fragmented, and Mother Earth was a literal reality.

The image of the classical seven-circuit labyrinth began to appear all over the Neolithic world about four thousand years ago. Carved into stone and into earth, this archetypal pattern surfaced simultaneously in the minds of many people widely separated from each other with no possible contact between them.

We can still see the labyrinth carved into stone and earth all over Western Europe: in Crete, in Troy, in Scandinavia, in Egypt, Africa, Peru and the British Isles. To the Hopi of the American Southwest it was the symbol of emergence from the Earth Mother. In France and Italy, Gothic cathedrals like Chartres have intricate but still unicursal or single-path labyrinths built into their floors. These were traveled by pilgrims in the Middle Ages, who crawled on their knees to the center and out again. This was known as "The Way to Jerusalem."

Sod Labyrinths, dug into the earth in Europe, Sweden and Britain can still be run today, as they have been for thousands of years. The English and Scandinavians call them Troy Towns, or the Walls of Troy, the fabled city, home of Helen, which was one of the last strongholds of the Mother Goddess. In the Welsh language, the labyrinth is called CAERDROIA— literally, "A Hill of Troy" or a "Hill of Turnings." The Labyrinth is, then, a "turning point," and the term "Troy Town" links the labyrinth to the feminine in another way. There are many ancient and persistent themes of the Goddess, or a woman, at the center of the labyrinths found in England and Western Europe.

Ariadne of Crete was one such Goddess, from the ancient matrilineal period of Mother Goddess worship. In Crete, she was known as the Mistress of the Labyrinth. Ariadne holds the thread that leads us to the center of the labyrinth, where we find her in ourselves. She represents the final holdout of an earlier Goddess-centered spirituality before Patriarchal Indo-European concepts and ideas came along and the Goddess no longer held her place at the center of the Labyrinth. Making the journey through the Labyrinth and out again traces the path of faith and mystery; both spiritual path and physical earth span. Walking this winding path mirrors the winding pattern of life, death and rebirth.

The Labyrinth can be thought of as an archetype brought down to earth, a literal pattern cut into the turf and danced into life. The Labyrinth is a connection to the Source, to the Sacred Mystery. To walk the Labyrinth is to trust there is guidance to help us live. It helps us to create inner sacred space: it reminds us that a loving presence or force behind the entire world urges us to risk our comfort and reach for meaning in our lives.

Using the Labyrinth as a part of your Counseling Practice

Walking the Labyrinth is a sublime reflective experience that moves us deeper into a coherent state of being. Though no research has been completed to date, anecdotal evidence suggests that the very action of walking in a spiral, to the right, left, and back again, inward and outward, has the effect of bringing Right and Left Hemispheres into balance, much like using your tuner dial on a radio to fine tune a frequency.

Labyrinth walking in many ways mimics the relaxation state that occurs in hypnotic induction or deep meditation. As the bodymind begins to still, and the client opens to awareness, the answers needed are revealed. In many ways, it is easier since the action of walking removes some of the self-consciousness many clients experience when trying to move into a meditative state. Using the Labyrinth is particularly helpful when the client's or practitioner's explorations have run into resistance of any kind.

Whether facilitating a group or working with a private client, the induction is the same:

*Set an intention.

Be clear on the issue you are exploring. Do you need a specific answer to a specific question? Do you need clarity concerning a troubling situation?

Are you seeking to connect with a "guide" or "inner healer?" Do you need to let go of grief or discover inspiration? You as the counselor should work with your clients to define the intention that would be most beneficial to their process. If you are having difficulty in coming up with an intention, and you have access to such skills as Specialized Kinesiology or the BodyTalk System, you can muscle test the client to refine the focus in order to serve the client's particular need.

*Take time to prepare.

Sometimes the Labyrinth isn't meant to be walked right away. Perhaps the client needs to participate in dream incubation for insight, write in their journal, or do some other form of "homework" to prepare for the event. Perhaps the healing process will be enhanced by having them help in the building of the Labyrinth or having them develop a particular ceremony or protocol for optimizing the experience. You may have the client create a drawing or sculpture to represent his or her feelings before walking the Path, which could be followed by making one after the experience. You may wish to begin the work with a prayer or meditation, or by reading a meaningful poem, or simply by spending some time in silence to gather one's thoughts.

If this is a group process, the group will need to be in agreement as to whether the process is undertaken in complete silence or whether it is OK for participants to chant, or to say a prayer, affirmations or mantra. Each one's journey is to be done alone.

The client herself created one particularly powerful session I experienced. She began by writing down a letter expressing her anger at an abuser. When she reached the center of the Labyrinth, she read the letter aloud and then burned it in a vessel provided for that purpose. As she returned she alternated repeating affirmations for her healing process with expletives of release. As she returned from her journey, she expressed feeling free of the weight of anger that had held her fast for many years.

*Walk with mindfulness.

I always counsel my clients, whether in a group or individually, to take all the time they need to walk the path. I ask them to be conscious of the contact they make with the Earth, to be aware of the sensations in their body as certain feelings arise, to walk in silence or murmur a mantra or prayer *sub voto*, if they must, but to be present to the process.

In a group process, mindfulness extends to basic courtesy about letting people pass, or being aware of your neighbor as you pass them coming or going. One may suddenly see a participating stranger in a very different light, literally seeing the God Source within them, or extending the heart of Compassion to them as a fellow human being on Life's Journey and want to extend a hug, bow, or some other form of recognition. Walking the Labyrinth as a part of a group is a very different process than an individual journey. Configuration made by the spacing of people can be informative to each one's process.

With a group process, the Labyrinth becomes a literal metaphor for the dance of life; people coming and going, walking parallel for a while, meeting each other on the path while going in different directions and having to let the other pass, following each other only to be separated as one goes faster or falls behind.

*Stop and deeply listen when you reach the heart.

Upon reaching the heart of the Labyrinth, take time to say a prayer, listen for your answer, begin the process of release, check-in with your body, and simply be aware. You might even have your client actually put their hand on their heart and imagine breathing through the heart in order to reach a coherent, integrated state.

When someone has reached the heart of the Labyrinth, all movement should stop. This, first of all, honors the person who has reached the center and honors their center. It allows them to commune without excessive distraction. On a practical level, it saves the group from creating a backlog of people waiting to get to the center. It does require some attention to others present.

*Release and return.

The journey out of the Labyrinth has often been described as faster and lighter than the journey in. I have watched clients dance and skip their way out of a Labyrinth in an expression of joy. Clients have said that they feel a literal shedding as they make each turning coming home. The mindful letting go process is a part of the power of the form.

*Process.

How you are most comfortable processing the client's experience is up to you. Whether through drawing, journaling, movement, play or simply discussion, it is important to put the journey into context, to explore the possible changes that have occurred, to explain sudden insights or simply give the client room to express their feelings in a meaningful way as needed.

It is especially important in a group setting to set aside extra private time to spend with clients who have reached an epiphany or extremely powerful insight and may need time away from the group to process fully. I have often presented a labyrinth program with one of my colleagues in order to have such a need covered. One of us can attend to a needy individual while the other facilitates the group's process.

Remember, the client has undertaken a mythic path of descent and return, and the story must be told and heard in order for healing to be fully accomplished.

Aesthetics and the Labyrinth

How many times have you heard the mantra, "I can't draw a straight line...I'm not an artist!" and yet, once a client has connected with the process of making marks, of manipulating line, shape and color, a light seems to go on behind their eyes! At first, expression is tentative, you can see the child who was told not to paint hair blue and skin purple in a coloring book emerge tentatively, waiting to be chided for drawing stick figures. Nevertheless, after a few attempts at expression are taken, once the client begins to realize the connection between the symbols and colors they marked and the healing of whatever issue they have brought to the table, a marvelous awakening occurs. Some of my clients have embraced continued artistic expression as an on-going process of living. If nothing else, they begin to see their world differently, observing the fragile beauty of a flower, or the glorious beauty of changing light during the course of a day. They begin to honor the beauty within themselves; they being to create beauty around them. As within, so without.

That particular statement paraphrases the ancient alchemical creed, "As Above, So Below," pointing to the interconnectedness of Spirit and Matter. If we cannot see the Divine Beauty within our souls, how can we possibly interact with the Divine Beauty manifest in all creation?

Clients come armored from the pains of life, whatever those are for them. The armor protects them from hurt but also blinds them to the Grace that naturally surrounds them and could be both their comfort and their strength. Left Brain, seemingly logical explanations and excuses continue to keep them boxed off from connection with the richness of dream, vision, and possibility that lies with Right Brain function. Without the balance of the Right Brain, imagistic functioning, and Left Brain manifesting functioning, clients experience the world through the lens of fear and restriction. Both hope and motivation are gone and they walk through life as through a maze, lost and confused, looking for the way out.

As Expressive Arts Therapists, we have found the Labyrinth an invaluable tool that can be used to bring a client out of themselves and into a reconnection with their world. It is a gentle and non-threatening way of balancing both hemispheres of the brain simultaneously and effortlessly, and has never failed to stimulate reaction that can be expressed through color and form. Working with the Labyrinth involves rhythmic movement, sound healing, meditation, ritual, and art to allow the clients to set their intention and actively work through a process and come up with their own insights. The clients become fully empowered in the process of their healing journey. They own their inspiration and the physical result, the art they create.

As a form or container of the healing experience, the Labyrinth is immensely flexible. It can be used to celebrate rites of passage, used as a meditative tool for centering, used actively to solve problems, inspire and increase awareness, promote peaceful interaction, team and community building, explore grief, balance energies, explore and heal addictions and be used both singly and for groups. Because the very action of walking the form balances both hemispheres of the brain creating brain synchrony, artistic expression seems to be encouraged to flow naturally. I liken the experience to lucid dreaming; symbols arise naturally and one experiences the feeling of being both here and not here at the same time. In this timeless container, one can connect with mythic archetypes for personal meaning.

The human being is a meaning maker as well as a toolmaker. Ancient cultures did not separate the use of an object from its beauty. I don't believe indigenous peoples struggled with the idea that, "I am not an artist because I can't draw a straight line," on a daily basis. I believe they simply lived within the flow of the very human need to be in connection with the beauty around them and reflect that beauty in the objects they created. To create is part of the human experience. The onus of "I am not an artist," that thought, that perception, shrivels our human experience and our world. The idea that someone out there, some professional artist, has the sole authority to create is, at its source, a modern economically motivated control, which creates a "Them vs. Us" schism in our perceptions and begins the separation of us from our souls, us from our surroundings, and us from our innate power to create. Whether we create an object of Beauty or a life of Beauty, both results are the same.

For Native Peoples of the American Southwest, the concept of Beauty, walking in Beauty, translates in to walking in Balance with ourselves, within, and all our Relations, without. I see the Labyrinth as very similar to the use of sand painting for healing as used by the Navaho. A mythic pattern is created which she who needs to be healed absorbs and identifies with, as a process to answering her own questions and returning to a healthful balance. The ancient origins of the Labyrinth constitute the mythic pattern. The client literally takes a walk within the myth and physically, as well as psychically, comes into balance. From that sublime set point, all answers are available.

Clients enter the Labyrinth looking for that which they already possess. They exit the Labyrinth with a gift, the gift of knowledge that they can create, be it a drawing, a poem, an idea, their health, or ultimately, their lives. The very action of meditative walking creates a mindfulness that transcends the outer world of worry and distraction to move pilgrims who walk the Labyrinth to a deeper and more personally meaningful understanding of their own life's journey. In this lies the power of this simple path that leads one to the center of one's soul and back home again.

IN SEARCH OF THE SOUL OF IMAGE: A COSMOLOGICAL THEORY FOR EXPRESSIVE ARTS THERAPY

PAULA ARTAC

Seven of the twenty-five years that I have been teaching art and the creative process have been devoted to focusing on the questioning, researching and expansion of the fundamentals and purpose of art therapy and expressive arts therapy into our personal, community and global lives. In all these years, I had not found an adequate answer to my question, "How have we neglected the importance of spirituality in the creative process, when it is such a vital component of human nature?" This question prompted me to search for answers in my doctoral work.

Fluid Energy Imagery, the process of spirituality-based creative expression that I have developed, is a postmodern, cosmological reverence for the creativity that flows within every soul, every being. This process physically transforms universal energy into the power of image. Fluid Energy Imagery reconnects body with soul, conscious with unconscious, heart with mind, individual with collective, humanity with Nature. This is a healing process that opens the imagination of the compassionate artist, increasing one's abilities for creative thinking, problem solving, collaboration, critical thinking, planning, design and holistic work practices. We will find that the eye, hand and heart become one in the process of replacing an outdated paradigm built on criticism and fear with innovation and imagination. Creativity is the light we bear within that births fresh ideas for re-inventing our life's work.

We can override the persistent psychological, spiritual, physical and emotional blocks that cripple our life choices with self-criticism, judgmental comparison, feelings of worthlessness and fear. The intent of Fluid Energy Imagery is to bring together the knowledge of the therapeutic and creative processes into an ongoing art-based research project that extends beyond the analytical restrictions of mainstream psychology. The intent of this essay is to ignite, inspire, renew and honor the creative energy that each one of us possesses. It acknowledges our noble responsibility to manifest our fullest potential as human beings, as spiritual beings in everything we do. We are on a spiritual course in the twenty-first century, charting our life experiences ultimately to return to our original source of oneness of mind, body and spirit. Creativity should be taken seriously as fundamental equipage on this transformative voyage.

Imagine our lives if creativity were the foundation of a community's activities—the "river's source" from which all healthy and meaningful work, prayer and play are generated. The precious gift of unlimited imagination would be recognized and nurtured as an essential part of human development from infants to seniors, rather than relegating artistic expression to a meaningless pastime when one has "nothing else to do." Imagine a world where expressive arts therapists are valued catalysts of wisdom, as artists and healers, by invigorating the healing arts with a sense of unlimited creativity.

Long before the beginning of formal religious institutions some 4,500 years ago, spirituality was an innate quality in the existence of human life. In its pure dynamic state, the nature of this gift invigorates the spirit to seek articulation and meaningful expression in our lives, beyond cerebral, rational and analytical boundaries. Spirituality is a powerful energy that circulates through the psyche, the Earth and the cosmos. The influence of Newtonian science and Cartesian philosophy heavily influenced our modern Western understanding of how life unfolds in the Universe.

Our fragmented world today needs deep spiritual healing through a reconnection of individual and collective mind, body and spirit. We continue to search for deeper spiritual meaning. The ideal model for therapeutic treatment plans still reflects a predominant Newtonian mechanistic habit of thought that a person resembles a machine with problems that should be treated as such. In the field of mental health, we have been largely ignoring our obligation to work with the soul, which is the translation of psyche, the root word of "psychology," relegating the scope of this work to the dictates of religion. The spiritual and transpersonal dimensions of creative expression in relieving suffering and promoting a proactive approach to health have been undernourished in the fields of art therapy and expressive arts therapy, which give us an incentive to look for new ways to define and understand wellness.

Throughout the past modern era, the inclusion of art as a vital element of an individual's spiritual development has virtually been ignored. In the era of modernism, the cultivation of fear and scarcity fragmented the mystical bond of the artist within each of us with his or her source of creativity, the spirit. Irrational imagination, which is beyond reason as the ultimate authority and births non-verbal, multi-dimensional images that are not found in certain places in space or time, clashed with the rational, linear world of words and ideas. Science and art were estranged. The mind, body and spirit could no longer function as the beautiful, mystical, interconnected whole that they were intended to be. Human beings were no longer filled with blessing, but reduced to powerlessness by their flaws (Fox, 1983, p. 83.)

There has been an ongoing attempt for many years to find a genuinely coherent theoretical approach that thoroughly encompasses all aspects of expressive arts therapy. Art as a therapeutic process continues to draw its identity from a variety of psychological theories ranging from Freud's psychoanalytical approach to Jung's use of imagery in therapy, from the influence of Gestalt and humanistic insights, to existential concepts. Art therapists and expressive arts therapists vary in their proclivity to either subscribe solely to one theory or draw from an eclectic synthesis of concepts. In 1987, art therapist Judith Rubin expressed in her book *Approaches to Art Therapy* an ongoing earnest desire to see the "development of meaningful theoretical constructs from the matrix of art therapy itself" rather than attempt to draw from different theories outside the realm of art therapy (Rubin, 1987, p. xvi.) It is her firm belief that creativity, of itself, propels a person to creative expression. When the flow of this positive creative impulse is blocked, the destructive forces of physical, emotional and spiritual imbalance affect the health and well-being of mind, body and spirit. To this day, the search continues.

It is now of utmost importance to develop a theoretical model that expands beyond the current secular mainstream of scientific method that appreciates the phenomenal properties of the created image, and returns the psyche to its spiritual origin, to its cosmology, to its creative "soul." A cosmological theory reunites humans with the sacred in nature and creativity of the cosmos, in what psychologist James Hillman describes as a psychology that can carry soul. He envisions a revolution in behalf of soul where there is "freedom to imagine, to be beautiful, to show pathologized oddity and variety [where] enthroned again is communion with soul in unspoiled nature, in the poesis of music, and in the evocation of Eros and the remembrance of death" (Hillman, 1975:219.) Spiritual writer and lecturer Thomas Moore alerts us in his book *The Re-enchantment of Everyday Life* to "never forget that 'analysis' means loosening, and the 'psyche' means butterfly, a beautiful but elusive being that should be glimpsed in flight but never pinned down. Quite literally, *psychoanalysis* means 'letting the butterfly go free'" (Moore, 1996:184.) Catherine Moon, a noted art therapist and author, writes in "*Prayer, Sacraments, Grace,*" that "the doing of art requires an openness to the salvific value in the accidental, and in this capacity to 'make do' with whatever is at hand" (Moon, 2001:32.) She believes in art making as prayer. Art becomes a means of transcending oneself—*beyond* the ego—going beyond the possible, the predictable, the ideological, and becoming open to mystery. Artist and art therapist Pat B. Allen's practice of cultivating the essential "unknowing" of the art process permeates both her personal and professional image work. She teaches how accessing the imagination gives voice to the soul as a way of knowing healing and transformation "making way for the new" (Allen, 1995:x.)

This essay introduces such a cosmological approach to expressive arts therapy, emphasizing the essential need in each person to love and create. A cosmological approach to creative expression, based on *cosmology*, the creative work of the universe and our conscious awareness of its beauty and grandeur, removes the constricting separateness, of subject and object, body and soul, matter and spirit, I and Thou, self and Self. This spiritual approach fuses both the ancient and contemporary wisdom of those who have been searching for, and found, plausible answers to understanding the essence of the psyche. It expands, however, beyond the mechanistic, anthropocentric and patriarchal limitations of modern psychological explanations and returns spirituality to the matrix. A cosmological path to wholeness revivifies a "spirit-filled way of living." Matthew Fox, theologian, modern day mystic and writer is a vital force for the re-invigoration of cosmology into our postmodern society. He affirms that "creativity and relationship, art and love, express our deepest beings, and what they share in common is empathy. Both art and love take us into the void and beyond in a kind of rhythm of birth and rebirth that never ceases" (Fox, 2002:33-34.) Empathy requires an understanding and mindfulness that through an attentiveness to the maternal heartbeat of the earth—the sound of waves, the wind, a bird's song, the touch of a leaf or rock—the birth of a deeper experience of the world and our relationship with it is once again possible. Through art and love, the ego opens to an undifferentiated, active relationship with the soul. Life inspired by renewed awe and wonder leads the imagination to a deeper healing relationship between the environment of the Earth and the environment of the soul. It is this liberation of the soul that brings healing creative energy through image to the mind and heart.

This rich spiritual language of image has given the soul of the Universe its earthly voice "speaking" non-verbally in images expressed through the undaunted creativity of countless cultures and civilizations throughout the course of Creation. The ageless spirit of the Universe emanates from the earliest "primitive" images of bison on cave walls to the colorful crayon renderings of a kindergartner. Image is the telling and retelling of the universal themes of a life story shared by all humanity, all creatures, every human being, all that exists in the conscious and unconscious. Images that have emerged through each millennium are all precious mosaic pieces that blend to describe collectively the continuous flux of humanity's relationship with the divine. Art is a symbolic communication that speaks of a reality beyond today's accepted stereotypes.

It is in response to this search for the soul of image, that this writer has developed a cosmological art therapy theory and expressive arts therapy modality, *Fluid Energy Imagery,* which emphasizes the restoration of awe and mystery through the power of image. This art process opens our minds to knowledge-learning, restores our sense of present-centeredness and eliminates the fear of realizing our fullest human potential. We are witness to the dawning of a new era, a shedding of the restrictive cocoon caused by a patriarchal hunger for *external* **power**, moving slowly from an uncreative machine to a creative cosmos. Contemporary philosopher and psychologist Jean Huston notes that there is an "acceleration of the psyche in our times" (Sheldrake, McKenna and Abraham, 2001:xiv.) Reaching deeper into the archetypal depths to understand the psyche, or soul, can be the bridge between the great force of nature and the force of spirit that have long been disunited. It is the re-birthing of the psyche's inner light of empowerment that takes wing in truth and creativity and bears the potential for wholeness. It is a time of counterbalance that takes us beyond the archetypal hero's journey burdened by adolescent notions of reality based on materialistic rationalism into a sacred life of unending, renewable possibilities. A qualitative energy shift matures the divine relationship between matter, our beings and the earth. It is the freeing of the Conscious Feminine in a complementary relationship with the Conscious Masculine to renew intuition, feeling, subjectivity, and relatedness. Feminine values such as caring, nonviolence and compassion can heal the wounds of deception and illusion that have fragmented the *anima mundi* for thousands of years. This creative process, a potential storehouse of wisdom, balance and spirit can function as a source of deep spiritual discovery, unity and transformation for our soul, and no one is excluded from this process. From a cosmological perspective, the essence of art and image, theory and practice unite in mystery and enchantment devoted to the service to the soul. "We follow it; we don't demand that it conform to our expectations and standards. We are its servant; it is not ours" (Moore, 1996:186.) Fluid Energy Imagery is soul-centered therapy that "aims at letting the soul sing, show itself, create a beautiful life"(ibid.,189.) It is how the body is able to speak the spontaneous language of its soul.

The advantages of a cosmological approach applied to art and wellness, as indicated in Fluid Energy Imagery, are numerous, which free the power of image to speak intuitively from the soul as ever-changing fluid forms are born from chaos. Recognizing that form creates order from chaos, just as the Universe continually creates from chaos, selected visible images can have a deeply psychological and spiritual impact on the dynamic workings of the mind, body and spirit. The work being done today in the field of fluid dynamics is applying a new multi-dimensional, interdependent vision of life processes to an understanding our purpose for existence. The growing use of the concept of *flow* is remarkable.

The media of tissue collage and watercolor enhancement are used effectively in this free flowing creative process, as can be seen in the sample artwork below. These particular media have been chosen specifically for their *fluidity,* a term also readily used in fluid dynamics, to compliment and reflect the energetic flow of change through color, line and patterns that are continually changing form in nature and the Universe. The experiential art that is the basis for this cosmological theory and practice utilizes a collage method that invites the artist within each person to play non-judgmentally with the random release, flow, and blending of color. Through a random arrangement of brightly tinted tissue paper, spontaneous images ultimately emerge. The artist/client is the receiver of these phenomenological images. Details of these images can be enhanced using watercolor or oil pastel. This postmodern theory is built around a spiritual receptiveness to the universal energy of the ancient Hindu chakra system, and recognizes how a physical, creative response with spontaneous images can bear the gifts of insight, healing and wellness. Through our imagination, we enjoy the power to partake of the wisdom of the universal imagination.

From our imagination and through our creativity we can capture a moment, interpret an impression, or feel an emotion within the continual flow of conscious experience. From an integrated approach, we can observe the process of creating with collage and watercolor from an entirely new perspective. The artist initiates this creative process in a seemingly chaotic flow of imagination translating the unpredictable forces of her world into flowing patterns of compelling beauty, perturbation, harmony, mystery and balance. The initial flood of color and water is formless and yet potentially attached to great amounts of soul information and muscle memory. The processes is releasing, simplifying, blending, creating mystery at the risk of letting go, create balance, form, substance and dimension, which provide deep psychic resolution. It is then evident that each time we engage in a creative process, we are flowing with the energy of the Universe, repeating a timeless creative process of inspiration and imagination, change, destruction, and rebirth.

At this point, we must take into consideration the role that the expressive arts therapist or art therapist fulfills as well as the preparation which is necessary to ensure that the personal experience of the client/artist is a spiritually transformative, optimal experience. Expressive arts therapists are being called to be today's contemporary prophets and mystics to assist in this healing transformation as we write the current, critical chapters of our human story. The postmodern practitioner as healer is a vital instrument in this critical time and in this new creation story, bearing a new heart and a new consciousness of wisdom and compassion. He or she transforms 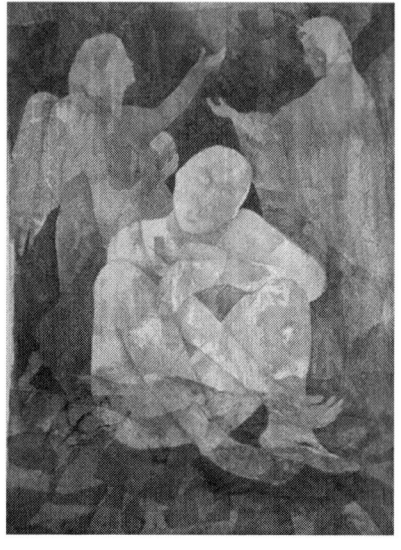 the art space into sacred space that becomes a safe and trusting environment open to the power of mystery and wonder. It becomes a space for individuals to become one within themselves and explore the mystery of the cosmos within and beyond the self/ego limitations.

This healer is grounded and rooted in the divine and inspires people to hope in themselves, assisting them as a midwife in discovering and birthing their power through their artistic expression. The art therapist or expressive arts therapist practitioner is artist, teacher and comforter; one who sits in mystery as well as ignites hearts with a passion for living. This person encourages every child or adult to explore the power and beauty of their imagination, allowing the image to speak, thus birthing form from potent chaos through their flow of creativity. Through visualization, healing images emerge, bearing renewed balance of mind, body and spirit. In honoring these creative abilities, the soul is fortified with deep spiritual strength.

An essential adjunct and quantitative accompaniment to augment the effectiveness of the non-verbal process within Fluid Energy Imagery is the inclusion of the Ingersoll Spiritual Wellness Inventory. The Spiritual Wellness Inventory is a measurement tool developed by Dr. Elliott Ingersoll of Cleveland State University, which provides continued "research and dialogues about healthy spirituality and [provides] a cross-culturally affirmed vocabulary for discussing spirituality" (Ingersoll, 1998:164.) The information that can be gathered by using Ingersoll's Spiritual Wellness Inventory along with the creative process is a powerful means of accessing core spiritual values and experiences. Confusion, alienation and frustration frequently accompany the process of the discovery of one's true spiritual Self. This trans-traditional vocabulary accompanied with art making can assist a client/artist in the verbal processing of the images that are present in their artwork. Resulting dialogue provides an opportunity for inquiry into the potent spiritual, psychic and archetypal information that an image bears.

As previously discussed in this essay, Fluid Energy Imagery moves beyond the mechanistic habit of thought that a person resembles a machine with problems that should be treated as such. From a cosmological-centered approach, the focus shifts from the treatment of the pathologies of people to the qualities within a person that creatively free their divine grace to reveal his or her soul. Fluid Energy Imagery validates the importance of the irrational, the mystical and the unexplainable manifested through the creative process.

Coleman Barks, author of *The Soul of Rumi*, describes the process as "Soul Art" (Barks, 2001: 232.)

> Soul artists guide the motions of energy that's given. How you love is the sky itself. When it rains (the grace of energy,) an individual roof with its guttering (the personal self) conducts water flow like skill with language [art and music.] Rumi says the most beautiful gardens grow from the rain collected in the barrel under your own roof, the one with your tears in it (ibid.)

For further information on the Fluid Energy Imagery art therapy modality, and the use of the Ingersoll Spiritual Wellness Inventory, contact information is available for Dr. Paula Artac on her website at: www.2dotsandaline.com.

References

Allen, P. *Art is a Way of Knowing: a guide to Self-knowledge and Spiritual Fulfillment through Creativity.* Boston, MA: Shambhala. 1995

Barks, C. *The Soul of Rumi.* New York: HarperCollins Publishers. Inc. 2001

Fox, M. *Original Blessing.* New York: Jeremy P. Tarcher/Putnam. 1983

—. *Creativity.* New York: Jeremy P. Tarcher/Putnam. 2002

Hillman, J. *Re-visioning Psychology.* New York: HarperPerennial. 1975

Ingersoll, E. "Refining Dimensions of Spiritual Wellness." *Counseling & Values,* 42:3 (1998) 156-165, 6

Moon, C. "Prayer, Sacraments, Grace." In Farrelly-Hansen, M. (Ed.). *Spirituality and Art Therapy..* London and Philadelphia, PA: Jessica Kingsley Publishers. Ltd., 2001:29-51.

Moore, T. *The Re-enchantment of Everyday Life.* New York: Harper/Perennial. 1996

Rubin, J. *Approaches to Art Therapy, Theory, and Technique.* New York: Brunner/Mazel, Publishers. 1987

Sheldrake, Rupert., Terence McKenna, and Ralph Abraham. *Chaos, Creativity and Cosmic Consciousness.* Rochester, VT: Park Street Press. 2001

"Elementary, My Dear, What's-On Tap for Children and Adults"

Sally Mathews

As the music began, each elementary art student closed his or her eyes and blindly drew a continuous line over the surface of a 12" by 18" piece of white drawing paper. No eyes were to peek, no pencil was to lift off the paper, and no talking, only listening, for sixty long music-inspired seconds.

They were fourth graders so we clocked another sixty seconds after "eyes open" for astonished cries as each student first disclaimed and then owned the weird results. Nevertheless, to validate this foray into the unknown, all the students were asked to hold up their work all at the same time for all to see, and bear the strangeness together. Though this activity was a warm-up for a more traditional drawing demand, the papers were collected. We don't throw away.

In the next art class when we passed our music-inspired scribbles back to be inserted into individual portfolios, two works were, despite my eternally severe directions, without names.

"Well, now," I said, thinking we'd experience an obvious lesson on the need for signatures on each and every piece of work, "to whom does this belong?"

The eyes I'm supposed to have in the back of my head secretly twinkled during the pause, when a child raised his hand and said,

"That belongs to Gregory. He's absent today."

I could feel my real eyebrows arching, "That's amazing. How do you know this?"

"Because I was sitting beside him."

I was now impressed but undaunted, I raised the other work.

"How about this one?" I waited, eyes twinkling; they'll learn someday to write their names on their papers.

A voice shouted, "That's mine…..but you're holding it upside-down."

We all had a laugh together.

Several years earlier, my Master's Degree professor had said to us, her adult students, that if you doodle during an emotional telephone conversation or during a class, out of boredom, when you see it again ten years later, you'll remember the physical setting and the emotions you were in. Recently at an arts and healing workshop, I saw a many-paged collection of doodles drawn from the patients of an Islamic doctor who, categorizing them over time, was able to diagnose illnesses from the patterns. An uninhibited configuration of marks will make a pattern unique to the person making them. Information, stored in the body, can make itself known through them. The expression of it is not obtained as an intentional activity of the mind.

A writer friend of mine, JoAnn Lordahl, with a PhD in Counseling Psychology, told me of a personal experience that echoes Candace Pert's theory that chemicals produced during extreme emotions can lodge in our muscles as memory. One time, submitting to a Rolfing session (deep massage,) she remembered, re-experienced, and realized an early childhood moment of being lifted out of her crib and vigorously shaken to stop her crying. This experience which she couldn't language, had registered itself chemically in her muscles, and the Rolfing pressure had released it.

The intermodal art technique, an intentional effort to use the body's knowledge to decipher what the body is expressing, moves the artist through various modes of art, bringing up material from the unconscious through, one might say, a series of sieves. For example, my professor of the doodle wisdom would first move us adult students through body exercises she'd learned in China (to detoxify us from the day,) then talk to us about theory, lower the lights, and on rice paper placed onto an inked slab, have us focus on moving our hands and fingers on the paper's surface (in a manner similar to the method the children used.) We made several monoprints this way. (I recommend numbering them.) After the papers were backed (to cover the wet ink) and taped to the wall, we'd stand in front of each other's work and look carefully, really attend, to what we were seeing. Then we'd write a few-word response onto a stick-um and paste it beside each work put up there by each person. Collecting the stick-um responses stuck onto his work, each artist would go back to the table and write a poem using those words. Often other people would see something that the artist hadn't seen regarding line, patterns, forms, repetitions, use of spacing, etc. And the artist responding with his images of experience could make his own connections.

The key word to each step of the process is "attending" so one may obtain clues for a later conclusion. Listening to the words used, seeing images but not labeling them, keeping open to the new use of an element to carry information, may trigger in the "attender" correspondingly revealed information which begins to make personal sense. Attending to one's images, impulses, and behavior in daily "doings" may help one toward healing or resolving issues carried.

After retirement, I found myself buying a thin white quilted bedcover for my bed during a time of renovating my home (an experience of intended expression.) I was interfacing some trendy ochre Herringbone material hanging over my bed with blue and white gingham. What was happening here? Finally, I realized that although I had discarded it years ago, I was reproducing a bedcover my grandmother had given me before I was old enough to be appreciative of the effort she had made for me. Instead of the gingham bonneted ladies going about their daily chores, labeled with embroidery as "laundry," "going to market," etcetera, I decided to sew a series of seven vertical spirals (in that blue and white gingham) in a sort of ladder form up the center of the coverlet, which would update my experience with days of the week and the idea of chakras. The act of sewing would reconnect me with my past in what I realized was needed at this time, a tribute and a thank you to my grandmother.

We are born into a cultural form, a ready-made construction with expected behaviors and their appropriate activities. In one aspect, culture can be like lava flowing from an erupting volcano, which upon cooling into a solid state forgets its origins. Germany during the Hitler years was not of a mind to question itself. It wasn't questioning its developing cultural behavior against pre-existing laws regarding the violence of some individuals toward others. These became real life and death matters to those who were violated. In a way, the survival of the self in any culture is a life or death matter. And art is related to cultural issues, personal issues, matters of justice, emergent birth of new views, new behavioral premises, and new freedoms. Art expresses an individual or cultural concern waiting to be given form. Cultural experience helps us grow. Our personal response to it helps us educate our intuition.

Attending to images with our conscious mind on the simplest level is how we in elementary school begin our steps in analyzing the artwork of established adult artists and in becoming sensitive to our own production efforts. Back in elementary school, after a class of cutting out paper shapes to glue into a work of art, some children stayed to help sweep up the paper scraps left on the floor.

"Look, Mrs. Mathews," a little girl called to me, holding aloft a small piece of paper.

"Somebody threw away a perfectly good shape."
"How wonderful of you," I called back. "You found it."
Her decision to use or not use a shape in her own work would depend on a conversation with her intuition, with which she is becoming familiar. It's very difficult for adults to "read" elements because we must take the time to find them. The process of questioning what is there is more difficult than comparing to find differences.

When my brother was five years old, he drew a pattern of train tracks into a circular design. Without being aware of his design, my son, at age five, drew a similar image. Though mounted in one frame, the patterns were unique, and obviously made by two different individuals. Comparing those sets up a conversation. Looking into the idea of a track pattern helps us begin to critique. A vertical track pattern may become a ladder, representing the climbing of a person, or the sequence of his spine, or the hidden matter in chests of drawers, or as Mircea Eliade in *The Sacred and the Profane*, suggests, it may connect the earth with heaven. Without knowing particularly why, I had hung a decorative vine ladder bought at a fair, on the interior of my front door. Two weeks later at the opening of a major art show I saw that Florida artist Mark Messersmith had also affixed big carved branch-wood ladders in front of several of his complicated artworks. Of course, I had to tap him on the shoulder and tell him I too had put a big ladder on my front door. He was nice about it. I felt I must be on the right track.

Steps, stairs, (ladders?)...absent on Egyptian pyramids because the surface is meant to reflect the sun and deflect others' touch, are present on Mexican pyramids to move people upwards. Their too-tall, difficult-to-climb, steps demand an effort that creates faster heartbeats and blood circulation, enhancing the quality of the activity taking place at the top. What took place there was a human sacrifice so that the relationship between man and the gods (invisible forces) would be upheld at least by Man. Man would give his all, his blood-flowing organ, to contribute to the victory of Good in the continually competing and demanding forces of Good and Evil, as well as survival.

Miles away from the (now Mexico City) Aztecs, the Mayans in the Yucatan Peninsula, who also practiced human sacrifice, refined their image of it by having royal persons drawing blood from particular members of the body (tongue, penis) so that the blood dropped onto a bowl of white papers and was burned, sending steamy messages to the gods. This variation in method (recorded in carved stone) allowed the involved royal persons not only to see if their prayers were answered, but also to be heard once again if the gods were of a mind to listen.

In our era, Mexican artist Frida Kahlo, prompted by her husband Diego Rivera, in order to resonate with historical Mexico, would include in her portrait of "The Two Fridas," a reference to the ancient Mayan stone image of bloodletting. We see her holding a clamped vein in one hand, drops of blood falling onto her white skirt, transforming into some flower patterns (pieces of paper?) at the pleated hem. The exposure of her hearts as real working organs instead of symbols is particularly Mexican in origin. The Mexican Indian, already subject to a hierarchy of set-in-stone laws and rules that favored the culture's more powerfully positioned, moved into Spanish hierarchical hands, and the "enslavement" continued, frozen positions culturally prescribed. And in the twentieth century, the cultural organization held the natives in their place as clearly as the American social order had held its "slaves." Diego Rivera's artistic expression meant to give voice and image to the Mexicans who needed to visualize consciously the cultural injustice for themselves. Ultimately, they would have to reject this injustice as a conscious demand, not as an acceptance of a forever fate, and help bring about a new organizing system of government that would go through a process of its own to emerge. Kahlo's presentation of her pain and suffering began as a personal means to give expression to her experience. Integrated into the Mexican cultural dimension, the questions of fate and the acceptance of reality were raised and visualized for the many. In my opinion, the place where honest self-awareness takes place is holy ground. Together, the artists Rivera and Kahlo spoke to the self-healing needs of a people, empowering these people as individuals in a shared cultural voice.

Teaching art in our public schools, and through it, our culture, means we are involved in the "selfing" process and healing processes as well as the growing and defining processes. Ideally, we are equipped to speak to the questions of creation, science, universal suffering, love, economics, historical eras, mathematics, astronomy, the arts, motorcycle maintenance, etc. In reality, we teachers may be busy with the processes of "selfing" and healing ourselves, which is where we ought to be.

I suggest we make a discipline of religiously attending to that process in ourselves, complete with time for consideration, reading, writing and other forms of expression, even making images for display, or, perchance to sell to somebody. For in our time we are becoming aware of the dimension of healing involved in self-expression, and religious awareness as a dimension of Creation consciousness helps prepare us for the concerns of others, past and present. In other words, believing in our unconscious growth in its individual uniqueness as being part of the intention of our universe, not as a separate result of the organism's growth schedule, raises the question of individual intention and also a Creator's intention.

Any teacher knows there will be instances when we are called upon to help children with primary concerns. In our elementary school, a first grade teacher's husband had died, and her class, led by a kindly substitute teacher who had apparently talked to the students, arrived quiet and pensive at the art room where classical music was softly being played. I had prepared ahead for them. Self-possession in children always makes an impression on me. A little girl, six years old, wearing glasses and nicely dressed, called forth from me the thought that here was an example of a child who had everything. Also in the class, a new student, a boy, consistently disruptive, set about to work on his art folder. From another teacher I'd learned a technique of having children draw their names with a marker, each letter wide enough to form a space to hold patterns. My variation was that each letter could be sideways, upside down, right side up, whatever, but it had to touch the preceding letter at least once, which meant the letters often connected with each other several times. This unified the design into a whole and left lots of room for unfettered decision-making. With the somber entry into a soft-music-filled room, making a design of impulse-driven patterns with markers, each child was involved in slowly choosing this or that set of lines or shapes to complete his folder cover, so I sat down beside the boy who at this time was quietly drawing and whispered a compliment about his working.

He continued to work. I watched, and then he said, "Of course you know that my father ran over my brother with his truck."

"Oh no," I said, "I didn't know that at all. I'm very sorry to hear that."

He continued drawing a pattern. "And my grandfather shot my father with a rifle."

I whispered more words of sympathy and he mentioned a few more of his distresses as he continued to work. Behind me, now stood the little girl I'd marveled at, and she announced,

"I've had a difficult life from the moment I was born. My father's divorced, he has a new family, and he doesn't come to see us, but my brother who is fourteen comes to our house and he is mean and scary. And I have to go to the doctor's and get shots…"

"Oh my dear," was all I could say, "oh indeed it sounds like you have had difficulties."

Then she said to the boy, "Perhaps you ought to keep a journal."

I was thankful that somebody had apparently assisted her with a plan for dealing with her concerns.

In all directions hands swung up into the air filling it with words like "divorce" and "left home." With the little girl back into her seat, I walked to the front of the room wondering what I would say. Something heartfelt drove my speaking to them, and I hoped they would get the message that I cared. I said the obvious, that we can see so many of us have worries and troubles, and life isn't easy, but maybe why we come to school is to learn how to have a better life for ourselves when we get older. Right now, so much happens to us without our permission that we really don't want to happen. We do have times with the guidance counselor and can learn how to help ourselves. (I hope I said this.) We need to be strong and be kind to each other. Soon the class ended, and I, walking in a zigzag line up to the office, asked our school secretary if all this was true.

"Oh yes," she said, and explained what she could.

I gave the boy a carved eagle on a solid wooden pencil from the Dollar Store and invited him to come to the art room before school to say, "Hello." He came several times, once to tell me he'd lost the pencil and could I get him another one. Certainly. Soon he was gone, the family moved away as abruptly as it had arrived. The little girl wanted to see *Cats*, the movie, so we collected a small group of girls and watched it after school, made purses, and began art-class connections doing other after school activities. Her health condition became worrisome, and she moved into home schooling, leaving the "gifted" classes she'd been attending. I have since retired from teaching and have never heard from her again. I do know that she has a loving family and grandparents around her.

We had experienced in that classroom intermodal art techniques which had allowed the boy to voice his concerns, concerns he had not adequately dealt with, concerns that had moved him unconsciously to perform classroom disruption. His problems may not be solved in art class, but the part of healing that accompanies recognition and voicing our unconscious distress can begin to take shape.

Distressed artist Vincent Van Gogh's "Starry Night" as a giant-sized poster was up on our classroom wall for critiquing. We began by describing 'what we saw for sure:' colors, lines, shapes, patterns, etc., anything that isn't preceded by "I think" or "That looks like a…" We saw a tree up close in the foreground on the left, brushstrokes, a horizon line, etc. Later on in our discussion, because we had previously looked at the yin-yang design, we saw that the swirls in the sky reminded us of a yin-yang design but the small centers of each of the two parts, were outside the design….in the sky around them. We were moving from naming elementary identifiable images and elements, to constructing a conclusion of meaning, which was based on them. Mike Venezia's DVD of *Vincent*

Van Gogh, funny and a good view for children and adults, handles the issue of his suicide with sensitivity at the end of the story. It is done well and doesn't become an issue of distress.

A kindergarten child, uninhibited by artistic intention after seeing the story, drew a big sunflower on the right of his paper with one petal extended upward into the top of the page. A rectangle representing a door was put in place at the tip of the upward extended petal. From the left bottom of the picture, a simple line drawing of zigzag steps moved diagonally up toward the bottom of the door and connected with it. It also touched the tip of the upward extended petal. Van Gogh was on the steps leading upward. The visual language was very clear. The child explained to me that the door was there so Van Gogh could go through it. Now I know why Picasso wanted to draw as a child does.

Drawing "The Line of Our Life" with the tip of a brush is easily done if the brush is held vertically with the palm of the hand or the elbow resting on the desk or paper. Fine lines, cursive lines, controlled comings and goings, can be thus accomplished by the youngest of children, much as they do in Japan where children learn to paint the brush-stroked word characters. Remembering or imagining our own birth, the sounds or breaths around it, our first words, our first steps, riding a bicycle, new siblings, can be indicated by a change in the line that can be interrupted, turned into dots, shapes, etc. by the use of pressure. This technique of pressing down on the brush is learned by outlining, then filling in the shapes of the spaces made by intersecting lines. Both conscious and unconscious material (as it probably always does) emerges as the activity progresses. To complete an exercise like this also teaches some staying power, as it will take several art periods, and will usually become owned by the young artist. (We used simple watercolor tray paints one can purchase in a drug store, but we also use very good brushes purchased at a discount through our county art department, which do come to a point when wet.)

Every year our elementary school participates in the Arts Center "Word and Image" contest. One year's theme was "Celebrate Harmony." In defining celebration, we thought of some examples: winning the Super Bowl so people run around outside, pushing over cars and spraying bottles of bubbly at passersby and making lots of noise, or gathering inside a house and singing Happy Birthday to your grandma and giving presents to her and lighting candles on a cake, or, as one child suggested, "celebrate Mass."

The Mass is a celebration by people gathered to share the belief that God is present with them. If a teacher's cultural understanding does not include religious practices as appropriate discussion, the subject might be avoided, but could also be simply acknowledged. If the subject has been investigated and found worthy of human consideration with known reason why, chances are it can be discussed in such a way as to include universal meanings understandable in children's words, or be historically instructive. We put it into the discussion. We decided that the thing all types of celebration had in common was the belief in our being given something, receiving a special boon from fate. Yes, a team deserved to win the Super Bowl, but we celebrate because it could have lost. Our response is ecstatic, a yippee, hooray. Grandma's Birthday is a gift of another day, we hope years, and the Mass is a celebration of the belief in the continuation of life itself in some good form, after death. (Didn't we study about that idea in Ancient Egypt?) And our response in gratitude is to celebrate. We are grateful for the occasion of realizing good fortune. In the religious dimension we are told to be grateful in all things, all the time. A culture may think life goes on after death, but those who recognize it as a belief in reality may find their daily decisions become based on this premise, and they may find a dimension to the symbols and images in works of art that a secular culture does not feel and therefore does not see.

In fact, if we are studying cultures in our schools today, or art history in our art classes, we need to have a capacity for recognizing what premises are driving cultural behaviors, expressions, or works of art…along with some discussion on what we consider works of art to be. One needs to be very careful in, for example, comparing the Mexican culture's Day of the Dead with "our" Halloween. Believing the spirits of ancestors live in one of a number of "Undergrounds" or "Heavens" (not any are a punishing place for life's transgressions,) the living can prepare gravesites as an elaborate invitation for the loved ones to return for a day of sharing. Incense and flower scent beckons the spirit, and paths of flower petals show the way to the desired destination. Favorite foods and pleasures are appropriately represented (Nov. 1 for "tender souls" such as children, and Nov. 2, for adults, hence the addition of cigarettes and tequila.) In pre-Columbian times, Aztec warriors fought "Flowery Wars" for sacrificial "victims" and real skulls have been replaced today with white decorated sugar skulls. Large marigold X's represent two opposing forces, as well as two integrating forces, and the two solstices, as well as the several Native calendars based on the sun, stars, and observations of the Milky Way. It is possible that the pre-Columbian configuration of cosmic dynamics stays in place because, though the Christian proposition regarding the cosmos has been accepted, the cultural reality has not made room for the recognition of the Indian psyche as an equal.

Families, children to grandparents, all work to prepare the gravesites and an "altar" or table to honor and be with the deceased. This experience isn't exactly Halloween that no longer includes its source of meaning for its continuation. Not in touch with its origins, we buy ready-made costumes, and our children beg, depending on the kindness of strangers, to fill their sacks full of sugar stuff, maybe Snickers bars or wrapped up Milky Ways. If we start with what the images represent (traditionally as in the Day of the Dead or open-ended, in assessing our own images,) we are in a position to enter their dimensions of meaning. We can "sleuth out" what's on tap for our own soul. In the presence of images from our sources, emerging and living, we should remove our shoes; we are on hallowed ground…hallowed ground as adults, "reading" our images, or as participants in others' resourceful presentations, or even as teachers helping students "self" themselves through self-disclosure.

Elementary images become our source, our self, our Universe.

References

Eliade, Mircia. *The Sacred and the Profane*, Orlando: Harcourt, 1957.
Pert, Candace. Interview by Bill Moyers. *Healing and the Mind:* PBS, 1993.
Venezia, Mike. "Van Gogh," *Getting to Know the World's Great Artists.* DVD, www.gettingtoknow.com,1989.

MANDALA: PATH OF PEACE

MELANIE CIRCLE

Mandala: Sanskrit for circle, sacred circle, both center and circumference.

Years ago, I used my own version of Mandala when working with "troubled" teens. I asked these kids who had little interest in art, and less in doing anything I suggested, to write their name on a 15"x22" sheet of paper. I asked them to write it again and again, large and small, turning the page, overlapping the letters, continuing until there was just a design of squiggles. I gave them oil pastels and suggested they fill the spaces with color. Although they each created colorful abstracts, nobody seemed too attached to their work. I told them to tear the paper into small pieces. There were a few startled looks, and then gleeful destruction. When each sat with a pile of colored bits, I gave them heavy pieces of Bristol board and glue. I suggested they make a mandala, using the colored pieces in any way they wished as long as the final image was within a circle.

The results were powerful and stunningly beautiful. I never quite understood why these collages were so universally "successful;" I suspected there was something about the form…

In 2002, during a trip to Northern India, I became fascinated by Tibetan Mandalas. I visited the traditional mandala workshops of Norblinka Institute outside of Dharmsala. The young men made their paints from pure powders and painstakingly copied the mandalas that had been copied for centuries. The peace in the workshop was palpable. Later, I stood silent and awestruck in the monastery of Alchi in Ladakh's Himalayas. An enormous bodhisattva and countless mandalas, busy with life and peace, sang out from the 13th century.

When I returned to Canada, I began to study, to practice, and eventually to offer workshops in Mandala. Following semi-traditional formats as well as creating mandalas in loose exploratory ways, I was amazed by the peace that accompanied the process. I was often surprised and sometimes informed by the images that arose within the container of the mandala. And, I've been continually delighted by the pleasure, surprise, insight and peace I notice in others who embark on the journey of creating a mandala.

-o-

Exercise 1.
Stand with your arms at your sides; place your feet on the floor (if they're not already there;) bounce softly, bending your knees a bit, maintaining your feet flat on the floor. Breathe deeply into your belly, finding the spot that is about two inches below your belly button and half way between your front and back. Feel the weight of your arms as they hang from your shoulders. Continue to breathe deeply, noticing what you feel inside your belly and inside your legs. Raise your arms to shoulder level. Reach far apart, savoring the feeling of your hands. As you slowly begin to spin around, notice all that you hear. Breathe deeply, and slowly turn until you are facing your original position. YOU HAVE JUST CREATED A MANDALA. With your body and breath as the center, your hands inscribe one ring, while the horizon of your vision forms the circumference. Center and Circumference.

-o-

Traditionally mandalas have been tools of meditation. Tibetan mandalas serve as idealized maps of the cosmos, within and without. The Chinese Yin-Yang holds the paradox and tension of apparent opposites in the unity of the circle. Native American medicine wheels form part of their traditional healing arts. The rose windows of European and American cathedrals bless us with rhythms of color and light. A labyrinth, seemingly infinite within its circle of containment, provides a path for deep meditation. Stonehenge still stands. Art within a sacred circle has appeared throughout the ages, around the world.

In the early twentieth century, Carl Jung pioneered the modern mandala. Whereas Tibetans and others selflessly, stringently followed rituals and existing formats, repeating what had been done before, Jung used the mandala in an entirely new and Western way. The Western mandala became a tool for self-expression and self-exploration.

As a personal practice, Jung created a mandala every morning. With the only requirement being the circle format, he allowed images to pour onto the paper. In this way he had insight into his own state of being, evidence of what otherwise could remain hidden or buried. Creating these morning mandalas became a personal fishing expedition, capturing rewards from the deep. Recognizing these healing and in-sightful diagnostic powers, Jung also encouraged patients to create mandalas.

Mandala has come to mean any art created within a circle. It can be formed with paint, with pencil, with sand, with butter, with stones, with bodies, with breath, with whatever you think of. In the West, mandala work has become a way of exploring the self: a way of orienting oneself within the world, a way of journeying inward. The mandala provides a container capable of holding the peace and the chaos, the disparate realities of life itself.

-o-

Why is the mandala so familiar? Why is the practice of mandala so apropos today? How does the creation of mandalas encourage peace?
Roundness of form and movement are everywhere. Body-wise, we begin as an egg. Pierced by sperm, we grow within the warm round womb. We enter this world through a tubular tunnel, landing in our mother's (someone's) circular embrace. Our breath is circular, a continuous in and out and in again. The horizon curves; "as far as the eye can see" is always round. We walk this spherical earth under the apparent dome of the sky. In community, we sit in circle, around tables and fires as we spin on this round earth around our sun. We cycle through the seasons: spring, summer, autumn, winter, spring, summer, autumn, winter, spring. Birth into death into birth…

-o-

Exercise 2:
As you read these words, notice your breathing. If the breath isn't reaching deep into your belly, to that spot a couple of inches below your belly button, midway between your front and back, let it flow there. Do you feel any warmth or aliveness there? If you're sitting, notice how your butt feels against the chair. Squeeze your anus and let it loose again. Wiggle your toes. Keep reading, but don't lose your awareness of all the messages your body is sending you. Being intellectually occupied is no excuse for cutting off the sensations in your body or the depth of your breathing. (Continue this exercise as you read. Actually, continue this exercise as you eat, as you think, as you walk, as you drive. Continue this exercise until it's no longer an exercise! The goal is to **in-habit** your body…always.)

As the center reaches out to the world, natural growth often shows us mandalas. Cut into an orange, look at the rings of a tree stump, stare at a daisy, watch a jellyfish swim, crack open an egg, gaze into a tidal pool containing sea urchins and starfish, flick water into a pond. Think of snowflakes. Picture the eye of someone you love. There are countless examples of mandalas around us.

-o-

In times of transition (when are you not in transition?) it is important to center yourself. As you reach out to the world, it's useful to remember the definition of the mandala: Center and Circumference. As I become more anchored within my center, I am able to function more effectively on the circumference. I can scan the horizon, but to give it meaning, I need to be anchored in my body—right here, right now. Center and Circumference.

Last week I was up a ladder picking cherries. The further I reached for those dark, dark red ones, the more I needed to anchor my awareness down, deep down into my feet, the ladder, and the earth far below. As my awareness moved downward, I could safely reach cherries further away. Balance. Center and Circumference.

Cherry:
Thin red protective skin

Around juicy dark mid-section, bursting with life,

dripping sweet, sometimes tart

source of dreams.

The seed: sacred center,

hard-core promise of life to come.

Mandalas are everywhere.

-o-

In these scary times plagued by polarized thought forms, the practice of mandala is more relevant than ever. Everywhere I look, I see people lined up on either side of seemingly unbridgeable gulfs. They stand staring with anger, disbelief, and ignorance; sometimes, not even staring, but studiously looking away. The extreme realities of poverty/wealth, ease/dis-ease, have's/have-nots, left/right, pious/heathen, "us and them" forever....We are stuck in patterns of polarization. Mandala practice offers a way to begin to deal with these seemingly exclusive extremes. In creating mandalas we form a container that can hold severely conflicting realities. Within the circle, all can be contained. In that containment, I can afford to accept and consider the existing realities. From there I can perchance begin to see ways of working with what is there and toward what I would like to see. Without the initial honest assessment, I don't have a chance. Simply beholding the disparities becomes a path of peace. Like many other things, peace is contagious.

Of the therapeutic possibilities of the mandala, Jung wrote:

"The fact that images of this kind have under certain circumstances a considerable therapeutic effect on their authors is empirically proved and also readily understandable, in that they often represent very bold attempts to see and put together apparently irreconcilable opposites and bridge over apparently hopeless splits. Even the mere attempt in this direction usually has a healing affect..." (1959)

-o-

Of the many ways to create mandalas, there are two that I practice and offer in workshops. Neither requires artistic experience or "ability." Both require attention to breath and the body. Both allow the exploration of self in relation to the world. They are peace practices in that they offer time and space to center, to focus, to make choices and to behold. They are peace practices in that they allow me to see what's happening along the inner path. That is the first step toward peace—turning my awareness within to notice and accept what I find.

Before any artmaking I make sure that my body and breath are engaged. Art, (like anything else) is best done with all of me. I don't paint with my hand tightly gripping the brush. The movement doesn't come from my fingers and wrist. It comes from my feet, my legs, my butt on the chair, my belly, my breath and my heart. All sensations and awareness of sounds flow into the art. The movement comes from all of me – the art is one edge of the dance. Qi gong and yoga-like exercises along with directed and free movement encourage presence in the process.

-o-

I work with "spontaneous mandalas" that utilize a process similar to that employed by Jung in his morning mandalas. Using ArtStix and squares of heavy paper, I ask people to start just moving colors on paper. With the only parameter being the emergence of something circular, I ask them not to think or direct their creation. I suggest they stay with the "not knowing" and continue to move the color around. After a while, some image will begin to emerge, or perhaps certain colors or shapes will intrigue them. I suggest they follow whatever they see and bring it further along. This exercise generally takes about twenty minutes. During the process, I remind people of their breath, their bellies, and their feet on the floor. We don't leave bodies behind.

Exercise #3
If you have the materials and would like to try it, follow the instructions above. But first, repeat exercises #1.

Some people begin with a looseness and willingness to not intellectually direct their mandalas. Others insist on preconceived symbols or images from the start. After practicing this type of mandala for a while, most delight in trusting the process, of initially surrendering to a non-directed color play and eventually noticing and coaxing whatever comes.

Inevitably, the "spontaneous mandala" is relevant and reflective of who they are that day. The mandala can be further explored individually or in a group, leading to strong team building. It can move into poetry or dance, or merely be gazed upon directly or peripherally. There is always a gift waiting to be received. Shaun McNiff sees "Images as angels" and suggests respect and hospitality for what emerges:

"In extending hospitality, we greet the person, spend time together, talk, enjoy each other's company, and afterward feel enriched or ensouled by the visit. Can't we extend this courtesy to the images we make?" (2004)

-o-

The more prolonged, intricate mandala that I work with is an amalgamation of a traditional Tibetan format with Western self-exploration and expression. It offers a different type of meditation and requires a larger commitment in terms of time, intention and focus. The potential learning is vast and the finished product is always wonderful. (Although the finished mandala is merely a by-product of the rich journey, it's nice to have something powerful at the end.) Anyone who stays with these processes of mind, body, heart and breath will end up with a beautiful piece of peace.

Embarking upon this type of mandala journey is similar to walking the Camino de Santiago (or any pilgrimage.) I may start out thinking I'm traversing a pre-set path with external challenges (as in paint and brush management,) but through intention, perseverance and focus, it soon becomes spiritual. The pilgrimage is then made one step (or brushstroke) at a time, hopefully with growing and expanding awareness. The creation of this mandala allows the consideration and contemplation of my world.

The painting is ritually done from the outer ring toward the center. First, a ring of fire is painted. Colors and symbols are chosen for this outer ring to provide protection as the painter/pilgrim travels inward. The second ring is a consideration of the material world. What does matter? In the third ring, the dream world is explored. This could be comprised of hopes and aspirations, sensed spiritual realities or literally dreams and nightmares. Next, the gates or portals to the sacred center are constructed. Within each gate is a guardian. These guardians can be fierce and intimidating or representative of qualities needed to pass through the gates into the Sacred Center. Having completed the mandala to this stage, it's time to turn back to the circumference, to choose one color that will hold it all together, and to paint a thin line around it all.

Colors and symbols only need make sense or have meaning for the painter. The repetition involved in painting each ring is a meditation and provides a chance for deeper and deeper exploration. Perfection doesn't matter. It is willingness, focus, awareness and intention that create the mandala. It is always beautiful.

-o-

This is not about making fine art. It is about the process of art-making. Expressive arts explorations have everything to do with how we've lived our lives and how we'd like to live. Expressive arts therapist Dr. Brian Nichols stated, "We can't always change our lives, but we can change how we make art." What we practice in making art becomes part of our way of being; it eventually moves out into how we live our lives. Taking time to create a mandala, to make art in a centered, conscious and focused manner shapes how we function when we aren't holding paintbrush or pencil.

"Let there be peace on earth, and let it begin with me....."

References

Jung, C.G., *Mandala Symbolism*. Princeton, NJ: Princeton University Press, 1959, 5.
Fincher, Susanne F., *Creating Mandalas*. Boston: Shambala Press, 1991.
McNiff, Shaun, *Art Heals*. Boston: Shambala Press, 2004.

A JOURNEY THROUGH TIME

FRANCES FALK

"The journey is the destination."
—Marilyn Ferguson

Each and every one of us has been on a long, long journey—nearly fourteen billion years long. We have come to a space now where we can rest before starting out again on the next lap of it.

We cannot help but be aware that there is in progress a global change in thinking which is moving us from the unidirectional straight lines we have been following into interconnected circles. Evidence is all around us that we are in a space that is like a pit between two worldviews. The road ahead is flavored with uncertainty because starting out from here is stepping into the unknown, and, as someone put it, like beginning to write a sentence before you know its ending. The sun is rising on a new day, though, and we have to pick ourselves up and move on whether we like it or not.

Within this larger picture, related to my work in the field of expressive art, I think of the metaphor of journey in the following two ways. First, a "journey through time" can be seen as the evolutionary journey of a model for health and healing which is in the process of emerging now as a post-modern, integral model. This holds great interest for me because of my many years as an expressive arts facilitator, helping cancer patients and others experience their creative process as a way to wholeness and healing. My work as a studio artist as well has involved me in projects devoted to art and spirituality and art and healing. Michael Samuels, MD writes, "Art, prayer, and healing: all come from the same source—the human soul. The energy that fuels these processes is the basic force of life, of creativity, of love." I cannot but strongly agree.

The second way I will make use of this metaphor of a "journey through time" is by introducing you to an art project that was displayed at the 18th annual conference of the National Expressive Therapy Association held in St. Petersburg, Florida in 2006. Later it became an exhibit, traveling in Florida and then to parts of New York and New England.

Presenting large scale paintings, sculpture, and an interactive labyrinth installment, the exhibit called "LifeDance: Our Journey through Time" uses the power of art to tell the great epic story of our universe and ourselves and, in doing so, becomes a site where cosmology, art, and spirituality come together on common ground to serve as a way of "healing with art and soul."

Integral Healing: a Journey into the Future

Crisis precedes transformation. The traditional model of western medicine has been in crisis. A post-modern integral paradigm for healing emerging today embraces all previous approaches including traditional, alternative, complementary, and integrative. At the same time, it transcends all it includes by creating a fundamentally new vision. Much more than just a therapeutic approach, it becomes an integral philosophy that goes from simply body, mind, and spirit to encompass scientific, social, political, economic, metaphysical, ecological and even cosmological dimensions of the person. It is biopsychosociocultural (Astin, 2002.)

In her essay "Towards a Post-modern Integral Medicine," Elliott S. Dacher, MD, writes about what will characterize the post-modern integral model that claims an expansion in consciousness as its foundation. Previous attempts to go beyond the traditional model caused a horizontal expansion of the scope of what already existed in medicine. The new vision, in the process of emergence, expands vertically. Embracing all previous outer approaches, it reshapes and weaves them into inner aspects of healing that have been rediscovered. Objective, measurable and subjective, and outer and inner now become inseparable. Each changes its opposite in such a way that both soon become two aspects of the same reality. That reality's components can be said to come together in a synergy and form a new seamless whole that is greater than the sum of its parts.

There have been several recent attempts to bring change to an entrenched health care system that is no longer effectively dealing with present day problems and is at odds with the post-modern viewpoint. One of these was the first wellness center that opened in the seventies. Dacher recounts how all the attempts, including that center, were eventually assimilated into the larger culture in a way that caused them to resemble traditional approaches and soon became packaged as wellness commodities with labels such as "holistic medicine." Old perspectives doomed the efforts, incorporating and reshaping them and accommodating them to the assumptions of the existing worldviews. As she says, "Without a defining leap in consciousness all we do is expand the range and scope of what is, deluding ourselves in thinking we are creating fundamental change... Wellness became prevention, holism became an empty word, alternative approaches became alternative treatments, and mind-body strategies became relaxation techniques" (Dacher, 2005.)

Two questions facing us now are: how do we give hospice care to what is ideologically dying and how are we to bury the dead? What we need to do first in order to take up the difficult task of being midwife to this new vision is to look for the seeds of new life in what we have. The older biomedical model came to its peak out of advances in science and technologies. With it, there existed a dualism between consciousness and matter, mind and body. However, it is the development of more outer technologies, informational and digital, that have actually brought us to a place that promises a transformation.

Meditation, contemplation, and mindfulness, which are called 'inner technologies,' along with a renewed appreciation for the sacred are hopeful signs emerging today. A concept of consciousness including the meaning of an expression of the direct experience of the sacred has transcended religion as we have known it, and a deepening of the capacity for self-reflection has put us in touch with the deeper voice of our souls. Dr. Dacher calls the new integral model "a seamless integration of the outer and inner aspects of healing."

LifeDance: Our Journey Through Time

Labyrinths are circular walkways created from sacred geometry. They are found in all religions of the world and in the art of every culture. Walking their paths, one becomes part of a large integrating mandala that reflects universal wholeness. They are said to have a unique transformative energy that somehow creates a harmonic vibration with healing energy. Since Medieval times, entering and walking the labyrinth has become a metaphor for the journey through life.

In the "LifeDance" exhibit, a twenty-five foot seven path Cretan labyrinth becomes the space for a cosmic walk through time. Surrounding this labyrinth are very large black fabric screens with paintings of galaxies, nebulas, and star 242 is order. As we walk the path and make our journey, they hold us, as if within the cosmic womb of Mother Universe, until we emerge as the first human beings. Telling the story of the universe in this way seeks to awaken awareness that this is our story, too. Although not yet in our human form, we were there from the beginning at the birthplace of the universe, rooted in the primordial fire and made from the contents of stardust. Small, solid painted shrines for markers reveal the proportion of the time sequence to us as we walk.

Making our way along the meandering path to the center, we hear the story told through earphones and are directed to stop at each of seven little shrines or stations that depict the main events along the way, starting with the birth of existence. Nearing the center of the labyrinth, we arrive at the seventh station that represents human emergence around 2.6 million years ago. Because it is too hard to wrap our minds around these billions and millions of years, we are asked to imagine all of this as one calendar year of our time. In May of that year, the Milky Way is formed. Only in September, exploding stardust begins to cool down and condense into a community of planets around our sun and our solar system is born.

We come to December and, on the last day of the year at 10:30 in the evening, the first human beings emerge with brains and nervous systems complex enough for Earth now to awaken into self-conscious awareness. Reaching the center, we are a few seconds before midnight on that last day of the year when Earth enters a new phase of consciousness through its human expression. It had controlled itself instinctively for those past billions of years but now it places itself in human hands and confides its destiny to human decisions. All creation trembles, waiting and hoping that human earthlings will accept their role with compassion, will drop their illusions of separateness, and integrate their lives into the life of the planet.

After a few minutes of quiet reflection at the center, we are asked to retrace our steps and come out of the labyrinth to view the eight paintings on the walls. These represent the human in the image of a feminine figure dancing in the two biospheres, the hydrosphere (pictured below,) geosphere, atmosphere, noospere (pictured on this book cover,) galaxy, and as a sundancer. This dancer in each painting is an archetype of woman, nurturing, being nurtured, and embodying Gaia, planet Earth as that living organism with a capacity to express its feeling and to celebrate.

Meaning: a Healing Force

One cannot overstate the important roles that meaning and purpose play in healing. Rachel Naomi Remen, MD, author, and founder of the Institute for the Study of Health, writes to physicians, "Meaning heals us by reminding us of our integrity, who we are and what we stand for. It offers us a place from which to meet the challenges of life" (2001.) The well known author of many books on consciousness, spirituality, and healing, Larry Dossey, MD, sees meaning as the most important aspect of healing. It is his belief that healing is about discovering our non-local nature, which is the infinite quality of our consciousness and its capacity to exist in space and time (Dossey, 2005.)

In terms of both the individuals and our whole culture, a sense of loneliness, isolation, and alienation seems to be the epidemic of our day. The social ties of previous times and the feelings of belonging to a community that came with them are lacking. However, the rate and ease of communications have accelerated and that actually should be connecting us. This is also a time when the planet is exploding in a destructive way and its amazing life system is withering. A "cancer of the spirit" seems to be affecting western culture, which affects the entire globe.

Considering all of this, what are the basic symbols representing human presence on the Earth in our times? Could one be the shopping mall? At times, we can get the idea that the role of the human is to obtain merchandise. Today the notion of "enough" is often laughed at and looked at as the mark of a simpleton. Cosmologist Brian Swimme, in a series of tapes called "The Earth's Imagination," shows how we are now becoming the greatest disaster to hit the planet in sixty-five million years. Biologists estimate that it will take ten million years to regenerate what we have already destroyed. Perhaps a million years into the future, humans, speaking about the Great Mass Extinctions, may be saying "…and the fifth one was caused by that strange species called the American consumer" (Swimme, 1998.)

The "Cosmic Species" Archetype

Is it possible to restore the balance and harmony that will bring about individual and collective healing and to reconnect with the universe and each other in a way that halts this downward spiral? What can help us transcend our culture and even move us into a greater sensitivity and capacity for awe? Duane Elgin, in an essay, "Archetypes of Humanity's Collective Future," says the images and archetypes that we visualize together and hold can act as a magnet and draw us into a future that will be meaningful for humanity. He writes:

> "We require tools of imagination that enable us to stand back from current crisis and see the human journey in a larger perspective. The most difficult challenge facing humanity is not devising solutions to the energy crisis or the climate crisis or even species extinction. It is bringing images and archetypes of the human journey into our collective awareness that will empower us to actualize who we think we are." (2008)

One of the powerful archetypes Elgin presents to help us collectively imagine a positive pathway into the future is that of a cosmic species learning to live in a living universe. It sees itself as part of a seamless fabric of creation and awakens to a sense of connection. No longer viewing ourselves as isolated beings whose identity stops at the edge of our skin but as interconnected beings immersed in an interwoven field of aliveness, we can discover a new sense of identity. A species of both biological and cosmic dimensions is taken in the spaciousness of a vastly larger journey.

I have found that the LifeDance cosmic walk and the visual art images support and lead to these insights and become a healing journey for individuals. Wherever I have taken it, the responses have far exceeded my expectations. A few examples of typical comments in the guest book demonstrate the impact the LifeDance project had on individuals:

> This is more than an art exhibit. It is an experience!
> Magnificent – mind and body expanding...
> I have never before experienced art in this manner. It is an experience I will never forget.
> It helps me to realize the immensity and spirituality of the universe...only gratitude can express one's feelings...
> Thank you very much for your passion in helping to tell people what life is really about.

After walking on the labyrinth and viewing the paintings, one comes to the Heartnet, a 6' X 4' banner with a large painted image of planet Earth and the poem of Tagore that begins, "The same stream of life that runs through my veins night and day runs through the world and dances in rhythmic measures..." Thrown over this banner is a big dark blue fishing net with the outline of a heart woven in red ribbon. Nearby, a table of art materials and a poster invite participants to express their reflections, experience, or heart wishes and attach these expressions to the Heartnet. One of these artistic attachments on the Heartnet had words in color within a heart shape that were arranged in a way that they spiraled into the center of the paper. The words express a deepening of meaning and indicate a new vision and perspective:

> In all my life, I have never felt before that I was ever in those 14 billion years in any way. Walking the labyrinth with the helpful words and art of the artist, was truly a tremendous experience and an awakening for me, helping me confirm my heart wish for our universe that we all walk

together, understanding our responsibility, not only doing no further damage but also restoring and enhancing.

Whenever the LifeDance exhibit is open to the public, I try to be a silent presence to hold a space that might facilitate a going inward and the final art experience. Largely this role is taken by the labyrinth itself as it lies within those maternal arms of the large black fabric paintings. After their walk, a number of individuals have often approach me to ask questions about the process of creating the labyrinth and paintings. Most just want to sit and share their experience or reflect on their finished art image. Sometimes flashes of self-discovery surface. I try to be totally attentive to the person as well as to what is happening inside of me. Respectfully, I ask if it will be all right to share what I experienced in looking and listening. In order to facilitate closure, giving a title to the art image may be suggested.

It is a challenge for me as an artist to be present in this manner without an agenda in my own head, and not trying to figure out what is going on. My role is just to provide a safe and open container in which something could take form if and when it needs to, and could find the passionate space to transform.

Prometheus of Greek mythology stole fire from the Gods and brought it as his great gift to humankind but he took away from us knowledge of the future. It is said he granted the gift of hope. Expressive art therapy always has been and is for me like a journey I am making, carrying these gifts of fire and hope. I like to think of this path as without a destination. I somewhat understand Marilyn Ferguson's thinking when she found it a paradox that a goal often betrays the process. The journey is the destination.

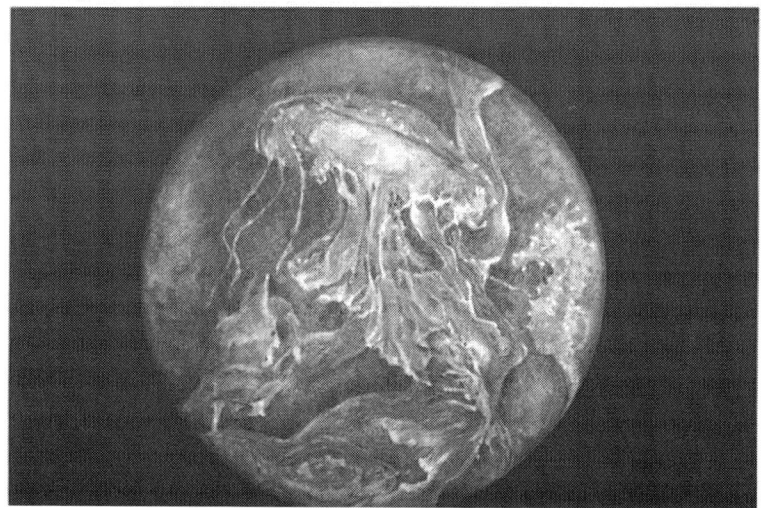

References

Astin, J. A. and A. W. Astin. "An Integral Approach to Medicine." *Alter. Ther. Health Med.* 8 (2002): 70-75.

Berry, Thomas. *The Dream of the Earth.* San Francisco: Sierra Club Books, 1998.

Dacer, Elliott. "Towards Post-Modern Integral Medicine." *Consciousness and Healing.* St. Louis: Elsevier Churchill Livingstone, 2005.

Dossey, Larry. DVD documentary for *Consciousness and Healing,* Elsevier Inc. California. Interview 2005.

Elgin, Duane. "Archetypes of Humanity's Collective Future." *Kosmos Journal* (Spring, Summer 2008.)

Halprin, Anna and Michael Samuel. *Returning to Health: with Dance, Movement and Imagery.* California: Life Rhythm, 2002.

Remen, Rachael Naomi. "Recapturing the Soul of Medicine." *The Western Journal of Medicine 74* (2001): 4-5.

Schlitz, Marilyn and Tina Amorok, Eds. *Consciousness and Healing: Integral Approaches to Mind-Body Medicine.* St. Louis: Elsevier, Churchill Livingstone 2005.

Institute of Noetic Sciences. *The 2007 Shift Report* "Evidence of a World Transforming" *The 2008 Shift Report* 18 (March-May): "Changing the Story of Our Future."

Swimme, Brian. *Earth's Imagination*. (a series of four VHS tapes,) California: Center for the Story of the Universe, 1998.

Swimme, Brian and Thomas Berry. *The Universe Story*. California: Harper, 1992.

West, Melissa Gayle. *Exploring the Labyrinth: a Guide for Healing and Spiritual Growth*. New York: Random House, Inc., 2000.

V: ENGAGING WORD

SOMETIMES WORDS ARE NOT ENOUGH

OLIVE M. "HOLLIE" ADKINS

I have always understood music and visual arts to be important elements of the healing process, but it was only when I began to use poetry, storytelling, and improvisation in my work in the arts in medicine program at a local hospital that I realized how powerful these modalities can be. At a recent Poet's Circle in the main lobby, a patient's wife came in and sat tensely in a chair as I read some poems and our harpist played. When we invited people to join us in creating a poem, she came over and began to tell us of her uneasiness and anxiety while her husband was undergoing a painful procedure. We started to think of words and phrases, moving them around on a magnetic board and before long, a very expressive poem was created. She looked at us with tears and told us how relieved she felt, no longer fearful, instead inspired and hopeful. This is the poem:

IN SILENT APPLAUSE

Like pain, the song eventually fades
on ripples floating silently away. ... .
comforting the soul
(all encompassed, all enraptured
accepted in silent applause)

Like joy, the melody remains
on strings of nature's harp. ... .
comforting the soul
(all encompassed, all enraptured
accepted in silent applause)

Like touch, the healing winds converge
on sweeping wings in corners of hope ... . .
comforting the soul
(all encompassed, all enraptured
accepted in silent applause)
Pain ... Joy ... . Touch ... Life ... Love . ...

Another time at Poets' Circle, the revolving doors of the hospital inspired a community poem as the group talked about issues of fear, anxiety, and learning to let go in order to live in the moment. The words came easily as we began to create this poem:

IN THE LOBBY

Walking through revolving doors
patients seeking patience
having lost our power
trying to find that well
of strength within.

With every revolution of the doors
focus lost and regained
learning to let go
to stop pushing doors
already turning
opening us to the day.

One day I received a referral to visit a patient who spoke only Spanish and whose cancer had left her face with a serious deformity. My Spanish is limited but I was able to determine that she and I were both grandmothers, "abuelas." I found an appropriate story on the Internet in both languages and was able to return and read it to her in Spanish and establish rapport with her.

At our evening open studio called "Night Out" a patient's family came in. The young girl went over to the magnetic words and began to create a poem. When she was finished, she let me read it aloud. We were all amazed by her talent and imagination. Her poem follows:

In a vision
I soar after dark
into a full moon
and memories blossom
like a beautiful storm
and a voice says
there is happy
but you must
dream the magic
to begin the story.

Artists trained in the expressive arts or Music for Healing and Transition Program understand that patients and caregivers cannot always express their concerns in words. There are times when paper and watercolor enable them to get in touch with their feelings. Other times just listening to music is helpful. We take our books of community art and poetry to the bedside where patients can enjoy just turning the pages. Occasionally a picture or poem will trigger a memory that they share with us.

Sometimes words are not enough
the body has to try
to speak its truth, to have its say ~
it sometimes wants to play
or dance or leap for joy ~
to spread its arms and fly
or sometimes beat its fists against a wall
too angry then to cry
or lie there crumpled in a heap
too miserable to die.

For those times words are not enough
the body needs to fly
perhaps to cry, and maybe even die
a little, and its cells
must sing their songs
its muscles weep their tears
its very bones to shiver
with their fears ~
and for those times mere words
are not enough.

During my years of psychodrama training, I became enamored with playback theatre and found yet another way to bring the healing arts to patients, families and staff at the hospital. Playback is improvisational theatre honoring personal story. It is performed by a troupe of actors, led by a conductor, who listen with their hearts to a person's story and then "play back" what they hear as its essence. Encouraged by our arts in medicine coordinator, I began to study the playback process, recruiting and training our own improvisational theatre troupe. We were invited to another hospital for a brief training course from their arts in medicine staff. Then we practiced, while studying everything we could find on "playback."

Now we prepare ourselves with a centering exercise, and travel to waiting rooms throughout the center with poetry, instruments, props and colored scarves, engaging people in warm-up exercises. Sometimes one of the actors will tell a little vignette and the troupe will play it back, just to get things started. Then we ask for conflicting feelings. "Does anyone have mixed feelings about the holiday coming up?" When we get some responses, we show these feelings in contrasting pairs. We then ask the patients for personal stories or vignettes that are played back for them with music and movement.

Our presentations can be light hearted and entertaining, but sometimes become deep and meaningful when a serious story is told, such as the one where an ex-patient volunteered to tell us her story. She was a foster parent who was called in to a hospital to spend time with a tiny abandoned baby girl who was dying. She came every day to rock her and talk to her and soon the baby began to improve. She was later able to take the child home and even later adopt her. That very week they had celebrated the child's tenth birthday. Our troupe acted out the key elements of the story as she watched, smiling through tears. At the end, they counted out all the years and sang happy birthday. We were all moved by that experience, and other similar stories. As we end each presentation, we find that people are talking to each other and the whole mood of the room has changed.

On another occasion when our troupe presented "Acts of Kindness" at a local church as part of a global playback theatre event, a woman told us about her friend, who was killed in a terrible automobile accident. A stranger came along, and finding the victim's cell phone, began to dial the numbers, letting his people know what had happened to him. She was moved to tears as she related the story. Our troupe quickly shifted into a somber scene, acting out the story and ending it with the family mourning together. A touching note was the fact that a little girl who was taking part in the playback experience was drawn right into the mourning tableau and added to its pathos. The woman was grateful that we were willing to move from an upbeat mood in order to honor her request.

Poetry is presented at the hospital in workshops or presentations in various ways. Sometimes we invite a guest poet to come and share poetry in one of the lobbies. Other times poems are woven into musical presentations. Every year I direct a workshop involving poetry, movement, music and dramatic interpretation, presented by our staff and volunteers along with guest artists. One woman, who has been a coordinator for an arts in medicine program, and who choreographs and dances her own version of American Sign Language, came to present her own workshop "See How They Dance ~ Her Hands They Dance."

This presentation included poetry and songs with flute and harp, original music by a double bass player, creative dancing with hand-painted scarves, as well as the 18 healing movements of Shibashi, all enhanced by the sign language interpretation. Much of the program was interactive with audience participation.

Often I am asked to compose poetry based on the themes of the hospital's conferences. An interesting experience occurred last year when I helped facilitate an expressive arts component at a Latino conference. Since most of the attendees spoke no English, I had my meditation (called "Loosing the Chains") translated and gave it in Spanish. Afterwards we brainstormed for relevant words and phrases and came up with a community poem, written in English and once again translated into Spanish. The participants loved the whole process, but were especially touched by the fact that I spoke in Spanish instead of having my words translated by someone else.

At a weekly "Scribes' Hour," a time of writing and storytelling, I asked one of the participants if he would like to write his story. When he explained that his English was too limited, I offered to write it down for him if he would tell it. He proceeded to give me a brief biography of his interesting life, including the courtship of his wife many years ago. When I typed his story and read it back to him, both he and his wife were very moved and grateful. His story, along with a copy of his painting of a Paris street scene, were included in a collection of hospital stories that were compiled as a means to encourage patients and families to write about their experiences as a part of their healing process. An interesting note is the fact that this man had never painted in his life until he developed a terminal disease. While at the residential facility owned by the hospital for patients in long-term care and their families, he painted and donated several pictures that were auctioned to help with the funding of the lodge.

Finding ways to reach patients, families, and staff at the hospital is a challenge that the arts in medicine team faces every day. The most important part of our work involves being present with the person and listening to what is being said as well as what is unspoken. If we remain flexible and allow the process to unfold, we can usually help the patient or family member get in touch with his or her own creativity.

Sometimes anxiety and fear have to be acknowledged before anything else can happen. Other times the person is ready to create a painting, a poem, even a greeting card that expresses love and concern. Recently we had grandchildren come in and paint loving messages on ceiling tiles for their grandparent in the hospital. Another vital aspect of this work is to remember that it is not about us. We need to leave our artistic egos outside the door if we are to be truly present for the people whom we are hoping to reach. It is therefore with a grateful heart that I find myself in my retirement years in the midst of a vital and exciting career, working with a talented and dedicated team of expressive artists. This hospital is one of the ones who are leading the way in the medical field by making every effort to meet the physical, emotional, and spiritual needs of its patients and families who come through its doors. Our arts in medicine program is proud to play a part in this effort to heal the whole person.

VOICES FROM THE CIRCLE: WOMEN'S RITUAL ART

LYNN CAROL HENDERSON

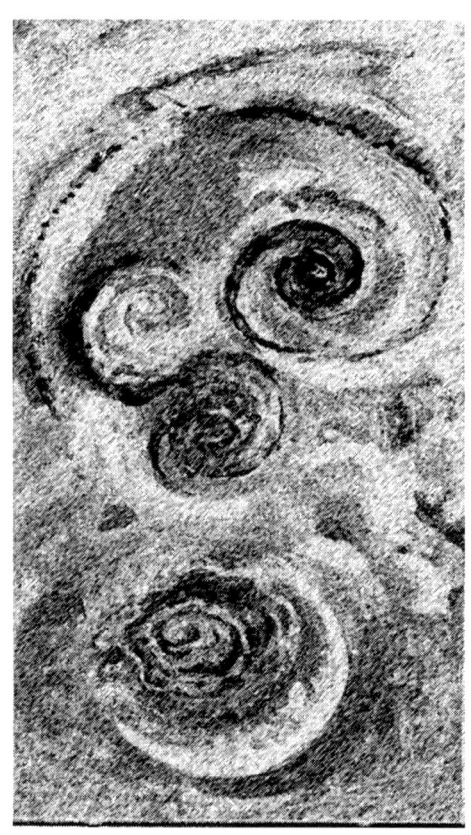

Lynn Carol Henderson (1949-)The Sacred Directions: Center/Spirit Blessing, 2003 (acrylic painting 5"x10")

This is a prose poem describing the ceremonies I create as a Ritual Leader of the Women's Spirituality Movement. It is designed to be performed in a circle of thirteen painted panels depicting elements of women's mysteries and followed by a meditation, expressive arts chalk drawings, and group processing.

> In the deep purple light that glows at the dawn of being comes
> She Who Thinks, the Hopi Spiderwoman (3.)
> From her own luminous being, she brings forth a silvery thread
> Which she casts to the East and the West
> And another which she casts to the North and the South.
> And there in the Center where the two threads meet
> She sings the Song of Life
> In a voice that is at once beautiful, deep and sweet.
> This is the voice of the Ancient Crone who still listens and responds.
> It is the voice in the mirror (4)
> Reassuring us that we are the fairest of them all,
> Granting even our harmful, destructive wishes.
> So that twelve strong sons may instantly become wild swans (5,)
> Only to be redeemed by the work of the maiden, Kore, Persephone (6,)
> The alchemical Rose (5) of Grimm's fairy tales.
> She re-ensouls her brothers with her weaving
> At the cost of her most precious gift,
> Her voice and her own destiny.

Women's Ritual Art reclaims women's voice. We are Maidens, Mothers, and Crones called into being by the forgotten litany: pure and white as the Maiden's breath; lips as red as the Mother's blood; hair as black as the Raven who comes to the Crone's command.

> We form our circles in the mythic time outside of time
> Where Art happens.
> We are birthed by mothers of every shape,
> Dark seers holding the serpent's wisdom (7,)
> Powerful queens who protectively love their princely sons so well that they will not share them,
> Mothers who cast their starving children to the mercy of the woods (8,)
> Mothers who nurture the orphans and whose wild wolf howls (9)
> Can be heard from the hillsides.
> There are mothers of monsters,
> Mothers of saviors, and
> Mothers of tricksters (10.)
>
> And there are those who would keep us safe:
> Warrior women and guardian priestesses (11)

Whose traveling suggestions we promptly ignore;
Our powerful sisters whose powers heal even the sun God's ills (12)
In return, of course,
for the power of naming.
This is the naming we use to restore serenity and balance
With our shape shifting between the worlds.

Intention is the key to our magical remaking.
We become the Great Goddess of Valiente's Charge (15)
...the beauty of the green earth, and the white moon among the stars and the mystery of the waters... (16)

Inanna lives among us

Impeccable intention.

We construct a boundary and animate its center of power.
It is our spirit of place, our sacred space (13.)

Around you is a theater of possibilities,
A circle dance of 13 panels with an altar at the center;
They wait to be charged in transformational ritual.

As we open our body-mind-spirit to the dynamic flow
We test the safety of our container,
all senses engaged:
Breathing, toning, chanting, drumming and movement
Even the most damaged may be carried into the inner light
Between and beyond the Cartesian framework (Called fretwork because we fret over it so much.)

Those that choose to make the passage return with renewed energy.
They return with a sense of empowerment and guidance for self-healing and growth.

And also with a heightened awareness of the preciousness of all creation.
Awestruck, attuned , we conjure ourselves
Protectors, co-creators, embodied incarnations of Gaia (14.)
This is the inspiration for my artwork:
The voices that speak in the Dark

Literally and metaphorically, they have called me to
A profound reverence for the earth,
A longing to enter her mysteries

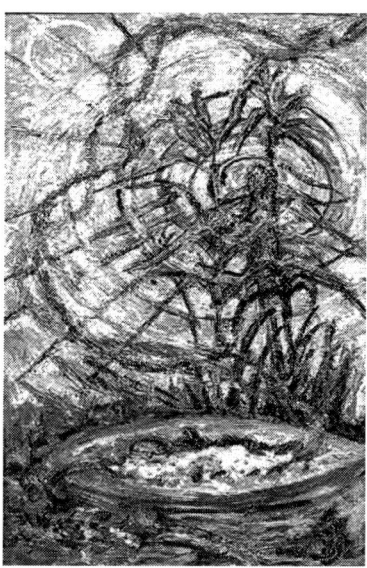

Lynn Carol Henderson (1949-) Origins: The Cycles of Growth 2003 (acrylic painting 5"x10")

Great Innana, beckoning, abandoning heaven, abandoning earth from the Great Above to the Great Below, guide and pilgrim on the inner quest (17.)
And a desire through ritualizing fantasy
To live within the feminist partnership paradigm (18.)

Women's rituals span the realms of science, religion,
archaeo-mythology, fantasy and folklore.

Like the Sufi's golden chain (19) its antecedents stretch deep into the past.
Matilda Joslyn Gage is our sister.
*We are the thoughts of our mothers and grandmothers,
embodied and made alive (20.)*

Marija Gimbutas (21,) Gerda Lerner (22,) Merlin Stone (23) Presente!

In one direction, there are descent mysteries
Whose common inheritance connect Eleusinian truths (24)
With the hydraulic high wires of Cirque du Soleil (25.)

In them is the reenactment of Eliade's eternal return (26.)

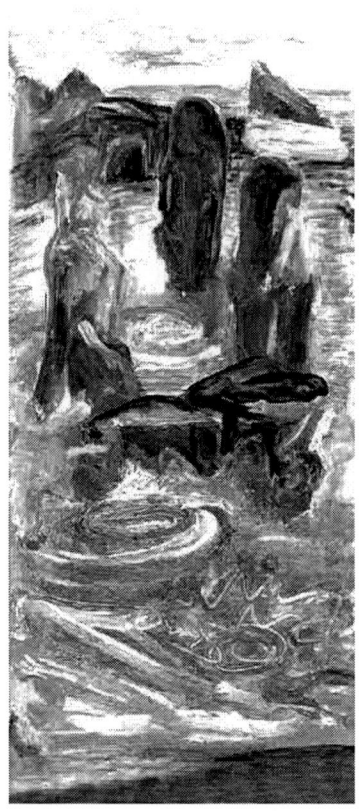

Lynn Carol Henderson (1949-) The Sacred Directions: North/ Earth Prayer 2003 (acrylic painting 5"x10")

The golden dream of creation,
Harrison's "words said over the deeds" (27.)
We wear the faces we wore before we were born.
We retrieve ourselves as the Other.
Now that we have revived a living tradition of pre-patriarchal collectivity
We carry its mantle through eco-feminism
To the struggle for preservation of seed banks and sacred lands (28.)
Ho! Mi' tak' oisin!
With my Lakota brothers and sisters, I respect you, "All My Relations."

The trance meditations I use follow paths opened by Jung's active imagination (29) and retrace his progeny:

Hardings' excavations of women's mysteries (30)

Beyond duality to Achterberg's healing imagery (31)
and finally now to Gotterner-Abendroth's matriarchal aesthetic (32.)

Other threads lead to spirit entities and animal allies
Through core shamanism (33) to Sandra's Ingerman's earth soul retrieval (34)
And homage to indigenous wisdom.
My medicine teachers
Dhyani Ywahoo (35), Josie Raven Wing (36), Brooke Medicine Eagle (37.)

Along the way, I have been schooled in the discourse of cultural appropriation —objections to ritual practice by those concerned for traditional wisdom (38.)
They caution about the dangers of neo-colonialism.
We must not arrogantly assume the availability of a universal body of direct experience.
We must not misuse indigenous cultural property.
This will undermine unique tribal teachings.

So I try always to remember to wake up differently
To make each choice wisely
Each decision for seven generations (39)
In the everyday sacred of the small details.

I rely on the loose blending of the rituals of the Women's Spirituality Movement,
mindful of my debt to the many traditions
from which they have been brewed.

You will recognize my simple guidelines as a mantra of respect:

Honor the ancestors,
Take only what is freely given,
Become a hollow bone,
Give back to the People,
Serve without attachment,
Listen.

Or if you prefer these words found carved on a rock in Minneapolis:

Accept fragility, Return love, Imagine justice, Breathe (40.)

I work with a pattern common to many rituals:

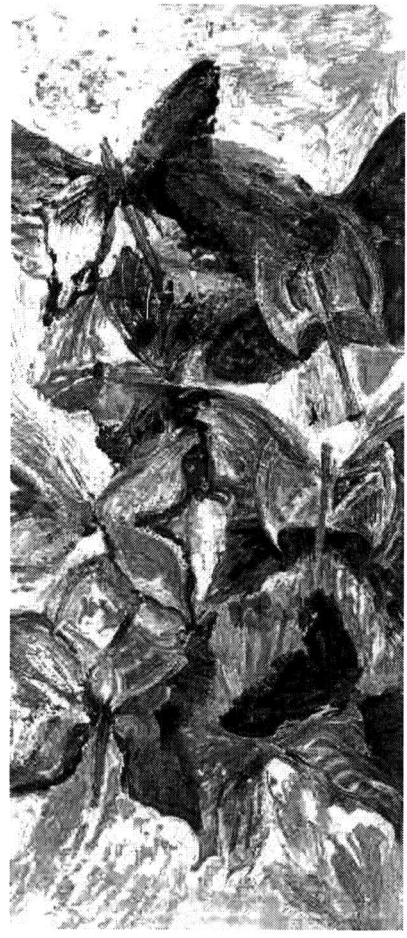

Lynn Carol Henderson (1949-) Women's Rites: Butterfly Rhythms Become Labrys 2003 (acrylic painting 5"x10")

A procession and purification,
Followed by invocation, storytelling and meditation.
These then give content to the Expressive Arts
Which are succeeded by sharing and personal commitment.
The final stages include releasing, grounding and celebration.

These elements have been honed at performance and pageant,
The eight pointed stars (41) of a half century of neo-pagan years;
I have found them at Irish séances of the Fellowship of Isis,
In the dells of Wisconsin with Priestesses of the Re-Formed Congregation of the Goddess,
In ritual circles of the Unitarian Pagans
In Pan-Indian 263isorder of the Daughters of the Earth.

With wild Wiccan women in my Florida home (42)
I have found communion
with tree-hugging dirt worshippers.

Battered and abused,
Communities of resistance,
We are communities of wounded healers.

We spark to Starhawk's spiral dance (43)
And in each place the veil is lifted.

We see women's circles
celebrate openly
The phases of the moon, seasonal cycles
And earth-based rites of passage.
Without fear of the Burning Times (44)
that may yet come again.
My paintings emerge from the circle.
They each hold one truth,
Obvious, clear, one literal idea with metaphoric overtones.

There are symbols of goddesses crossing time and story maps,
Archetypes from women's experience, and practical aspects (45) of ritual.

They are portals for the uninitiated and way stations for seasoned travelers
We rename ourselves, reclaim ourselves,
The panels are filled with dancing, laughing, furious and passionate beings.
Powerful beings in visionary worlds.

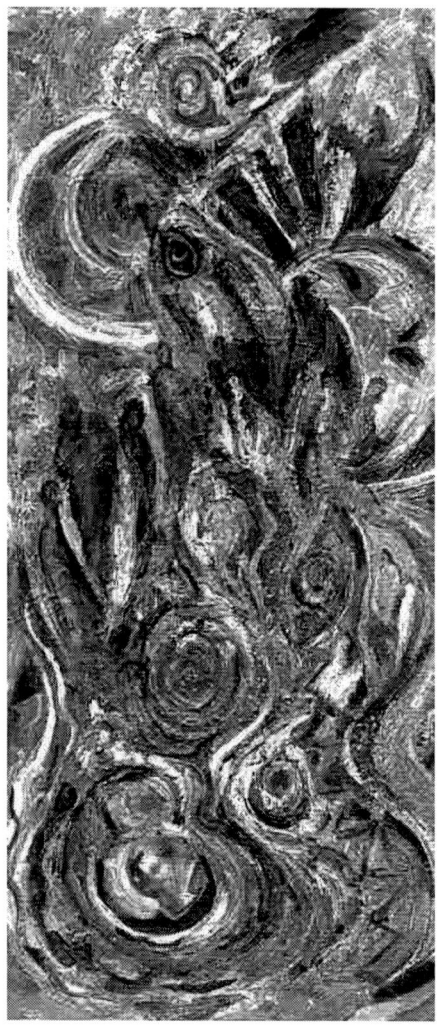

Lynn Carol Henderson (1949-) The Sacred Directions: South/ Fire Dance 2003 (acrylic painting 5"x10")

Each contains a spiral: it is the journey through the womb
Inward and outward
Passage of memory
A path demanding flexibility and the acceptance of uncertainty.

Spin the wheel and take your chance,
each time deeper
subtly changed..
She changes everything she touches, and everything she touches changes
(46.)

The images' forms hold intrinsic meaning.
There are overlapping and disconnected edges of volumes
Distortions of scale
The transformative mythic herstory.
They hold the numinous.

Figures fade and emerge in such a way
That when the viewer is ready, the multiple layers appear.
They hold the thresholds.
These images are fragmented; they call to us to complete them.
They hold the symbols of memory. They come to us and through us.
They hold our stories.

Sources for Further Reading about Names, Quotes, and Concepts in Numerical Sequence:

1. Carol Christ:
Christ, Carol. *Rebirth of the Goddess: Finding Meaning in Feminist Spirituality.* Reading, MA: Addison-Wesley, 1997.
2. Expressive Arts:
Rogers, Natalie. *Creative Connection: Expressive Arts as Healing.* Palo Alto, CA: Science and Behavior Books, 1993.
3. Hopi Spiderwoman:
Allen, Paula Gunn. *Grandmothers of the Light: A Medicine Woman's Sourcebook.* Boston: Beacon Press, 1991.
4. The mirror reassuring us that we are the fairest of them all:
 The Brothers Grimm. "Snow White and the Seven Dwarfs." *Tales of Grimm and Anderson* Ed. Frederick Jacobi Jr. New York: Random House, 1952.
5. Wild swans and the alchemical Rose of Anderson and Grimm:
Anderson, Hans Christian. "The Twelve Wild Swans." *Tales of Grimm and Anderson*. Ed. Frederick Jacobi Jr. New York: Random House, 1952.
6. The Maiden, Kore, Persephone:
Spretnak, Charlene . *Lost Goddesses in Early Greece: A Collection of Prehellenic Myths.* Boston: Beacon Press, 1978.

7. Dark seers holding the serpent's wisdom...Powerful queens who protectively love their princely sons so well that they will not share them
Stone, Merlin. *Ancient Mirrors of Womanhood: A Treasury of Goddess and Heroine Lore from around the World.* Boston: Beacon Press, 1979.
8. Mothers who cast their starving children to the mercy of the woods:
The Brothers Grimm. "Hansel and Gretel." *Tales of Grimm and Anderson.* Ed. Frederick Jacobi Jr. New York: Random House, 1952.
9. Mothers who nurture the orphans and whose wild wolf howls can be heard from the hillsides:
Estes, Clarissa Pinkola. *Women Who Run with the Wolves: Myths and Stories of the Wildwoman Archetype.* New York: Ballantine, 1992.
10. There are mothers of monsters, mothers of saviors and mothers of tricksters: Walker, Barbara C. *The Woman's Encyclopedia of Myths and Sacred Objects.* San Francisco: Harper & Row, 1983.
11. Warrior women and guardian priestesses whose traveling suggestions we promptly ignore
Fraser, Antonia. *The Warrior Queens: The Legends and Lives of the Women Who Have Led Their Nations in War.* New York: Vintage Books, 1988.
12. Whose powers heal even the sun God's ills: The story of Isis and Ra
Wolkstein, Diane. *The First Love Stories: From Isis and Osiris to Tristan and Iseult.* New York: Harper Collins, 1991.
13. Spirit of place, our sacred space:
Christian Norbert's "genius loci"
Korp, Maureen. "The Earthwork: A Sacred Art." *Sacred Art of the Earth: Ancient and Contemporary Earthworks.* New York: Continuum, 1997.
14. Gaia:
Spretnak, Charlene. *Lost Goddesses in Early Greece: A Collection of Prehellenic Myths.* Boston: Beacon Press, 1978.
15. Great Goddess of Valiente's Charge:
Valiente, Doreen. *An A.B.C. Of Witchcraft Past and Present.* London, England: Rovert Hale and St. Martin's Press, 1973.
16. Starhawk. *The Spiral Dance: A Rebirth of the Ancient Religion of the Great Goddess.* San Francisco: Harper & Row, 1979.
The Charge of the Goddess
(Excerpt from Starhawk's adaptation of Doreen Valiente)
I who am the beauty of the green earth, and the white moon among the stars, and the mystery of the waters, I call upon your soul to arise and come unto me. For I am the soul of nature, who gives life to the

universe. From Me all things proceed, and unto Me they must return. Let My worship be in the heart that rejoices, for behold—all acts of love and pleasure are My rituals. Let there be beauty and strength, power and compassion, honor and humility, mirth and reverence within you. And you who seek to know Me, know that your seeking and yearning will avail you not, unless you know the mystery: for if that which you seek, you find not within yourself, you will never find it without. For behold, I have been with you from the beginning; and I am that which is attained at the end of desire.

17. Inanna lives among us:

Wolkstein, Diane and Samuel Noah Kramer. *Inanna Queen of Heaven and Earth: Her Stories and Hymns from Sumer.* New York: Harper Collins, 1983.

18. The feminist partnership paradigm:

Eisler, Riane. *The Chalice and the Blade: Our History, Our Future.* San Francisco: Harper and Row, 1987.

19. Sufi's golden chain: The chanted litany of the names of the Sufi masters

20. "We are the thoughts of our mothers and grandmothers, embodied and made alive":

Gage, Matilda Joslyn (1972): Woman, Church and State: A Historical Account of the Status of Woman Through the Christian Ages: With Reminiscences of the Matriarchate. Reprint of 1900 edition ed. Ayers, Salem NH.

21. Marija Gimbutas:

Gimbutas, Marija. *The Language of the Goddess.* San Francisco, CA: Harper, 1991.

22. Gerda Lerner:

Lerner, Gerda. *Women and History: The Creation of Patriarchy.* Vol. 1. New York: Oxford University Press, 1986.

23. Merlin Stone:

Stone, Merlin. *When God Was a Woman.* New York, San Diego: Harcourt, Brace, Jovanovich, 1976.

24. Eleusinian truths:

Stone, Merlin. *When God Was a Woman.* New York, San Diego: Harcourt, Brace, Jovanovich, 1976.

25. Cirque du Soleil: modern combination of the shamanic magic tradition blending elements from theater and circus: Turner, Victor. *The Anthropology of Performance.* New York: PAJ Publications, 1986.

26. Eliade's eternal return:

Eliade, Mircea. *Myths, Dreams and Mysteries.* New York: Harper, 1957.

27. Harrison's "words said over the deeds":
Harrison, Jane Ellen. *Mythology*. New York: Harcourt, Brace, Jovanovich, 1963.
28. eco-feminism...the struggle for preservation of seed banks and sacred lands:
Orenstein, Gloria, and Irene Diamond, eds. *Reweaving the World: The Emergence of Ecofeminism*. San Francisco: Sierra Club Books, 1990.
29. Jung's active imagination:
Jung, Carl. Gustav. *Memories, Dreams and Reflections*. New York: Vintage Books, 1963.
30. Harding's excavations of women's mysteries:
Harding, M. Esther. *Woman's Mysteries: Ancient and Modern, a Psychological Interpretation of the Feminine Principle as Portrayed in Myth, Story and Dreams*. 1971 ed. London: Rider and Company and C. G. Jung Foundation, 1955.
31. Achterberg's healing imagery:
Achterberg, Jeanne, Barbara Dossey, and Leslie Kolkmeier. *Rituals of Healing: Using Imagery for Health and Wellness*. New York: Bantam Books, 1994.
32. Gotterner-Abendroth's matriarchal aesthetic:
Gottner-Abendroth, Heide. *The Dancing Goddess: Principles of a Matriarchal Aesthetic*. Trans. Maureen T. Krause. Boston: Beacon Press, 1991.
33. core shamanism:
Harner, Michael. *The Way of the Shaman*. New York: Bantam Books, 1980.
34. Sandra's Ingerman's earth soul retrieval:
Ingerman, Sandra. *Soul Retrieval: Mending the Fragmented Self*. San Francisco, CA: Harper San Francisco, 1991.
35. Dhyani Ywahoo:
Ywahoo, Dhyani. *Voices or Our Ancestors: Cherokee Teachings from the Wisdom Fire*. Boston: Shamblala, 1987.
36. Josie Raven Wing:
Raven Wing, Josie. "Jaoa De Deus, the Miracle Man of Brazil." The Shaman's Drum Spring 2001: 34-35.
37. Brooke Medicine Eagle:
Medicine Eagle, Brooke. *Buffalo Woman Comes Singing: The Spirit Song of a Rainbow Medicine Woman*. New York: Ballantine Books, 1991.
38. Objections to ritual practice:
Messenger, Phyllis Mauch. *The Ethics of Collecting Cultural Property*. Albuquerque: University of New Mexico Press, 1989.

39. Each decision for seven generations:
Allen, Paula Gunn. *The Sacred Hoop: Recovering the Feminine in American Indian Traditions.* Boston: Beacon Press, 1986.

40. Or if you prefer these words found carved on a rock in Minneapolis:
Gateway art project sculpture in the Lyndale Park Peace Garden, Minneapolis Art in Public Places Program: www.gardensforpeace.org

41. The eight pointed star:
The eight major sabbats of the Celtic Year: Samhain, Yule (Winter Solstice), Imbolc, Oestar, Beltane, Lithia (Summer Solstice), Lammas, and Mabon

42. Wiccan /wiccen (meaning wise) women in my Florida paradise:
I live in St. Petersburg Florida on three acres of cultivated jungle where I own and operate Enigma Growth and Life Center in my geodesic dome art studio

43. We spark to Starhawk's spiral dance:
sparking: "speaking with tongues of fire: igniting the divine spark in women; lighting the fires of female friendship...": Daly, Mary. *Webster's New Intergalactic Wickedary of the English Language: Conjured in Cahoots with Jane Caputi.* Boston: Beacon Press, 1987.

44. Burning Times:
refers to the witch burning of the Middle Ages and Renaissance

45. Practical aspects of ritual aspecting is to take on the role of the Divine:
Leavy, Lynn, ed. *Dianic Wiccan Cella Healing Program of the Re-Formed Congregation of the Goddess.* Madison, WI: RCG Reformed Congregation of the Goddess, 2000.

46. *She changes everything she touches, and everything she touches changes:*
Chant adapted by Shekhinah Mountainwater: Mountainwater, Shekhinah. *Ariadne's Thread: A Workbook of Goddess Magic.* Freedom, CA: Crossing Press, 1991.

POETICS OF THE NIGHT:
THE TRANSFORMATIVE POWER OF DREAMS

KATHLEEN M. SANDS

Monsters and mayhem, longing and betrayal, blunders and mishaps, intrigue and sorrow, adventure and romance. This is the stuff life and dreams are made of. Whether pauper or prophet, royalty or riff raff, sinner or serf, our collective imaginations have been captivated for centuries. We may delude ourselves that our waking life operates under conscious control, but our dream life—now that's another story.

Universal and cross-cultural, it is something we all do. Of course, we may not always remember. Or even want to. But still, we all dream. Unbidden, they come to us in many shapes and sizes. Some in color. Some in black and white. Some are accompanied by sound while others remain silent. A precious few will stay with us forever. Others, perhaps most, seem to evaporate even as we become aware of their presence quietly slipping away. Some may startle us awake, trembling and out of breath, momentarily unsure as to our surroundings, temporarily disoriented in time and space. Others may taunt us as we find ourselves unprepared for an important exam, falling helplessly off a tall building or haplessly strolling naked through a downtown mall. Still others leave us excited and aroused, blissful in the memory of an encounter with an old love or in erotic anticipation of a new or forbidden one.

For some people dreams may appear telepathic or even prophetic. An arrival or departure is sensed. The telephone rings. A loved one has died. "It was only a dream," we tell ourselves, not entirely convinced of our own words.

However varied our dreams may be, most of us have wondered where they come from and what, if anything, they mean. As with most phenomena, one's view is influenced by the context of one's particular life history. In ancient Greece, for example, pilgrims traveled great distances to visit sacred temples where they hoped to incubate healing dreams. Little more than a century ago, Native American adolescents ventured into the woods on vision quests during which they would fast and pray while awaiting a dream to reveal their life mission. Then again, if you were born Hindu, you would be taught that it is this life, our waking life, that is the illusion—the one dream from which we will all someday awaken. At the turn of the century in Western Europe, a Victorian patient would recline on a leather couch free-associating to a recent dream while her analyst sat in a chair behind her quietly taking notes. Today, a small group of friends gathers in a participant's home, form a circle and share their stories. Then serve as their own experts.

Dreams have been both revered as messages from the gods and dismissed as electro-chemical waste material. Rich in imagery and metaphor, they have been analyzed to death, picked over, interpreted, categorized, intoned, dreaded, prayed for and poeticized. Whatever the framework, it is something we all do. And with only two notable exceptions, so do all other mammals as well as some birds and reptiles. Despite the amount of time spent on this activity, for the most part it remains beyond our consciousness. Some of it is pleasant, but much of it is not. Since our muscular skeletal system is shut down, we could not escape even if we wanted to. Meanwhile, our minds, which were previously thought to be at rest, are most definitely not. For something we can't even explain and frequently forget, we actually spend several years of our lives in its grip.

And so, we continue to ask. Do dreams matter and if so, what is their significance? For materialists whose concept of reality begins and ends with the physical realm, dreams represent little more than random psychic discharge. However, for those with a more metaphysical bent, one that allows for or acknowledges a realm beyond the empirical, dreams can prove to be one of many possible avenues to the transcendent. As such, they do indeed matter. As Gregg Levoy remarks in *Callings,* "Some things can only be seen when it's dark" (1997.)

Whether in the stillness of a cave, the silence of a church pew or during an unexpected pause in the midst of an otherwise frenetic day, we are soon reminded "...the real questions in life are all existential" (David Engle, 1994:4.) To that end, we have historically looked to religion, to the arts and even to our nightly visitors for guidance.

> "The processes of dreaming and of creativity are similar, and both are unlike the way we think in ordinary waking life. The dream language is similar to the way we made sense of the world before we learned to speak – through image and metaphor. It mimics the way we think when we create. Freud called this kind of thinking primary process, and believed it was essential for any kind of creative work."
> —Veronica Tonay (2006:64)

In my own life, it was while working with a Jungian analyst that I began to experience powerful dreams. There was an element of irony at play here as when I began my search for an analyst I first met with another woman, also a Jungian. She, however, immediately informed me as to her two requirements prior to taking on a client. And those were the production of dreams and artwork. The latter was not going to pose a problem, but the first would, as I was not big on dreaming at the time. This eventually led me to Sylvia who remained my analyst for many years.

Once I made my descent to the underworld, after all the inevitable reluctance and reservations, a rich supply of dreams appeared on its own. One of the most profound dreams that I experienced during this time I entitled, "Snow White Meets Spider Woman." It is the story of a dream embedded in a fairy tale.

> "Archetypal images serve to take us out of the realm of the mundane and personal...Because these images are the language of the Soul, they give us a sense of what is possible. Dreams are our major personal access to this realm. Fairy tales and myths fascinate us for the same reason. It is the interplay between the personal and the archetypal in our dreams...that gives them their juice."
> —Sylvia Senensky (2003:21)

All summer Sylvia and I had been working with the story of Snow White. For centuries, this Grimm classic has remained one of the most beloved and best-known pieces of European folk literature. In the opening scene, we find the young Queen sitting by a window hoping for a child. Her wish is soon granted. I, too, had been a much-wanted child. In fact, contrary to the social prescriptions of the day, my mother prayed that her firstborn would be a girl. The young Queen dies in the process of childbirth. In a year's time, the King remarries. The new Queen is very beautiful, but also proud and vain.

Anyone familiar with the tale knows that Snow White's only crime is to be of good nature and fair of face. In time, this unwittingly poses a threat to the new Queen who regularly checks her magic mirror to make certain she is still the "fairest in the land." This remains so until Snow White reaches the age of seven at which time she begins to eclipse the Queen. Narcissistic and violent, the wicked stepmother plots the demise of her stepdaughter who has now become her foremost rival.

Unable to bear this natural challenge and process, let alone support the young child in her development, she chooses instead to eliminate her. For this, she selects a hired hand, who she orders to kill Snow White. When the two meet, Snow White begs to be spared, promising to flee into the forest and never return to the castle. Not having the heart to carry out his mission, the huntsman slays a young boar instead. We hear nothing of the King in all this. Clearly absent, he fails to protect his daughter, let alone come to her rescue.

"In Snow White's story the father-huntsman fails to take a strong and definite stand. He neither does his duty to the queen, nor meets his moral obligation to Snow White to make her safe and secure. So Snow White must fend for herself when she is abandoned by the hunter in the forest."
—Brunno Bettleheim (1977:205-06)

For a time Snow White finds a safe haven with the seven dwarfs for whom she keeps house. Upon learning that Snow White lives and continues to outshine her, the Queen becomes consumed with rage and jealousy. The huntsman has failed her as well. Now she must take matters into her own hands. Dressed in a variety of disguises, the wicked stepmother pays the child several visits. Ignoring the dwarfs' instructions not to let anyone in the house, the naïve and trusting girl allows the old woman to enter. Using all her cunning plus a dash of witchcraft, the Queen attempts to trick Snow White with a variety of attractive wares. However, it is not until her third visit with the tantalizing yet poisoned apple that she apparently succeeds.

After months of exploring parallels and connections between this story and my own, I had an amazing dream. Fortunately, it took place in the morning and I remembered it well. Just to be sure, I immediately got up and took copious notes, knowing from past experience the ephemeral nature of dreams, and how quickly details slip away.

The dream begins in the upstairs bathroom of my childhood home. I am sitting on the toilet. I am also quite grownup, probably a young woman in her twenties. My mother is sitting to my left. Later she is joined by my father who sits beside her on the edge of the bathtub. At this time, I look up and notice a large, fuzzy, black spider in the upper right corner of the ceiling. Somehow, I know it is meant for me. And sure enough, down it comes, landing on my right forearm. My eyes remain fixed on the spot. I am more mesmerized than horrified. Then clusters of grey, fluttery creatures form a circle and dance around the giant spider. "Get it off. Get it off!" I finally scream.

In an attempt to do so, my father picks up a white plastic kitchen spatula. "That's not going to kill anything!" I exclaim. Then my mother, using a metal spatula swats the bug off my arm, but not actually killing it. Next thing I know, the spider is perched on my left shoulder looking up at me. At that moment, I awaken and find myself pelting the bed with my pillow.

> "The body's images are like those of a dream. There can be no thesaurus of body imagery. This is what a symptom is: body and life falling together as if by accident. The response is to contain that coincidence."
> —Thomas Moore (1992:163)

Upon learning of my nocturnal adventures, Sylvia was as excited as I, later referring to it as a "healing dream." During one of our subsequent sessions, I remarked that I saw myself as having come more or less half way in this life. Had I remained at home, played the role of the devoted firstborn, ever-solicitous daughter, perhaps my mother would have suffered less. However, that would have required the sacrifice of my own life. Instead, I married young and left. One could actually say fled. Of course, there was a price to pay for my freedom. There always is.

However, like Snow White, I did not actually swallow the poison. While some toxin did manage to trickle down into my system, I did not die. My mother, however, chose to die decades before her actual death. So great was her need to escape, that she swallowed the poison, drop by drop, pill by pill, day after day, year after year.

Collectively speaking, women have been taught for centuries to remain chaste and pure, wait for the prince to show up, produce offspring, and then live happily ever after. My mother had done all the right things. She married her handsome boss, had two beautiful children, and kept a lovely home. But there was no happy ending.

In the Grimm version, Snow White remains in her glass casket for a very long time. On it have been inscribed the words, "the King's daughter." Her body does not decay. She appears asleep. Then one day as the crystal coffin is being carried away, it hits a bump in the road. Snow White spits out the piece of poisoned apple lodged in her throat and wakes up. Sylvia says that is what I am doing now. Starting to spit out the poison, claim my life, write my own fairy tale.

> "Here is a dream depicting negative Feminine energy as it has been passed through the generations. The dreamer, a woman in her fifties, was raised by a severely mentally ill mother who would go into rages. Negative mother complexes often show themselves in dreams in the form of spiders, in this case the most poisonous form, a black widow. The dreamer has struggled all her life to free herself from this poison. In addition, she has recently been a passenger in a serious automobile accident from which she sustained severe injury to her right arm. At the time of the dream, she continued to struggle with considerable pain and physical limitation.

Interestingly, her mother had lost complete use of her right arm after a falling accident in the home. At the time her mother was also in her early fifties from which point on she gradually became an invalid...Upon subsequent reflection, the dreamer came to realize that the "Dark Feminine" was a shared place, one both she and her mother had known.

At the time of this writing, the dreamer has almost entirely recovered the use of her arm. She has also come into her own creativity, which in addition to offering its own rewards, has become, for her, a place of positive connection to both her mother and her grandmother."
—Sylvia Senensky (2003:99-100)

Few dreams present themselves as an over-sized sunflower — loud, bright and clear. Often they arrive striated, multi-colored and complex. While there are those that crouch in a shaded corner reluctant to display themselves, others are thorny, spiky and just plain scary. In addition, some simply lie there – a seeming massive tangle of weeds.

"As for dream material itself, some of it is like junk mail. Only a small percentage is truly useful and worth slogging through."
—Gregg Levoy (1997:83)

So what's an attentive dreamer to do? Well, paying attention is an excellent start. Treat the dream as you would a friend, lover or work of art. Welcome it, listen to what it has to say, ask a question or two – like, "Why have you come?" or "What do you have to tell me?" Cultivate an interactive, reciprocal relationship. In order to enhance the experience even further, one could give the dream form in another medium such as dance, poetry or music.

Dreams are myriad and diverse and open to multiple levels of meaning. While interpretation can certainly be of value, one need not necessarily understand in order to be moved – just as one can be by a work of art. In fact, dreams and art occupy the same realm and speak the same language. Many, perhaps most, are little more than a collection of easily forgotten fragments. A precious few, however, are so powerful that they are long remembered.

Early on in therapy with my Jungian analyst, we appeared to have hit a snag. More than once, Sylvia remarked that I had not yet cried in session. Seldom given to real bouts of tears, I began to feel pressured, and then resentful. Finally, one day I arrived with some of my poetry. After reading several aloud, I handed the papers over to her and heard myself say, "This is the place where I cry." She never brought the matter up again.

In our search for direction and guidance, it might be best to think more in terms of aspiring to wholeness rather than seeking a cure for what ails us. As Connie Kaplan notes in *Dreams Are Letters from the Soul*, "Healing means bringing something or someone into full alignment with the level of soul, while also rooting them more deeply in the level of form. A healed being is one who experiences unity consciousness and sees the interconnectedness of all beings, awake or asleep" (2002:143.)

There are many paths. There are many guides. Some people sit cross-legged on pillows in silence. Others twirl and spin in wild abandon. Some people pray. Others drum. Some people celebrate the mystery in community. Others quietly light a candle before a makeshift altar at home. And some do both. As Rumi, the twelfth century mystic poet so beautifully noted, "There are a thousand ways to kneel and kiss the ground."

So I say to you – find the place or places where you connect to your Source. The manner and ways in which you awaken. Then dwell within and you will be blessed – by day and by night.

Suggested Readings

Alvarez, A. *Night*. New York: W.W. Norton and Co., 1995.
Barasch, Marc Ian. *Healing Dreams*. New York: Riverhead Books, 2000.
Bettleheim, Bruno. *The Uses of Enchantment: The Meaning and Importance of Fairy Tales*. New York: Vintage Books, 1977.
Boa, Fraser. *The Way of the Dream*. Boston: Shambhala. 1994.
Bosnak, Robert. *A Little Course in Dreams*. Boston: Shambhala, 1988.
Brehony, Kathleen. *Awakening at Midlife*. New York: Riverhead Books, 1996.
Campbell, Joseph. *The Power of Myth*. New York: Anchor Books, 1991.
DeSalvo, Louise. *Writing as a Way of Healing*. New York: Harper Collins, 1999.
Engle, David. *Divine Dreams*. Anna Maria, FL: Christopher Books, 1994.
Epel, Naomi. *Writers Dreaming*. New York: Vintage Books, 1994.
Hall, James A. *Jungian Dream Interpretation: A Handbook of Theory and Practice*. Toronto: Inner City Books, 1983.
Hobson, J. Allan. *Dreaming*. New York: Oxford University Press, Inc. 2002.
Hollis, James. *Creating a Life*. Toronto: Inner City Books, 2001.
Johnson, Robert A. *Inner Work: Using Dreams and Imagination for Personal Growth*. San Francisco: Harper & Row, 1986.

Jung, Carl. *Memories, Dreams and Reflections.* New York: Vintage Books, 1989.
Kaplan, Connie. *Dreams Are Letters From the Soul.* New York: Harmony Books, 2002.
Levine, Ellen. *Tending the Fire: Studies in Art, Therapy and Creativity*, Toronto: Palmerston Press, 1995.
Levoy, Gregg. *Callings.* New York: Three Rivers Press, 1997.
Mellick, Jill. *The Natural Artistry of Dreams.* Berkeley, CA: Conari Press, 1996.
Moore, Thomas. *Care of the Soul.* New York: Harper Perennial, 1992.
Rock, Andrea. *The Mind at Night: Exploring Dreams That Can Transform Your Life.* New York: Basic Books, 2004.
Senensky, Sylvia Shaindel. *Healing and Empowering the Feminine: A Labyrinth Journey.* Wilmette, IL: Chiron Publications, 2003.
Siegel, Alan B. *Dreams That Can Change Your Life.* Los Angeles, CA: Jeremy P. Tarcher, Inc., 1990.
Tonay, Verónica. *The Creative Dreamer.* Berkeley, CA: Celestial Arts, 2006.
Van DeCastle, Robert. *Our Dreaming Mind.* New York: Ballantine Books, 1994.
Wakefield, Dan. *Creating From the Spirit.* New York: Ballantine Books, 1997.
Wolf, Fred Alan. *The Dreaming Universe: A Mind-Expanding Journey Into the Realm Where Psyche and Physics Meet.* New York: Simon & Shuster, 1994.

THE ART OF CHOICE THEORY

LAURA JJ DESSAUER

Change occurs for multiple reasons throughout our life cycle. Perhaps the choices one is making are no longer effective in their attempts to meet one's needs, or perhaps others have noticed one's ineffective behaviors and the individual is influenced by how the behaviors are impacting others. To be open to change, an individual must move from contemplation into the preparation and action (Prochaska, 1999.) Change is only possible if individuals become aware that what they are choosing to do no longer meets their needs. When they reach this point they are ready to move into action, whereby they seek therapy to help them find solutions to their problems.

However, what a client may see as a problem may vary from what a therapist may see as the primary problem. To help individuals understand how their behaviors are affecting them and the important relationships in their lives, it is imperative that a clinician offers new insights to influence how the client perceives the problem. To truly help clients become aware of their ineffective attempts to meet their needs, a therapist must build a relationship of trust, compassion, understanding, humor, and safety unlike any other relationship that the individual is currently experiencing in their lives. Almost all individuals seek therapy or are referred to therapy because they are experiencing problems with the important people in their lives. In order to help a client, the therapeutic relationship must be a safe place for discovery, connection, and co-creation. It is within the alchemy of this relationship that the client often discovers the "ah-ha" moment.

To help facilitate change it is important to work from the client's and family's strengths as Pledge (2004) suggests. "What are the client and family already doing well that can be adapted to help them be more successful in the therapeutic task at hand?" (2004:97) Interventions that come from the client's frame of reference provide an opportunity to integrate change more successfully. In order to develop cognitive integration, the information can be presented via multiple experiences that connect with the client's particular strengths of intelligence as suggested by Gardner (1993.) It is essential to present information via multiple intelligences, such as verbal/linguistic (talking,) interpersonal (role-playing,) visual/spatial (creating art,) intrapersonal (journaling,) logical/mathematical (problem solving,) bodily/kinesthetic (creative play,) musical (creating songs,) or naturalistic (collecting and grouping objects.) Therefore, the expressive arts can strengthen integration of new information by providing the clinician with tools to encourage client change.

Moreover, for the integration of new information a therapeutic trusting relationship must be developed. This is the foundation for all change. Glasser (2004) suggests that the source of all problems stem from unsatisfactory or non-existent connections with people we need. Reconnecting essentially starts with the clinician first connecting with the individual and modeling how the disconnected person can reconnect with the important people in their lives.

Choice Theory explains that all behavior is purposeful and it is our best attempt at the time to meet our basic needs, given our current knowledge and skills. These needs drive all of our behaviors and are part of our genetic structure. We have one physiological need, survival, but more psychological needs: love and belonging, power, freedom, and fun (Glasser 1998.) Basic needs are generalized concepts; they become personalized and specific when they enter into our Quality World. Our Quality World is like a photo album of images of people, things, ideas and systems of belief that increase the quality of our lives (Glasser 1998.) Each person's Quality World is individualized. What we put in our Quality World are pictures associated with strong positive feelings when our needs are satisfied. This World consists of what we want the most and meets one or more of our basic needs.

The client's Quality World may be the most essential tool in understanding their perspective and helping them in treatment. Once a picture is in our Quality World it is very difficult to take out. In order to remove a picture, a satisfying alternative needs to replace it. Pictures that we put in our Quality World are unique to us and our experience. They have value for the individual alone.

All information is just that, information. It has no specific good or bad value until it passes through our Total Knowledge Filter. We decide if it's not meaningful, if we need more information, or if it has meaning to us. If it has meaning, it passes through our Valuing Filter. As it passes through our Valuing Filter, we decide to place one of three "values" on the information. Value refers to the importance we place on the information, not necessarily moral or ethical value. If the information that enters our Valuing Filter is something we have learned is need satisfying, we place a positive value on it; if it is something we have learned hinders our ability to meet our needs, we place a negative value on it. If it neither helps us nor hinders us in meeting our needs, we may place little or no value on it, so it remains neutral.

As information passes through our Valuing Filter, it enters our Perceived World. How we perceive information is highly subjective based on individual culture, experience, education, age, and gender. It is unique to us. It is subjective to change; new information and new experiences equal new perceptions. Knowing we have control over the perceptions we choose, we can seek more information and/or ask ourselves which perception is better to hold (Glasser, 1998.)

Unless we truly understand what is in our client's Quality World picture we cannot develop a helping relationship. We will be operating from a place of trying to meet our need and we will be imposing our perspective and values on the client. The individual's Quality World is essential to understand so we can help clients make choices that will meet their needs. Unhappiness arises when individuals attempt to meet their needs but may be choosing behaviors that are not helping them to meet their needs. Glasser calls this the Comparing Place, like a set of scales we compare what we want (Quality World) with what we have (Perceived World.) When your scales are out of balance, you feel the frustration signal, which is the urge to behave to get more of what want. Glasser (1998) believes that all behavior is Total Behavior, made up of four components: thinking, acting, feeling, and physiology. All four components of total behavior are present at all times. Like the wheels on a car, by changing the direction of one wheel, the others will follow, and the car will move in a new direction.

Glasser (1998) believes all behavior is internally motivated, chosen, and purposeful and is our best attempt, at the time, to satisfy our Basic Needs. By changing what we are doing (acting) and thinking, we can change our feelings, emotionally and physically. By teaching Choice Theory to our clients, we will give them tools to understand that they have the power to change what they want, change what they are doing, or change both. We provide them with the opportunity to learn more effective ways of meeting their needs and help them to be the driver in their own car.

The expressive arts can be used to help clients to see their total behaviors (thinking, acting, feeling and physiology) as a choice, instilling a sense of hope. Glasser (1998) suggests, "If you can make one choice, you can make another-better-choice." Moreover, "to be depressed or neurotic is passive. It happed to us: we are its victim, and we have no control over it" (1998:77.) Introducing choice theory and helping individuals and families to understand that they choose their behaviors empowers them to assert control over their lives to find more effective ways to meet their needs. "If it is a choice, it follows that you are not a victim of a mental illness; you are either the beneficiary of your own good choices or the victim of your own bad choices" (1998:77.)

Moreover, Choice Theory can be beneficial to individuals and families throughout the life cycle. For instance, when children/teens are choosing ineffective behaviors they have not learned other ways of expressing their needs. Glasser (1998) suggests that individuals chose to depress in order to restrain anger, ask for help, control others, and avoid taking action. To help children and teens move from inactivity and passivity into action and responsibility, helping them to understand their Quality World is imperative. In addition, exploring their relationship with others is essential. Introduce the idea that unhappiness comes from one's perception of their surroundings and how it relates to their Quality World. With this new knowledge a child can change what they want or change their behaviors. For children in the concrete operations stages this needs to be presented in a variety of kinesthetic concrete activities. For teens, it can develop into a coaching relationship, helping them to develop and move toward outcomes they would like in setting goals and creating action plans. In younger children choosing depressive behaviors often manifests in acting out, clinging, somatic complaints, and avoidant behaviors (Pledge 2004.) A new way of behaving can be introduced.

Treatment would involve teaching Choice Theory to the children and parents, using art to explore what is in their Quality World and what is happening in their Perceived World. For children it would involve developing coping skills to meet their needs, such as developing a workbook of choices, using clay to creatively play out choices, helping them to identify "big feelings" and ways to diffuse anger/ aggressing (for example: "blowing out anger," or "waving your magic wand and counting to five.")

Noteworthy, an individual who chooses anxiety or frustration has not yet learned other ways to change their total behaviors. Choice Theory would be taught. Children and teens that use art materials are often able to work through anxiety/frustration behaviors. In such a session, an initial baseline for the feeling is established for children at the beginning, with a 1-10 scale. A number is again identified at the end of the session to rate the amount of felt frustration. This allows the child to understand that taking action (attending the session/ creating artwork) typically will reduce choosing anxiety/frustration/depression and increase feelings of well-being.

Furthermore, using clay, paint, or pastel allows for self-soothing opportunities, eliciting an emotive response to the materials. This is helpful for clients to integrate self-soothing behaviors outside of the session. For example, painting with pink, a client's favorite color, can be accessed as a cue when the client feels they have become overwhelmed/anxious. Moreover, if developmentally appropriate, a song about pink can be made up and a visual image of playing with pink paint can be incorporated into a hypnotic-type suggestion.

In the sessions, clients can identify times that they have felt anxious, how they overcame it, and what resources they chose. Using body outlines helps a client understand what the body is feeling as they become more anxious and how they can choose to reduce those feelings. For teens developing a book or a physical "tool box" are ways to identify resources they can choose instead of anxious behaviors.

Glasser does not subscribe to psychopathology as a way to determine treatment for clients; instead, Choice Theory is used to assess the behaviors the client is choosing. To help the client in treatment the clinician may evaluate the underlying needs the client is attempting to meet. This may be helping the client to identify ways to meet their need for survival, safety, love and belonging (relationship issues,) or perhaps power (feeling a sense of mastery/ competency.) Depending upon the need, they are attempting to satisfy the clinician may create art activities to help them move towards behaviors and thoughts that help the client meet their needs. For example, if a child was feeling powerless and was choosing behaviors of aggression/ depression, akin to cycling (up and down) behaviors, the clinician could help the client explore ways to develop a sense of power in his/her life.

The clinician may prescribe art activities that challenged the client and focused more on developing a skillful product rather than an emotive "process- based" intervention. This might include hand building with clay, painting with acrylics on a canvas, or carving a wood project. The goals is to help the child, "evaluate the behavior that he is choosing, learn that he is responsible for his choices, and to help him develop the skills to make more effective choices" (Passaro, et al., 2004: 506.)

Furthermore, adults can benefits from the learning the tenants of Choice Theory and using the expressive arts to reinforce these constructs. Lambert (1992) researched therapeutic factors that influence client improvement in treatment. He found that more than a specific theory or even expectancy, the client-therapist relationship accounted for 30% of successful outcome in client treatment. As much as the specifics of

Choice Theory influence client outcomes, what may be of most significance is the understanding of the client by building relationship.

Therefore, unless the clinician truly understands what is in our client's Quality World picture, we cannot develop a helping relationship that facilitates change. Many expressive therapeutic interventions allow the client to share what is important to them. Such interventions may include creating a Quality World picture album, creating a picture/poem/dance/story of what's important to them, explaining the concept of Quality World and asking the client what they would include, asking the client to create a collage or words by answering questions. "What people do I most want to be with"? "What things do I most want to own or experience?" "What ideas, beliefs, or values are important to me?" In addition, we can create "Workbooks" with our clients by asking the client to create artwork/images of their Basic Needs, Quality World, and their Total Behavior to explore how to meet their needs more effectively.

To teach the five basic needs and help the client identify what needs they are meeting they can use words or images to create a circle representing their basic needs. Ask the client to create a second circle on a separate piece of paper of what they would like their basic needs to look like. Finally, use a third piece of paper to join the two circles together. On this paper, create a "needs highway" choosing a color to represent each of the five Basic Needs and labeling what actions the client would take to get where they want to be. The clinician can use this is an opening activity to help the client identify what is important to them, actions they can take to meet their needs, as well as establishing a baseline for treatment.

Moreover, the clinician can teach the client about the Comparing Place by asking the client to create a picture of a scale and adding images on each side to compare what they have with what they want in their lives. The clinician can use this artwork to dialogue about what the client can do to balance the scales. By exploring the concept of the Comparing Place, the clients can evaluate what is in their Perceived World and what they desire in their Quality World. The clinician can provide a large piece of paper, asking the client to draw two circles, one on each side of the paper. Label one on left "what am I doing now;" label one on right "what do I want." Ask the client to fill in each circle with images and words. Another way of exploring the Comparing Place is to ask the client to draw a picture of what they want and what is happening in their life right now that is causing them frustration. Choices can be explored by asking the client to verbalize what they might do or think differently, and imagine how this will affect them emotionally and physically? The clinician can ask the client to make a road drawing including their past, present and their future choices and use this to dialogue about overcoming obstacles & future goals.

In addition, to teach Total Behavior the clinician could ask client to make a car (or provide a drawing of a car) and label the wheels with what they can do or think that will help them to get to their future goals.

In conclusion, by teaching Choice Theory to our clients using the expressive arts, we will give them tools to understand that they have the power to change what they want, what they are doing, or change both (Glasser, 1998.) We provide them with the opportunity to learn more effective ways of meeting their needs, and we help them to be the 'driver in their own car,' in control of their life choices.

References

Berk. L.E. *Landscapes of development: An anthology of reading.* Belmont, CA: Thomson/Wadsworth, 1999.

Corsini, R. J. and D. Wedding. *Current Psychotherapies*, Itasca, IL: Peacock, 1995.

Gardner, Howard. *Frames of mind: The theory of multiple intelligences*, New York: Basic Books, 1993.

Glasser, W. *Choice Theory: A New Psychology of Personal Freedom,* New York: Harper Collins, 1998.

—. *For Parents and Teenagers: Dissolving the Barrier between You and Your Teen*, New York: Harper Collins, 2004.

Lambert, M. J. "Implications of Outcome Research for Psychotherapy Integration." In J.C. Norcross & M.R. Goldfried (Eds.*), Handbook of Psychotherapy Integration.* New York: Basic Books, 1992:94-129..

Passaro, P. D, M. Moon, D. J. Wiest, and E. H. Wong, "A Model for School Psychology practice: Addressing the Needs of Students with Emotional and Behavioral Challenges through the Use of an In-school Support Room and Reality Therapy." *Adolescence, 39* no.155 (2004), 503-517.

Pledge, D. S. *Counseling adolescents & children: Developing your clinical style.* Belmont, CA: Brooks/Cole, 2004.

Prochaska, J.O. "How do People Change, and How can we Change to Help Many More People?" In M. A. Hubble, B. L. Duncan, & S. D. Miller (Eds.*), The Heart & Soul of Change: What Works in Therapy.* Ann Arbor, MI: Sheridan Books, 1999:227-255.

THE GOOD AND THE BEAUTIFUL: AESTHETIC CONCEPTS AND EXPRESSIVE ARTS THERAPY

JOAN FOREST MAGE

Introduction

Expressive Arts Therapists are led to several questions regarding the relation of aesthetics to our work. "What is art? What is the purpose of art? What is beautiful? What is beautiful art?" Is art to be produced only for its own sake, its inherent "beauty?" On the other hand, if art's purpose is to produce a beneficial social result, do we define the art that produces such a "good" result as beautiful?

Should Expressive Arts Therapists even be concerned with aesthetics? Some would define Expressive Arts Therapy in terms of its purpose: it is a form of healing which may include related purposes such as teaching, community-building, personal growth, spiritual expression, etc. Why don't we simply define Expressive Arts Therapy in terms of producing good social purpose, rather than producing beauty?

A final question is whether we need to separate the good from the beautiful. A central debate in the history of Western aesthetics is whether the purpose of an artistic activity should be considered as part of that art form's aesthetic. In this paper, we will look at various opinions on aesthetics. We will also discover cultures that include art and aesthetics as part of larger cultural activities such as healing or community bonding. We will see how Louis Sullivan's theory of "form follows function" and Ellen Dissanayake's theory of the common basis of play, ritual and art provide a link between good purpose and beauty. I believe that Expressive Arts Therapy can find a home in such an aesthetic theory.

This paper is an overview of aesthetic concepts that I see as relevant to the field of Expressive Arts Therapy. It is not an exhaustive research paper in the fields of philosophy, art history or anthropology. I hope it will be of value to Expressive Arts Therapists as we continue to develop individual and collective approaches to our work, and to explore the ways Expressive Arts Therapy can contribute to society.

Aesthetics: What's Included?

One of the big debates in the field of aesthetics is whether the purpose or "reason" for art should be part of what constitutes the beauty of that art form. Webster's dictionary (1993) defines "aesthetics" as:

> A branch of philosophy dealing with beauty and the beautiful, especially with judgments of taste concerning them. The philosophy or science of art, specifically the science whose subject matter is the description and explanation of the arts, artistic phenomena and aesthetic experience.

"Taste" is defined as:

> The power or practice of discerning and enjoying whatever constitutes excellence, especially in the fine arts and "belles letters:" critical judgment, discernment or appreciation.

Aesthetics, therefore, is a philosophy of beauty and the arts, and especially discernment or judgment regarding what constitutes beauty and art.

Peter Abbs (1991) points out that the word "aesthetic" derives from the Greek *aisthe,* meaning, "to feel, to apprehend through the senses." The opposite is our word "anesthetic", meaning "loss of feeling or sensation." Anesthetic commonly refers to the drugs given during surgery to create numbness to pain. To increase the aesthetic sense implies increasing and sensitizing one's feelings and awareness.

The word "aesthetic" is associated with the feeling or sensation created from experience, more than with our intellectual understanding of experience. To have an aesthetic sense means that a person is alive, feeling, and conscious of experience.

Beauty Separate from Purpose

In aesthetics, different authors vary greatly on what should even be included in the topic. Some say that aesthetics is about beauty *as separate* from purpose. Immanuel Kant (trans. 1951) brilliantly articulated this viewpoint. In *Critique of Judgment,* Kant draws a distinction between the good, the pleasant and the beautiful. He says that "pleasant" has to do with the sensation an individual feels; it is an individual's reaction to a thing that is enjoyable and delightful. "Good" means that a thing serves a useful purpose. For example, Kant says that if we asked the 18th century thinker Rousseau if the king's palace is beautiful, Rousseau, the champion of the common people, might say the palace was not beautiful because it was built by heavily taxing the poor. Kant says that this is a question of good, not beauty. One can say that the palace is not good, because it causes suffering for the people. However, whether the palace is beautiful is an entirely different question, according to Kant.

Kant says that beauty is not based in either logic (like the good) or sensation (like the pleasant.) Beauty is based in subjective reflection on an object, which is beyond mere sensation: it originates in *reflective judgment*, which is a deep, underlying sense of the rules and principles of "beauty" which the observer perceives in the object. Kant says that reflective judgment is *a priori*, meaning that it is an inherent faculty in each person. In other words, each person has a "sense of beauty" that it is not possible to explain further.

Even though beauty is subjective, it often has the characteristic of universality. It is not limited to the sensation that a particular individual has. Rather, many people using their reflective judgment will agree that a certain object is beautiful.

Kant's ideas were very influential throughout the 19th and early 20th centuries. A group called the aesthetes took these ideas to a logical extreme. Their philosophy was "art for art's sake"—they believed that art need serve no purpose outside of its own existence.

Philosophers such as Bullough (1912/1984) with his concept of "psychical distance" also built on Kant's idea. In psychical distance, the observer must contemplate the artwork or other aesthetic experience in a detached way in order to truly understand and appreciate its beauty. The observer should not be influenced by other factors, such as fear or distaste of the situation itself. This holds true whether the other factors are based on personal opinions, cultural tradition or even biological imperative, such as the safety of the observer. For example, Bullough says that passengers on a ship in foggy weather who were truly cultivating their aesthetic sense would focus on the beauty of the fog's mysterious, misty grayness, rather than worrying that the ship may run aground because of the lack of visibility.

Kant's *Critique* has its critics. Several authors (Dissanayake, 1992; Leuthold, 1998) point out that separating the good from the beautiful encourages the idea of aesthetic detachment, which has not been the norm in most cultures throughout history. It is peculiar to our modern technological society, where people learn to take an objective stance towards many aspects of life. Dissanayake (1992) quotes Jane Ellen Harrison as saying that, if we stick to this meaning of aesthetics, then if you are in a boat and a fellow passenger falls out and begins to drown, instead of going to the rescue you would merely admire the play of light and color on the waves created as the person flails about! I believe Kant would say that this situation requires a different branch of philosophy: it calls for ethics, which is about evaluating morality, rather than aesthetics, which is about evaluating beauty.

What constitutes aesthetics differs from one writer to another. Some writers are concerned with how the sense of the beautiful arises within the human being; some talk about what constitutes an ideal of beauty within a specific art form; others try to find an overriding principle that can serve as an assessment tool for the "success" of art. Leo Tolstoy addresses the question of artistic success in his essay *What Is Art?:*

"To evoke in oneself a feeling one has once experienced and...then by means of movements, lines, colors, sounds or forms....to transmit that feeling so that others experience the same feeling – this is the activity of art....If a man is infected by the author's condition of soul, if he feels this emotion and this union with others, then the object which has effected this is art; but if there be no such infection, if there be not this union with the author and with others who are moved by the same work – then it is not art. And not only is infection a sure sign of art, but the degree of infectiousness is also the sole measure of excellence in art" (Tolstoy, trans. 1930.)

Comparing Kant's to Tolstoy's views, we come to a central question. Is aesthetics about beauty, or is it about art? For example, should beautiful natural phenomena, like sunsets, be included in the study of aesthetics? Or is the study of aesthetics limited to those things and experiences crafted by humans? Again, we find differing opinions. Hofstadter (1965) states his belief that any object in nature can be aesthetically beautiful. Art is not the aesthetic object, but rather a statement of the aesthetic experience that the object brings forth in the observer. "It [the art work] is, in the strict sense, not an aesthetic *object* at all, but rather an aesthetic *symbol,* part of whose content is an aesthetic object, since it articulates aesthetic experience" (Hofstadter, 1965:184.) In other words, the artwork is art because it comments on the human reaction to the aesthetic impact of a natural object.

Twentieth century artists further questioned the aesthetics of human-formed vs. natural objects. By displaying common objects as artworks, artists raised the issue of whether simply displaying an object in certain contexts transmuted it into a work of art. Arthur Danto presents an interesting idea: it is the art world itself, as a community with particular beliefs and concepts that makes an object art:

> "To see something as art requires...an atmosphere of artistic theory, a knowledge of the history of art: an art world.
> Suppose a man collects objects (ready-mades,) including a Brillo carton: we praise the exhibit [and the collector] for variety, ingenuity, what you will...True, we don't say these things about the stock boy. However, a stockroom is not an art gallery, and we cannot readily separate the Brillo cartons from the gallery they are in...
> What in the end makes the difference between a Brillo box and a work of art consisting of a Brillo Box is a certain theory of art....It could not have been art fifty years ago. But then there could not have been, everything being equal, flight insurance in the Middle Ages, or Etruscan typewriter erasers. The world has to be ready for certain things, the art world no less than the real one. It is the role of artistic theories, these days as always, to make the art world, and art, possible. It would, I should think, never have occurred to the painters of Lascaux that they were producing art on those walls. Not unless there were Neolithic aestheticians."
> —Danto, 1964/1984

Art As Human Behavior: Purpose as Part of Aesthetic

Danto's comment about Neolithic painters leads us to the other side of the debate about whether art should serve a purpose beyond creating "beauty." Architect Louis Sullivan created the famous maxim "Form follows function:"

> "...shapes express the inner life, the native quality, of the animal, tree, bird, fish....Unceasingly the essence of things is taking shape in the matter of things, and this unspeakable process we call birth and growth.......Whether it be the sweeping eagle in his flight or the open apple-blossom, the toiling work-horse, the blithe swan, the branching oak, the winding stream at its base, the drifting clouds, over all the coursing sun, form ever follows function.... It is the pervading law of all things...that life is recognizable in its expression, that form ever follows function" (Michel, 1997.)

Here we see an aesthetic that connects purpose and beauty. For Sullivan, each thing born or created strives to reveal itself in a form corresponding to its very essence. The task of the artist is to follow and manifest this form. As Expressive Arts Therapists helping our clients to develop their individual potential, we can embrace Sullivan's aesthetic that art's purpose is to manifest the inner being.

Victor Turner was an anthropologist who studied the connections between play, ritual and art (Ashley, 1990.) He created a new field called Performance Studies, which looks at human activities such as religious ritual, civic ceremonies and performing arts as all arising from the human need for symbolic action (Schechner, 1993.)

Steven Leuthold and Ellen Dissanayake focus on the *reasons* humans make art. Both of them discuss art in indigenous cultures. An indigenous culture is a traditional way of life—language, religious beliefs, economy, social structure, arts—that has developed in a specific group of people over hundreds of years. Both Leuthold and Dissanayake comment that debating whether the purpose of art should be included in aesthetics is peculiar to Western culture. In his book *Indigenous Aesthetics,* Leuthold points out that the term aesthetics originated in the West, with its autonomous view of life:

"In an autonomist view art has several attributes: artworks are "unique," non-utilitarian, ego-identified (with the artist's intention,) self-validating in a psychological sense, innovative, "without rules," and for sale or exhibition as a commodity or an independent object that extends beyond a community. These attributes of art are tied to other experiences and problems in the West such as the nature of materialism versus spirituality, the development of capitalism, the value placed on individual freedom, and so on.

"Many of these attributes of art run counter to the attributes associated with art in indigenous cultures...many indigenous cultures did not identify their traditional expressive works as "art"; natives often believe there are social rules or guidelines for expression that must be followed and guarded; expressive objects and events are community-oriented; art is both useful and beautiful (its functioning is a part of beauty;) the artist is not above or separate from society (not "different" or "eccentric;") and there is no pressure towards innovation for its own sake."
—Leuthold 1998:6 - 7

Leuthold argues that we need a systems approach to understand the aesthetics of indigenous cultures:

"How is art integrated into or a part of a total system of belief and actions?...A difficult assumption for many Euro-Americans to question is that the artist's intention is the basis of aesthetic experience, a central element of autonomist views of art. A systems approach shifts the focus

from the private intention of an artist to an environment of information and experience: the entire environment as ready to become a work of art."
—Leuthold 1998:7

Leuthold states that "art is both useful and beautiful (its functioning is a part of beauty)...Aesthetic experience is bodily, sensory; it is not just abstract and theoretical. Our value systems are rooted in our experience of the world....beliefs and values are lived and embedded in social relationships."

Strange: don't these ideas of "value systems embedded in social relationships" and "the entire environment as ready to become a work of art" sound a lot like Danto's idea of the "art world?" In designating objects from the environment (such as Brillo boxes) as art, contemporary artists seem to be coming full circle to the larger, integrated concept of indigenous cultures, where art is often about creating ritual consciousness of relationships to the entire environment.

Danto says that a Brillo box would not have been art fifty years ago, but progressions in the theory of art now identify it as art. Whether an indigenous tribe or the modern art world, communities express their beliefs and values through their art.

Another concept is that art should serve to teach positive values in society. Many indigenous cultures have storytelling and songs that explain the history of their people, and the proper relation of humans to the spirit realm (Abram, 1996.) Clothing, adornments, tattooing, piercing and other body decorations are used to advertise or to signal changes in social status or membership in particular groups, thus ensuring the stability and safe transitions of status within the community. In Zambia, boys practice the *mukanda* dance, which helps them develop relationships with their peers to replace their childish dependence on their mothers (Dissanayake, 1992.)

While art in ritual contexts can have a positive effect in building relationships and communication among community members, some say that too much focus on conveying traditional values through the arts can have a stifling effect on society. The ancient Greek philosopher Plato wrote in *The Republic* that the purpose of art is to instill virtue in the young, and he recommended a type of censorship so that the arts would encourage young people to be virtuous (Plato, trans. 1892.) Karl Marx felt the arts should reflect the realities of society and show how to win the class struggle, thus creating the ideal society (Marcuse, 1978/1984.)

Marcuse says artistic aesthetics should not demand the demonstration of a particular system of social values:

"A devaluation of the entire realm of subjectivity takes place...of inwardness, emotions and imagination. The subjectivity of individuals... tends to be dissolved into class-consciousness. Thereby, a major prerequisite of revolution is minimized, namely, the fact that the need for radical change must be rooted in the subjectivity of individuals themselves, in their intelligence and passions, their drives and their goals."
—Marcuse, 1978/1984:521

Expressive Arts Therapists perform their work in contexts such as healing, education, social development, civic and religious ceremony, rather than in an "art for art's sake" environment. In that way, Expressive Arts Therapy is part of an ancient tradition found in many cultures, in which purpose—creating positive social value—is considered part of art's aesthetic.

Art As Energy Work

Many Expressive Arts Therapists ground their practice in the concept of healing through transforming energy. This concept of energy healing is shared by many indigenous cultures, as well as the Asian world. For example, the acupuncture and herbs of Chinese medicine and Indian Ayurvedic medicine are based in balancing energy.

In healing from an energetic standpoint, we focus transforming the energy to a positive, healthy state. Peter Abbs (1991) proposes a similar line of thinking in his aesthetic field model:

"Art should not refer to a series of discrete artifacts or what some critics call "art objects" but to a highly complex web of energy linking the artist to the audience, and both artist and audience to all inherited culture."
—Abbs, 1991:247- 248.

We may also recall Sullivan's statement "Form follows function." According to Sullivan, everything in existence has an inner essence that strives to become manifest in a form peculiar to that essence. If we think of this inner essence as energy, "Form follows function" is a wonderful statement of an energetically based aesthetic.

Art in indigenous cultures is often intertwined in spiritual ceremonies. From the Hawaiian hula to the Kung healing dance of Africa to Indian dancing of the Shiva mythology, dance is used as a means of channeling spiritual energy. Song and chant are used from Australia to North America to invoke the gods and spiritual power, as are visual art forms such as costumes, masks and sand painting (Dissanayake, 1992.)

Throughout history, writers on aesthetics have talked about art as being inspired from a spiritual or energetic source. In his work *Ion*, the ancient Greek philosopher Aristotle (trans. 1925) differentiates between the training and skills needed for the technical aspects of one's art, such as learning techniques of singing or dancing, and the inspiration for the art, which Aristotle says comes from possession by the spirits. The artist receives the inspiration from the spirits and then passes it on to the audience. Aristotle gives the analogy of a magnet (spirit) magnetizing one piece of iron (an artist,) which in turn attracts many other pieces of iron (the audience.)

Anthropologist Victor Turner said that both art and ritual are liminal. Liminality is a state of changing structures and identities, "of ambiguity, even paradox, outside or mediating between customary categories" (Ashley, 1990.) Just as a tribe might employ a ritual as a liminal process to create the shift from boyhood to manhood, so art is often a liminal experience, helping the audience and artist make energetic shifts to new perceptions and even identities.

Lev Vygotsky (1971/1984) was a 20th century Russian psychologist who spoke of art as energy work. For Vygotsky, art creates catharsis, or transformation, through awakening contrasting affects (emotions) in the observer. He relates emotions to rhythms.

"We can say that the basic aesthetic response consists of affect caused by art, affect experienced by us as if it were real, but which finds its release in the activity of imagination provoked by a work of art …[art delays] the motor expression of emotions and, by making opposite impulses collide…initiates an explosive discharge of nervous energy."
—Vygotsky, 1971/1984:518

In Vygotsky's description, we see the artist as creating a transformational container through the artwork. This form becomes so powerful that it can transform the emotions (affect) of the audience.

Arts-Based Community Development (ABCD) is "arts-centered activity that contributes to the sustained advancement of human dignity, health and/or productivity within a community" (Cleveland, 2002.) Cleveland's article explains that arts-based community development encompasses many approaches to the arts, from artists creating murals about a neighborhood's history, to using the arts to teach children conflict resolution. Cleveland has created a model for ABCD that shows its four fundamental purposes: educate and inform; inspire and mobilize; nurture and heal; build or improve the community. He says, "Historically, we see ABCD as a modern iteration of perhaps the oldest 'field' with a lineage that stretches back to prehistoric shamanism." The shaman's role is to heal through shifting energy, and shamans often have used the arts to accomplish this goal.

A Common Bond: The Imaginal World

Ellen Dissanayake's book *Homo Aestheticus* (1992) points out that though people are called *Homo Sapiens* ("thinking man") art is as omnipresent a behavior for humans as thinking. Virtually every human being in every human culture for all of human history has participated in the arts.

Dissanayake says that art must have evolutionary survival value for the human species, because no behavior is universal in a species if it does not have survival value for that species. Dissanyake then asks what is the difference between three common types of human behavior: play, ritual and art. She gives a most profound answer: *"other" worlds [are]...invented in play, invoked in ritual or fabricated in the arts"* (Dissanayake, 1992:51.)

Play, ritual and art all deal with the imaginal realm. But the purpose of play is to invent a non-ordinary realm; the purpose of ritual is to invoke its spiritual or energetic power; and the purpose of art is to fabricate the imaginal realm into physical form. The artist takes materials in the physical world – paint, movement, sounds, and words – and causes them to manifest the energy the artist perceives.

Dissanayake's theory has great potential as part of an aesthetic for Expressive Arts Therapy. It aligns with the way many Expressive Arts Therapists guide their clients from initial exercises (play) to energetic catharsis (ritual) through various media (art.) Of all the theories about art and beauty, it answers the most basic question of how art is able to create transformation. It does not create an aesthetic in terms of defining which forms are considered more beautiful than others are, but provides a fundamental definition of art's purpose. Expressive Arts Therapy, which unites good purpose and beautiful form, can benefit from such an aesthetic theory.

Conclusion

Aesthetics, the philosophy of beauty and the arts, has engendered numerous theories throughout history and cross-culturally. Two major branches of aesthetics are those that include the purpose of the artwork as part of the definition of the aesthetic, and those that define beauty as separate from other purposes the art might have. Such Western authors as Kant, Bullough and the aesthetes define beauty as separate from good purpose. In contrast, the aesthetics of many cultures consider how well the art helps fulfill social, religious or other purposes.

Expressive Arts Therapy, which deals with healing and other social and spiritual purposes, may be considered as more aligned with aesthetic concepts that include good purpose and beautiful form. Such authors as Victor Turner, Steven Leuthold and William Cleveland explain the impact the arts have in fulfilling social purposes.

Many Expressive Arts Therapists define their work as healing through utilizing art to shift energy. This is similar to the spiritual healing practices of many indigenous cultures. Artists and thinkers from Aristotle to Vygotsky have included the spiritual/energetic component in their definition of aesthetics.

Louis Sullivan theory of "form follows function" and Ellen Dissanayake's theory that sees play, ritual and art as having a common basis in the imaginal world, both have great potential to serve as the basis of an aesthetic for Expressive Arts Therapy.

References

Abbs P. "Defining the Aesthetic Field" In R. Smith and A. Simpson (Eds.), *Aesthetics and Arts Education,* Urbana, IL: University of Illinois Press, 1991: 245 – 255.

Abram, D. *The Spell of the Sensuous*, New York: Vintage, 1996.

Aristotle. "Poetics." In S. Ross (Ed.), *Art And Its Significance: An Anthology of Aesthetic Theory.* Albany, NY: State University of New York Press (Original work translated 1925,) 1984:68 – 78.

Ashley, K. Introduction. In K. Ashley (Ed.), *Victor Turner and the Construction of Cultural Criticism.* Bloomington, IN: Indiana University Press, 1990: ix –xxii.

Bullough, E. "Psychical Distance" as a Factor in Art and as an Aesthetic Principle." In S. Ross (Ed.), *Art And Its Significance: An Anthology of Aesthetic Theory.* Albany, NY: State University of New York Press (Original work published 1912,) 1984: 458 – 468.

Cleveland, W. *Mapping the field: Arts-Based Community Development.* [Online]. Available: http://www.communityarts.net/readingroom/archive/intro-develop.php. 2002

Danto, A. "The Artworld." In S. Ross (Ed.), *Art And Its Significance: An Anthology of Aesthetic Theory*. Albany, NY: State University of New York Press (Original work published 1964,) 1984: 469 – 482.

Dissanayake, E. *Homo Aestheticus*. New York: The Free Press, 1992.

Hofstadter, A. *Truth And Art*. New York: Columbia University Press, 1965.

Kant, I. "Critique of Judgment," In S. Ross (Ed.), *Art And Its Significance: An Anthology of Aesthetic Theory*. Albany, NY: State University of New York Press (Original work translated 1951,) 1984: 98 – 144.

Leuthold, S. *Indigenous Aesthetics*. Austin, TX: University of Texas Press, 1998.

Marcuse, H. " The Aesthetic Dimension," In S. Ross (Ed.), *Art And Its Significance: An Anthology of Aesthetic Theory*. Albany, NY: State University of New York Press (Original work published 1971,) 1984 (pp. 519 – 529.)

Michel, J. *Form follows WHAT? The modernist notion of function as a carte blanche*. [Online]. Available: http://www.geocities.com/Athens/2360/english-only.htm. 1997

Plato." Ion." In S. Ross (Ed.,) *Art And Its Significance: An Anthology of Aesthetic Theory*. Albany, NY: State University of New York Press (Original work translated 1892,) 1984: 47 – 58.

Schechner, R. *The Future of Ritual,* London: Routledge, 1993.

Tolstoy, L. "What Is Art?" In S. Ross (Ed.), *Art And Its Significance: An Anthology of Aesthetic Theory*. Albany, NY: State University of New York Press (Original work translated 1930,) 1984: 179 – 183.

Vygotsky, L. "The Psychology of Art." In S. Ross (Ed.), *Art And Its Significance: An Anthology of Aesthetic Theory*. Albany, NY: State University of New York Press (Original work published 1971,) 1984: 516 – 518.

Webster's Third *New International Dictionary of the English Language.* Springfield, MA: Merriam Webster, 1993.

VI: VIEWING A FIELD OF LIFELONG LEARNING

INNER HEALING: THE CO-CREATION OF EMOTIONAL TRANSCENDENCE

BENJAMIN B. KEYES

"Inner healing" has been co-opted as a psychological technique used primarily in spiritual communities to connect to memories of pain, hurt, or trauma in an effort towards cathartic resolution. The purpose of this abreaction is to work through deep-seated and repressed feelings and memories, and to enable the present day effects of such to dissipate.

We know that memories include feelings, concepts, patterns, attitudes, and tendencies towards actions that accompany the mental pictures that arise during the process of creative visualization in the abreacting of a memory (Seamands, 1985.) Whole actions and not just distorted pictures, that is to say our stored visual memories, particularly those of a traumatic nature, tend to draw us towards certain behaviors and actions, often leading to dysfunction when not confronted and worked through. The process of inner healing is a form of counseling which focuses the healing power of God (in AA terms God as you perceive God; in Christian terms, God embodied in the Trinity, Father, Son, Holy Spirit; in Judaic and Islamic terms, the One God, etc.) on specific areas of emotional and spiritual problems. This creative force allows individuals literally to co-create with God, through tapping emotional boundaries and entering new landscapes for our psychological wellbeing and our very lives. We are only limited by our own levels of creativity, insight into the conditions and problems, and our faith in being able to connect with a power beyond ourselves.

It has been said that time heals all wounds; however in a case where emotion and memory has not been sufficiently addressed, the leftover feelings are often repressed or compensated for in ways that allow the person to bear and manage the problem situation. For instance, in the area of childhood sexual abuse, a child may learn to dissociate or disconnect from the actual feeling of the sexual violation in order to cope with the traumatic situation. Later, because of that disconnection, the child may continue to idolize the perpetrator, especially if the perpetrator is a close family member, because the affective memory of the trauma has been effectively blocked. Over time, this can and will cause significant cognitive distortion in this child's perception of relationships.

Our minds act as a protective defense mechanism, not only in significant trauma situations, but also in times of hurt, shame, or humiliation. These mechanisms become a way of protecting ourselves from difficult emotions and, wonderfully, preserving an essence of self. Situations for which techniques for inner healing are particularly useful include: death of a family member, severe trauma, the effects of war, the horror of child abuse, perceived hurts and slights by others, family of origin issues, and traumas from manmade or natural disasters, to name but a few. When our emotional reactions and feelings become overloaded, we literally experience the sensation of a "fuse blowing out." The result is that problems and feelings often sublimate to the subconscious and later reappear as physical illnesses, unhappy marital situations, or significant psychological distress. These conditions may spiral into recurring cycles of defeat.

Theory

Cartesian theory separates the mind from the body and does not address the spiritual nature of human beings, since the latter nature is not seen as something that is tangible, nor can it be measured. Recently Descartes' theories have been challenged by quantum physics and the postulation that the spiritual self can be quantified through electromagnetic energy (Ross, 2009.) We do not know if this is "true," but it raises an important question about the nature of our spiritual selves. Religions around the world, and man himself, have been wrestling since the dawn of thought with ideas about the essence of who God is, who we are spiritually, and what our purpose in life is. Each has devised his/her own theory. I believe that the one place where the three energies of mind, body, and spirit converge is in the heart. Not the literal organ, but the soul we often refer to as the heart. The heart, in Jewish tradition, incorporates the wholeness of the self, all that the self is; the seat of emotion, love, and transcendence. In Hindu tradition, the heart is the gateway to the higher self. The ability to give and receive love unlocks the gifts of insight, true knowledge, and spiritual awakening. In the heart sits the ultimate battle between the higher and lower selves, good versus evil, heaven versus hell.

The good news, I believe, is that there is a way out of hell, out of the lower self, and a way to avoid evil. The tough news is that all of us have to work at it, to work through it. The hurts, pains, and traumas of our lives often hinder our continued growth. They affect all areas of our "self" in various ways, and it is the processing of the affect or feelings, which have been held back or repressed, that allow both release and freedom to continue our growth. Thus, when we process through the heart, we know continued growth and spiritual development.

My personal work with traumatized patients has spanned nearly twenty-five years. It has encompassed hospital, partial and residential treatment, outpatient, and field settings. I have worked with the entire dissociative spectrum, including Borderline Personality Disorders, Post Traumatic Stress Disorders, and a variety of Dissociative Disorders. All hurt and trauma, whether emotional, physical, or sexual, becomes encoded, because of dissociation, into mind and body. This happens at various levels based on the degree of severity, duration, and perception of the trauma. With children, these experiences and feelings become encoded from a childhood framework and are often frozen in time. Time literally stands still in their internal state, and if the trauma is not processed from the very moment of the trauma, the child will be forced to adapt or integrate the experience, complete with feelings, sensations, thoughts, and secondarily beliefs, into a concept of how the world is. The paradigm that is formed often causes distortions of thoughts and behavior in later life.

The New Testament states that the Kingdom of God is in the heart and to enter this Kingdom we must enter as children (Matt 19:14; Mk 10:15.) I would like to look for a moment at both of these aspects before exploring the inner healing process. If the heart is where the Kingdom of God is, it must incorporate all that we are and the totality of self, again the place where mind, body, and spirit are perceived as one. The early Greeks had a theory that has shaped much of our Western thinking about the division of physical and spiritual identity. They separated each aspect of the self. From this framework, when we are encouraged to have a change of heart or take heart, it literally means to change or take stock of all, the whole of who we are. The Greek word metanoia translates as "repent," or "turn around." Figuratively, it means to have a change of heart or a change of wholeness.

The inner healing process and the model that we will be discussing is a journey to the depth of our heart or the depth of our wholeness to experience change. Generally, we human beings are not complete, not full of wholeness; most of us are in process, unfinished; we find that we have parts that are infirm or incomplete. Unexpressed hurts, traumas, and weaknesses have a tendency to distort our ability to function. They become qualities of our personality that predispose or incline us to not become all that we are capable of being. They are weakened places in our defenses that undermine our resistance to our lower or baser self.

Think for a moment about the world of a young child. If it is nurtured well, it experiences wonder, awe, and growth. Many of us were born into a world where our parents expected us, cared for our needs, and answered our cries. However, many do not have that experience. If the child is shut down, that child experiences hurt, pain and frustration. Think about the world into which you were born. Most of you can say that your parents planned for you, nurtured you, some were breast-fed, you were changed regularly, and given attention to grow and develop. This type of experience in early childhood leads to growth and the development of a sense of gratefulness, awe or grace. Take for a moment, a child born to a mother who was addicted to crack cocaine, who prostitutes to support herself. This child is often neglected, left alone, not changed, or properly cared for. The child may be physically harmed or malnourished. These children experience the world as cold, unbending, and in turn develop distrust because their needs have not been met. They expect the world not to meet their needs.

The Greeks used two words to identify aspects of childhood. The first is "nepios" which literally means childish and would be used to categorize the results of an unhappy childhood. It also denotes someone who is spiritually immature. A healthy childhood however is described as the word "pation," literally, childlike. A healthy child is teachable, humble, accepting of others, and has faith. The process of inner healing, especially when we consider the heart-centered model, can restore and transform part or all of an unhappy childhood. By co-creating with God, as you understand God to be, co-creating within a basis of faith, a healthy "adult child" emerges, capable of being taught and seeing the wonder in life.

Certain theories of trauma, especially that of Jack and Helen Watkins (1993,) who wrote so much regarding ego-state therapy, hold that most people are multiplicities at some level whether they be covert or overt. Personality segments called ego states represent specializations of functions that have been initiated and developed for better adjustment, and in some cases for the very survival of the individual. We all have ego states. Currently I am in the role of a writer, but when I answer the phone and speak to my wife, I am in the role of a husband, and when I talk to my son, I am in the role of a father. Each of these is an example of ego states. When I experience feelings of anger, sadness, ecstasy, or joy these are also ego states. Alternatively, I can recall situations in my own life, such as when I was 17 and hated school, or when I was five and was frustrated at a party due to illness. These, too, are ego states. Qualities such as vulnerability or strong will are also ego states. Another way to look at this is that we do not feel, think, perceive or act the same way all of the time. A music fan may shout or scream at a concert but at home be perceived as shy or conservative. A laid-back mother may become fierce or warrior-like if her child is threatened. To quote Jack Watkins:

> "Such differential responses are common and are taken for granted. What perhaps is not so recognized is that these different response patterns result not only from different precipitating conditions, but also from differing internal organizing systems of feeling, motivation, and cognition within the individual. Sometimes the same internal conditions will provoke a very different response because a personality segment has been activated and for the moment becomes activated or controlled by the individual." (1992)

In non-technical language, it simply means that parts of ourselves can and are often segmented, isolated, or disconnected from our conscious self. The inner healing process is used to reconnect to those places, with the goal of achieving a greater sense of wholeness. I believe that this reconnection is not only a journey to our past, but must be done with a sense of faith in God for completeness. There has been an age-old conflict between psychologists, scientists, and physicians, against with those who come from a theological frame of reference. Regardless of which religious reference you use, Jewish, Christian, Islam, Hindu, Buddhist, etcetera, or even the AA term of "Higher Power," I believe that a sense of something greater than yourself is essential to healing and transformation. Several years ago, my daughter read a book during a time when she was exploring her theological boundaries. The book said in essence, 'There is a God and you are not Him.' This seemed profound at the time; it met her at a teachable moment. I believe that we have to connect beyond ourselves, even if that is reaching out beyond ourselves to others like us; when we do, we will see the total of others is greater than ourselves. Folks in AA often start out this way, seeing the group as greater than the self and, more importantly, as being more powerful than they are themselves, in isolation. The "canvas" of co-creation we can paint in life is only limited by our creativity. We can use our creative force and our connection to others, moving through our spirituality as a vehicle for healing, growth, wholeness, and beauty.

Methodology

The technique for inner healing itself is a systematic process that utilizes creative visualization and can incorporate some hypnotic technique and/or guided prayer to allow the individual to clearly see and recreate the experience of the submerged memory. The experience of reconnecting to difficult and sometimes horrific situations may cause a re-experiencing of an affective response that often needs to be talked out, worked out, and processed using therapeutic counseling interventions. The issues of repressed anger, hurt, and deep-seated emotion quickly may come to the surface and can be confronted and worked through towards resolution. Often in these situations, clients have blamed themselves when the blame was not in any way theirs. As for their spiritual situation, issues with their view of God may have formed a distorted framework for thinking, and must be confronted. A victim may feel that God did not protect them or rescue them from the situation. In most major religions, God's promise is one of presence, that is, God promises to be with us through difficult times, not to rescue us with the immediate, hoped-for change. To realize that God has been with us at time of trauma, hurt, etcetera, and that God continues to be with us, up to and including the present time, often represents a significant paradigm shift for many dealing with ongoing spiritual and psychological issues. The spiritually based therapist's task is to somehow communicate and demonstrate this presence of God. The change, when God's presence is known, is often enough of a shift to be able to foster hope and renewed purpose in life as the client works towards resolution of ongoing issues.

The inner healing process moves through a series of events in order to allow the adult self in present time to emotionally and spiritually reach back and rescue the child or younger adult self from the time of hurt or trauma. From a Judeo-Christian context, since God is not a God of time, we literally allow God to travel with us back to the memory and work towards healing that memory and bring back a change to our awareness in present time. In a very real sense, we are allowing our adult self to reach to our inner child (Bradshaw, 1990.)

Often the issue of forgiveness becomes a primary component of the healing process. Interestingly, however, the issue is focused on the self, that is, forgiving ourselves, not so much forgiving any perpetrator that inflicted the hurt. While this last issue may be an appropriate avenue to pursue in counseling, forgiving others is not a necessary component of the healing process. Forgiveness of self, though, is essential. The final stage of this process has to do with reconnection, or in Gestalt terms, "the parts becoming whole." By combining techniques of creative visualization, creative relaxation, and visual color therapy, the feeling of wholeness can be achieved with a corresponding pleasant affective response. For the sense of wholeness to be realized, it is not just a connection to the self, but also a connection to God, that completes this process. While I have not defined God in this article, I have a particular Judeo-Christian bias, which is the framework that defines my work. I am also aware that not everyone shares my worldview, so I have left the definition of God to the way the individual defines God to be, such as AA terms, a "Higher Power." From this writer's perspective, however, it is essential that the individual begin to experience God (again how they understand God) as truly loving, caring, and supportive. This is essential to long term healing. Having such an agenda may bring up, in the course of working, this individual's distortions of God. These may cast a negative light on the Higher Power, and create spiritual distance for the hurting person. As in the working through of personal issues in the case of their trauma, the same must be done in their issues with God if they are to know full healing. A connection to God as well as to self is necessary for their wholeness to be complete.

The process of inner healing can be done in the course of one therapeutic session (i.e. one to two hours.) It is more common however, for this process to occur over a period of time, which for severe trauma may take several months or even years. Issues surrounding hurts, shames, humiliations, etcetera, can often be worked out in a matter of a few sessions or weeks.

I have heard it said that some people are not visual. While it is true that some people do not engage in a visualization process easily, memories are primarily visual. They incorporate so much more than visual images, however, and the process of abreacting may occur through any of the other senses. It may take a little time to discern the learning and encoding style of the individual before healing work can begin.

While the step-by-step process listed below may seem somewhat simplistic, I would like to sketch out the model as a systematic process. The title of the model is Healing Emotional/Affective Responses to Trauma (HEART) and incorporates the following ten steps (Keyes, 2008):

1. Create a safe environment.
2. Reconnect to and anchor memory.
3. Process affect and/or cognitive distortions.
4. Dialogue: do emotional negotiation between adult self in present time and adult self and/or child at time of hurt or trauma.
5. Facilitate forgiveness of self.
6. Facilitate awareness of spiritual higher power or God. Process possible distortions of Higher Power or God.
7. Facilitate forgiveness of self in relation to Higher Power or God.
8. Merge the split parts.
9. Merge split relationship between self and Higher Power or God.

10. Refocus to life with new insight, purpose, and hope.

Any spiritual processing, whether from a counseling framework or as a spiritual intervention, needs to provide safety for the person doing the experiencing. This safety aspect is not only physical but encompasses a level of trust and rapport with the practitioner; its purpose is to provide a place of emotional safety for the client or the one who is on the spiritual journey. The process of inner healing starts with trust and then focuses on reconnecting to memories, being attuned to them. We are sometimes not consciously aware of those memories while abreacting or reliving the experience. In working this process, it is important to anchor to the memory, bringing it to fullness, by expanding the perceptual hold on it. This is done by using all five of our senses and locking in, possibly using a signal, the awareness of prior experience. Many will find this similar to hypnosis, neuro-linguistic programming and other regressive techniques; however, a clear distinction, that of including the use of prayer, is essential. The prayer becomes a focus or guiding path for dealing with the inner pain or trauma. In the third stage, we deal with feelings, allowing the full expression(s,) reaction(s,) connection(s,) to feelings past and present, as they currently are experienced in the situation. David Grove (Grove and Panzer, 1991) describes the processing of trauma in the following manner:

$$T-1 \rightarrow T \rightarrow T+1.$$

In other words, going to a time before the trauma, and then working through the trauma, and on to a time just after the trauma. This stage brings up many feelings, reactions, and cognitive distortions. The encoding of the trauma is in pictures, in whole concepts, because there has been no time to sectionalize, compartmentalize, or categorize. It is just this process that the false memory people have criticized in the work with traumatized children because of their belief in the ability to create false memory. It is therefore essential that a therapist's questioning process not have any iatrogenic quality and that any information revealed comes from the individual's process.

The next step of this process negotiates between the adult self of present time and the adult or child self at the time of the hurt or trauma. This often brings up tremendous cognitive distortion around issues of self-blame, regret, or self-condemnation. Sometimes issues around exoneration of the perpetrator attached to self-blame become present. Discussing and working through the issues might take a considerable portion of time, but is necessary in the healing process. The goal of these negotiations is to find a way for the adult self to forgive and not to seek some type of repayment from the earlier adult or child involved in the trauma. Self-forgiveness is essential for someone to open up to a spiritual dimension because self-blame and other issues often block a person from openness, freedom, and spontaneity. The latter qualities, exemplified in a healthy personality, are the qualities for living an artful life.

We have what may be called a sixth sense, which allows us to intuit, discern, or sense a presence. Have you ever walked into a room and started to feel uneasy, later to find out that there had been an argument or disruption of some sort in that room? In the same way, we can sense or know the presence of God. We feel, emote, connect; it goes beyond words. That connection often brings up distortions in our image of God. When these distortions come into play, they can create tremendous turmoil, confusion, and/or frustration. The distortion pattern works this way: we confuse my father who abused me, with my God who allowed me to be abused, or worse yet, God who abused me. Or, my friend, brother, mother, etc, who died, with God who killed or allowed my friend, brother, or mother to die. Until we have a mental picture of God, as we understand God, as a truly good, healing, and gracious presence, there can be no lasting spiritual victory in our lives (Seamands, 1985.)

Our failure to trust and love a Higher Power/God stems from a picture of that Higher Power/God as unlovable and/or untrustworthy. Our anger therefore is not at God, but in reality, it is at our wrong concept and perceptions of God. Our pictures and/or perceptions determine our paradigm of the ways things are, and that belief determines how we behave. We can find, through experiences of love and acceptance by our Higher Power/God that God's presence abides: it has always been there. This Spirit of God therefore bears witness to and within our spirit. Allowing a sense of love, freedom and forgiveness from the Devine to flow to us releases self-forgiveness and offers us hope and freedom in the future. We can have freedom from our distortions and freedom from a refracted belief system.

The rest of the inner healing process is both a solidifying of pictures and emotions of present times and the time of hurt and trauma. Bringing the adult self-of-now together with the adult or child self-of-then, and then allowing our awareness of our Higher Power/God to solidify with the united parts of ourselves is when much of the healing occurs. This merging and blending is done through guided visualization and is supported with prayerful intentions of healing by both the practitioner and the individual. When we allow the images/picture of the memory to blend and merge into one image and allow our spirit to connect fully to God's Spirit, we become whole, complete, and a vital force both in the memory of the past and in present time. We can then connect to present time whole, together, and renewed. It becomes important then, and only then, to share the experience. Sharing further validates the transformation as we continue to grow and develop spiritually.

Conclusion

In this process of inner healing using the HEART model, we do not change the past but we reframe and restructure the present in regards to the past with our Higher Power/God's help. There is a song in pop culture by the Indigo Girls titled Galileo in which the question is asked, "How long 'till my soul gets it right? Can any human being reach that light?" (1992) The song manages to capture humankind's age-old struggle to affirm existence by attempting to attain insight and enlightenment. Reworded, it cries to us, "do we ever finish?" or "do I ever get the full understanding of myself or my purpose in life and be able to move on?" And "do I ever get to be free of the binding trappings that take away from who I am and who I want to be?" It is important to know that our life is a process and a journey, not a destination. The journey will last our lifetime and will move us to higher levels of consciousness and awareness, a greater sense of self, and ultimately, true freedom. This path starts with our willingness and intent, and ends in love. It is the path of HEART.

References

Bradshaw, J. *Homecoming- Reclaiming and Championing Your Inner Child*. New York: Bantam Books, 1990.

Grove, D.J. and B.I. Panzer *Resolving Traumatic Memories – Metaphors and Symbols in Psychotherapy*. New York: Irvington Publishers, Inc., 1991.

Keyes, B. B. *Healing Emotional Affective Responses to Trauma (HEART), A Christian Model for Working with Traumatized Clients*. Pre-Conference Workshop Presented at the 6th Annual Mid-Year Conference on Religion and Spirituality, Loyola College in Maryland and Division 36 of the American Psychological Association, Columbia Md. (February, 2008.)

Ross, C. A. *Human Energy Fields- A New Science and Medicine*. Richardson, TX: Manitou Communications, (In Press)

Saylors, E. "Galileo." Sung by the Indigo Girls, on *Rights of Passage*. Epic Records, Bearsville Studios, Woodstock, N.Y. 1992.

Seamands, D. A., *Healing of Memories*. Wheaton IL: Victor Books, 1982.

Watkins, H. H. and J. G. Watkins. "Ego-State therapy in the treatment of dissociative disorders," In R. P. Kulft & C. P. Fine (Eds.), *Clinical Perspectives on Multiple Personality disorder* American Psychiatric Association, Washington D.C., 1993:277-299.

Watkins, J. G. *Hypnoanalytic Techniques*. New York: Irvington Publishers, Inc., 1992.

ARTWORKS IN TIMES OF CRISIS: TRAUMA & TROUBLED TEENS

POPPY MOON

Sand Tray Exposure Therapy and PTSD

Sand Tray Exposure Therapy (STET) is a form of exposure-based therapy for treating Posttraumatic Stress Disorder (PTSD.) STET has been used as an effective treatment for returning American Iraq war veterans diagnosed with PTSD. STET requires the client to focus on and recreate the details of traumatic war experiences in a sand tray with miniatures. Sand trays allow clients to confront their fear stimuli in a safe, therapeutic environment. STET continues until anxiety is reduced.

Sand Tray Exposure Therapy with American Veterans of the Iraq War Diagnosed with PTSD

"Nothing in my simple, suburban, Starbucks coffee drinking life prepared me for the horrors of what I would witness and experience in Iraq," Mark stated, shifting in his chair. "The worst part is these memories continually play over and over in my mind. My wife tells me to just forget about it, but she doesn't understand."

Mark, like 15 to 17 percent of returning veterans suffers from Posttraumatic Stress Disorder, or PTSD (Hoge et al., 2004.) PTSD is a psychiatric disorder that results from experiencing or witnessing events that are extremely traumatic or life threatening. Soldiers in Iraq, who experience firsthand military combat and terrorist threats, are especially at risk for developing this disorder. A study by the Department of Defense found that one in six soldiers returning from Iraq reported symptoms of PTSD, such as depression and anxiety (Epstein & Miller, 2005.) It is important that counselors educate themselves about current treatment methods to help this growing population. Exposure therapy is thought to be one of the most effective treatment methods for PTSD (Foa et al, 2000.) "Sand Tray Exposure Therapy" (STET) can be used as an innovative exposure therapy technique to treat PTSD in American veterans of the Iraq war.

PTSD

PTSD, or Posttraumatic Stress Disorder, is listed in the in the DSM-IV-R as an emotional disorder that results from experiencing an event that elicits a severe stress reaction (American Psychiatric Association, 2000.) Individuals suffering from PTSD relive the traumatic event(s) repeatedly in their minds, through nightmares and flashbacks. These thoughts can become so realistic and severe that the individual begins to dissociate, become estranged from friends and family members, and experience reduced functioning in daily life. PTSD is comorbid with other illnesses, such as depression, physical and mental problems, and substance abuse.

The medical profession believes that PTSD is the result of chemical changes in the brain that occur after an individual has experienced extreme stress (Tyre, 2004.) In a high intensity war situation, a soldier's body releases large amounts of adrenaline into the bloodstream. The adrenaline heightens awareness, speeds up the heart, and prepares the body for a fight or flight situation. When the soldier is in this state of hyperarousal, the amygdala, or fear center of the brain, is stimulated for long periods of time. His mind memorizes the sights, sounds, and smells of the moment. After the soldier has returned home, these sense memories can be triggered if the veteran is exposed to similar situations. Although the situation is no longer harmful, the brain still registers it from a fight or flight perspective.

History of PTSD

PTSD is not a new disorder; it has affected people since the beginning of human civilization. In 490 B.C., the Greek historian Herodotus recorded symptoms of PTSD in his writings on the Battle of Marathon. Egyptian and Roman historians also noted PTSD symptoms in their records related to various wars (Bentley, 2005.) PTSD is not solely linked to war trauma. Any type of traumatic experience such as rape, a motor vehicle accident, or physical abuse, can trigger PTSD. Samuel Pepys, an English journalist from 1666, described the Great Fire of London in his writings. He wrote "A most horrid, malicious, blood fire.....so great was our fear....it was enough to put us out of our wits" (Bentley, 2000.) Although his home and possessions were not destroyed, he reported characteristic symptoms of PTSD, such as anger, anxiety, nightmares, and flashbacks after the incident.

How PTSD Affects Returning Iraq Veterans

When a soldier returns from war, he usually experiences a time of intense relief and joyous reunions with family and friends. However, after this initial honeymoon period, life settles back into a predictable pattern. The family unit may have changed while the soldier was away, and he may have difficulty assimilating back into home and work life. Many soldiers find that they are unable to let go of their war memories. Veterans may have trouble sleeping, experience vivid dreams and nightmares, and/or become plagued with distressing thoughts and unwanted memories. Depression and anxiety symptoms may manifest. Along with these conditions, many soldiers report increased anger, irritability, and emotional numbing. All of these signs indicate PTSD.

Treatment for PTSD

For the past 15 to 20 years, exposure therapy has been effectively adapted and applied as a treatment method for PTSD (Foa et al., 2000; Rothbaum & Schwartz, 2002.) Rothbaum and Schwartz (2002) provide a complete review of exposure therapy and PTSD. In exposure therapy clients are exposed repeatedly to their own personal fear stimuli. Over time, exposure to these stimuli diminishes fear responses. The main goal of exposure therapy is to help the client gain control over memories and the resulting negative emotions, recognize faulty perceptions of danger, and learn coping skills to deal with distressing conditions (National Center for Post-Traumatic Stress Disorder, 2004.)

Initially exposure therapy techniques can cause heightened anxiety, which can result in avoidance behaviors. The client, with the help of the counselor, must press through these feelings of discomfort. Allowing the client to use avoidant behavior teaches escapism as a coping technique, which is not conducive to therapy. Most exposure therapy techniques involve having the client describe traumatic events over and over until he is able to tell the story without distress. Common techniques include having the client say the story aloud repeatedly, writing the story, or telling the story to a tape recorder and playing it continually.

Sand Tray Exposure Therapy

Veterans in therapy often find that the monstrosities of war cannot be adequately expressed through words. Veterans may find that they need more tangible ways to express their thoughts and emotions. STET is a therapeutic tool that requires the client, in a therapeutic setting, to focus on and recreate the details of a traumatic experience. This is done by having the client create a three dimensional picture of the events in a sand box with toy miniatures. Sand tray work provides a way for veterans to symbolically express emotion and events. Although sand tray therapy is considered a play therapy technique, it is effective with adults (Sandplay Therapists of America, n.d.)

Miniatures

General Miniature Collection

Clients are provided with collection of miniatures that they can use to create "worlds" or scenes in the sand. Miniature collections should include "everything that is in the world, everything that has been, and everything that can be" (Amatruda & Simpson, 1997:8.) The general collection to be used consists of several pieces from the following categories: animals, insects, birds, sea creatures, half-human/half animals, reptiles and amphibians, monsters, eggs and food, fantasy figures, plants, rocks, shells, and fossils, mountains, caves, and volcanoes, buildings, barriers, vehicles, people, fighting figures, and spiritual figures. Author (2006) provides a detailed list of miniatures and how they are to be displayed in the sand tray room.

Military Miniature Collection

Counselors who work with military veterans will need to provide a collection of war related miniatures. U.S. Military miniatures should include soldiers, helicopters, tents, barricades, barbed wire, military buildings and vehicles, and various weapons (bombs, grenades, guns, etc.) Iraq miniatures need to include houses, stores, children, infants, women, men, soldiers, terrorists, old cars, bicycles, roads, bridges, and local animals. Rocks, twigs, and other natural materials can be used for landscaping. Other miscellaneous miniatures, such as fire, rocks, sticks, red candles, sparklers, matches need to be included. To simulate blood, the wax from a red candle can be dripped on the sand or figures. Sparklers are hand-held fireworks that emit colored flames and sparks. These can be stuck in the sand tray near explosion/fire related incidents. The client can light the sparklers to show the counselor the intensity of the situation inside the tray. A list of sand tray resources is located under Reference Books at the end of this essay.

Creating Miniatures

Counselors can make their own miniatures if they cannot find suitable war toys. Iraqi soldiers can be made with fabric, people miniatures, small plastic weapons, and hot glue. There are guides available for how a man miniature can be transformed into a terrorist. Tiny tents can be made with canvas fabric.

Sand Tray Exposure Therapy Method

The sand tray is a rectangular box approximately 28 ½" x 19 ½" x 3" or 57 x 72 x 7 cm, painted or colored blue on the bottom and sides (Amatruda & Simpson, 1997.) The tray is filled with play sand, which is readily available at local hardware shops. Sand play sessions are 50-60 minutes in length. After an initial welcome and brief check in with client mood and pressing issues, the client should begin working on a tray. Most trays need 30-45 minutes to compose and create. When the client completes the tray, the therapist should encourage him to verbally explain and process the scenes in the tray. Clients may become anxious creating and discussing painful events. The therapist needs to reassure the client that he is safe, that the event is not happening now, and that memories can be mastered. Some clients may be so traumatized that they not only refuse the tray, but also they refuse to touch miniatures that are associated with their trauma. In this situation, the counselor needs to encourage the client to hold the object(s) in their hands for 5 minutes, 10 minutes, and over time build up exposure until the stimulus fails to trigger a fear response. At that time, the tray should be reintroduced.

Difference between STET and Traditional Sand Tray

STET is different from traditional sand tray therapy. Traditional sand tray therapy allows the client to create on different trays during each session. In STET the client is asked to recreate the same scenes repeatedly until they can be recreated and discussed without anxiety or fear. As a homework assignment, counselors should take photographs of the scenes to give to the clients so they can review them during the week. Once the client's anxiety levels began to decrease, clients may want to start sharing the photographs and stories with trusted friends and family. Sharing helps the client form a support network of caring individuals who want to understand and help the veteran.

In traditional sand tray sessions, the scene is never dismantled in front of the client. Most sand play therapists believe the tray is a "sacred creation" that should never be destroyed by the creator. In not allowing the client to take their tray apart, it shows the client that their work is important and valued. However, in STET the client needs to dismantle the tray. Dismantling the tray is a symbolic act, a way of consciously destroying the power the scenes and memories have over the client. When the figures are removed, they should be placed back in the exact same position on the shelves. This creates a semblance of permanence and safety in a constantly changing world.

STET Case Studies

To illustrate the use of STET with returning Iraq war veterans, this article will highlight three case studies where sand tray was an effective treatment technique.

Casey: A Case Study

Casey was referred to me for treatment by her family physician due to depression that was not responding to medication. Casey had served in Iraq for almost a year. In the initial interview, Casey reported that she felt depressed and was having trouble "getting back into family life." She stated that her mother had taken care of her two children while she was away. "Now I feel like the kids like her better than me. They say things like 'grandma didn't make us do that' or 'she didn't make us do chores.' It's like I have been replaced and I am not welcome in my own home." Casey also noted that she was having trouble fitting in with friends. "Being a soccer mom with a Coach purse seems silly now. After seeing death, poverty, and devastation, material goods are almost meaningless."

Next to my sand tray, I had a tub of military toys, which included green and tan military men, army trucks, helicopters, and other military related items. I had made a collection of Iraqi soldiers complete with Iraqi clothing and head coverings. Each soldier was holding a large rifle. Casey asked if she could arrange the toys in the sand. Her completed tray consisted of two different worlds that were divided with a picket fence, barbed wire, and a globe. Casey explained to me that the left side represented Iraq on one side of the globe and the right side portrayed her current life in the U.S. The side that depicted Iraq was a picture of destruction. Cars were overturned on the bodies of soldiers. A fire burned over the bodies of women and children. Satan stood in the corner, calmly observing the scene while Death brandished his scythe from the opposite corner. Life on the U.S. side was peaceful and happy. Children played under the watchful eye of caring adults. Well kept homes, white picket fences, and a church completed the scene. Lady Liberty overlooked the quiet town, her torch burning brightly.

Through this medium, Casey was able to show me the radical difference between the two places. She stated that the tray had helped her show me her situation without having to explain in words. In the next session, Casey asked to create another tray. She said that she had been thinking about the sand tray all week, composing images in her mind. In the second tray was a little girl holding a naked baby. A shabby hut and barbed wire fence were placed behind her and three soldiers stood in front of her. "This was a village. Every day we made rounds to several villages. We liked to give the children candy. One day this dirty little girl came up to me with a baby. The baby was covered in some kind of scabby rash. He looked more dead than alive, and he was whimpering. The little girl begged us for medicine. All I had in my pack were some alcohol wipes. I gave them to her, knowing that they wouldn't be of much help. She looked so grateful, as if I had really given her something that would save that baby. I felt so sad and so helpless. It was awful. Now I look at my own children, who have so much by comparison. I get angry when they whine for new toys at the store. I tell them they don't know how good their lives are. They tell me that I am mean, and I just want to smack them."

Casey continued to create the same trays over and over. After seven sessions, she said that she was less anxious and "jumpy." Occasionally Casey would bring in her own miniatures that she had created for specific scenes. "Making my own miniatures really helps me show you my experiences in a unique way." Casey continued to use the tray throughout her therapy sessions. She stated that she liked thinking about and planning trays she would make in upcoming sessions.

Paul: A Case Study

Paul came to me for PTSD treatment following his return from Iraq. His fiancée urged him to seek treatment because he no longer could express affection or emotion. Our first four sessions were punctuated with long silences. Despite my best efforts, our sessions seemed stagnant. Paul would discuss trivial issues; however, he seemed unable to go any deeper than the surface level. During one session, I offered him the use of my sand tray and miniatures. The mood of the session changed instantly. He immediately began to touch the sand, feeling the texture and weight as it slipped through his fingers. Then he collected all my military figures and started to create a scene. It took him almost the entire session to complete the tray. At the end of the session, I asked him if he wanted to tell me about his tray. Paul pointed to a section of the tray where five children laid face down in the sand, dead, unmoving under several army trucks. He said that these tiny bodies had been plowed over by American army supply trucks on a mission in Iraq. The children had been part of a human barrier preventing supplies from reaching our troops. Despite the fact that they were children, the orders were clear – "deliver the goods at all costs." He stared at the image, strangely detached and unemotional. "I was driving one of those trucks." Through the sand tray, he was able to describe to me the horrors of war that he had previously unable to share with me verbally.

Mark: A Case Study

Mark came to see me at the insistence of Anna, his wife of six years. "He's just not the same. I miss the old Mark." Mark angrily told me that his wife wanted me to "fix" him. He stated she expected him to act as if the war had never happened. I decided to use sand play in their sessions as a way for Mark to show his wife what he had experienced in his time in Iraq. Mark was initially resistant. "I don't play with toys." At his wife's insistence, he agreed to create a tray. In his tray was a scene that consisted of a man underneath a military truck. A fire blazed next to the truck. To the side of the truck was a male figure that was gazing at the wreckage. "Our truck hit a bomb and it exploded. My friend's face was burned beyond recognition." He died instantly. "I had never been that close to death. It was so raw, so real, and so hopeless." Mark dripped red wax all over the face of the miniature he had chosen as his friend. He wanted to use a sparkler in the tray to depict the fire from the bomb. We took several photos until he was happy with the image. He handed the photo to his wife and burst into tears. In a choked voice, he told her about the picture, his feeling of devastation, loss, and fear. His wife looked pale and scared. She pulled him into her arms and they wept together. Anna was slowly beginning to understand why her husband could not simply forget these raw memories.

Conclusion

The purpose of these case studies was to offer a different approach to the treatment of PTSD, specifically for American veterans of the Iraq war. This approach uses the veteran's need to express feelings of guilt, anger, depression, and anxiety through a modality (STET) that allows symbolic, rather than verbal, self-expression. Through the sand tray, clients are able to reenact, relive, and reconstruct their war experiences.

By using STET, the veterans were able to resolve underlying fears, anger, and frustration in a safe, therapeutic environment. Within the sand tray, the veterans were able to explore and master these situations. Recreating the same scenes over and over and sharing the scenes with a caring spouse and/or a counselor helped clients reduce negative feelings and fear reactions. STET offers the mental health counselor a viable intervention with American war veterans diagnosed with PTSD. Most counselors can easily add this type of innovative, effective therapy into their practices.

Reaching the Tough Adolescent through Expressive Arts Therapy Groups

Our group of teens stared at us with angry eyes and hands crossed tightly across their chests. One girl primped and applied lipstick while another adjusted her hot pink thong so it showed just over the top of her jeans. "So", Brad, my group co-leader said to the group, "what's up with you guys today?" No one answered. It looked like the group had an unspoken agreement that we would be getting the silent treatment. "Well Brad," I said in my sweetest voice, "I guess since no one is talking then we need to make puppets." The kids looked dubious. Brad agreed, "Poppy, what a great idea! The puppets can talk for the kids!" Brad and I started pulling out supplies — felt, hot glue, sparkles, google eyes, shells, marbles, Mardi Gras beads, yarn, markers, and scissors. We spread the materials out on the floor and went to work making puppets. Slowly, our surly group of adolescents slid out of their seats onto the carpet, fingering the materials with interest. "Can I use these black sparkles to make a pimp puppet?" one teen asked. "Whatever you think is cool," I replied. The boy quickly grabbed up the black sparkles before anyone else could claim them. Brad and I glanced around the room. Now instead of a room full of angry adolescents, we had a room full of industrious teens busily creating puppets. The girl with the thong was happily adding a pink thong to her puppet. Another teen was deep in discussion with another group member about how he could add a do-rag and braids to his puppet with the hot glue gun. Ah, the magic of art therapy works again!

Adolescents are perhaps the most difficult group to counsel. Neither child nor adult, teens are in a kind of developmental limbo. They are too old for time out, yet too young to shoulder grown-up responsibility. Many therapists are reluctant to work with adolescents in therapy because they require a great deal of personal energy and patience. This is unfortunate, because adolescents benefit greatly from therapy with a counselor who understands the special needs of this unique group of young people. This part of my essay will (1) describe how group therapy is an ideal therapy to use with adolescents, (2) demonstrate how expressive art therapy groups can be used effectively with teens, and (3) give hands-on examples of art activities that can be used with different adolescent groups.

Adolescents and Group Therapy

Teenagers are used to being in groups. In school, they learn in groups, most sports are played in groups, and they hang out with groups of friends. Therefore, group therapy is an ideal choice of therapy because it is a setting that is safe and familiar. Bandura (1989) believes that social interaction is key to the developmental process. Adolescents learn by watching each other interact and seeing the results of these interactions (Bandura, 1989.) Most teens are referred to therapy because they are having trouble with interpersonal relationships (e.g. parents, peers, teachers, authority figures) (Leader, 1991.) The group setting provides a safe space where the adolescent can learn and practice social/interpersonal skills, such as cooperation, turn taking, and anger management.

Selecting Group Members

When creating adolescent groups, the therapist should consider the needs, abilities, and diagnosis of the potential members. Kymissis (1996) notes in his book *Group Therapy for Children and Adolescents* that groups that are matched according to issues and development bond faster than groups that are simply created based on age.

Art Therapy with Teens

Teens, unlike adults, often need more innovative ways to express themselves than through "talk therapy." Expressive art therapy groups are a perfect way to allow teens to communicate difficult thoughts and feelings through various artistic mediums. Art therapy assists teens in solving problems, increasing self-esteem, building social skills, and behavior management. The process of art therapy helps adolescents chart their therapeutic journey from start to finish, helping them see where they have been and how far they have come. Many counselors have to work with open groups, groups where new members are continually accepted and there is no set starting point or completion point. Art therapy is excellent for these types of groups because it allows members to participate at their own level, rather than forcing them to "catch up" with other group members.

When creating art therapy groups, the counselor should try to limit the group to six to twelve members. Groups of this size allow members to gain a sense of kinship and togetherness. In smaller groups each member is guaranteed time to share their thoughts, feelings, and artwork. Members can maintain visual contact with other members at all times, thus creating a safe space for therapeutic work. For teenagers, structured art therapy groups are best (Liebmann, 1986.) Structured groups have planned activities for each session that revolve around a theme, such as "painting your depression" or "creating a personal portrait with string." Unstructured groups, which allow members to create random art, are not suitable for teens. Teens, although they are almost young adults, still need limits; they thrive in supported environments (Riley, 1997.)

Planning for Art Groups

Art therapy groups require much more preparation than talk therapy groups. The group leader is responsible for planning the session topic, obtaining the necessary materials, and structuring the session so that members can complete their artwork with time for discussion. Expressive art therapy groups run from 1 ½ to 2 hours. A typical session usually begins with 15-30 minutes of "warm-up" time. During warm-up members meet and greet each other and briefly check in with their current feelings and problems. The next 20-45 minutes are devoted to the art activity. The group ends with the follow- up and discussion, where members can share their creations, discuss feelings about the activity, and recenter before they go back into the real world.

When selecting art activities the therapist should consider not only the logistics of the room, but also the level of mess they can handle. For example, paint and paper mache are both very messy media. A roomful of teens armed with wet glue and paint might end up worrying the counselor so much that she is unable to be fully present in a therapeutic sense (because she is concerned about paint on the lovely white carpet!) Of course, the more open the therapist can be to messy media allows teens to have a much broader experience with art materials. Therapists may have to come up with novel solutions to deal with group room situations. Group rooms with carpet can be covered with tarps purchased at the local hardware store. If there is not a sink in the room, buckets of water can be brought in to wash brushes, activate watercolor paints, and to clean sticky hands. Another problem is presented if the room must be immediately cleaned up for the next group where will group members place their wet artworks to dry? When planning activities, the therapist should be sure that all members have enough personal space in which to work. Teens with anger management and boundary issues sometimes become upset if another member is "intruding" in their work space (even if it is accidental.)

Most teens will want to have a snack or at least a soda during group. Is the room suitable for food or can you set up a space where snacks and open drinks can be kept? Since you are dealing with teens, the issue of music will come up. Teens enjoy listening to music while they are creating. If you can stand it, let them listen to their favorite music — this will automatically give you instant "cool points" with the kids. One counselor who does art therapy dislikes most rap and heavy metal music because of their explicit lyrics and derogatory remarks towards women. She tells her clients that art and jazz are a classic combination. Not only do the kids love the music, they are probably the only teens on the planet who know the music and identities of Charlie Parker, Etta James, Billie Holiday and Miles Davis. In fact, they ask for Miles Davis when they are working on art relating to depression and request Ella Fitzgerald for sessions that are more upbeat!

When setting up your initial space you will most likely want to have the following materials on hand at all times:

- Paint: acrylic paint is cheap and does not need to be mixed, cups for paint, brushes, brush cleaner, plates for mixing colors, spoons to stir paint, plastic garbage bags for kids to wear over their clothes
- Dry media: wax crayons, felt tip pens, oil pastels, charcoal, colored pencils, markers
- Paper: construction paper, white paper, tracing paper, brightly colored paper, cardstock – white and colored, scraps of unusual paper (found at craft stores), rolls of newsprint (ask the local paper to save you the ends of the rolls), and art paper of various sizes (watercolor paper, Biggie Scribble paper, etc.)
- Cutting materials: scissors, x-acto knives, circle cutters, hole punches (with different punch designs – stars, hearts, etc.), edge punches
- Collage materials: old magazines, fabrics, textured materials

- Miscellaneous: bits of thread, embroidery floss, beads, hemp rope, stickers, ribbon, old and unusual buttons
- Adhesives: collage glue, craft glue, fabric glue, rubber cement, glue sticks, spray adhesive, tape
- Clean up supplies: rags, paper towels, newspaper to cover the art surfaces, plastic bags, tarps, drop cloths, Windex

Group Warm-up

Group warm-up should be a fun time where members reconnect with each other and transition from the outside world into the safety of the group. A basic warm-up activity is to have the members introduce themselves and tell one good or bad thing that happened to them during the previous week. This is especially important in open groups where new members are present at each meeting. To help the members remember each other's names, use a simple name association game. For instance, have each member describe him/herself using the first letter of his or her name. Hello! My name is Poppy and I like popcorn, my favorite dessert is popsicles, and my favorite animal is the panda. Teens feel more included and in control when other members address them by name instead of "Hey you — the new kid".

Once the group has completed the warm-up activity the group leader should spend a few minutes going over group rules and boundary issues. The rules and boundaries need not be lengthy or set in stone. However, it is important to give teens limits for their behavior within the sessions so they know what is and is not expected of them. Common group rules include: (1) attending sessions on time, (2) no talking when the leader or another member is talking, and (3) not interrupting other members. Most teen group leaders need to set limits on bathroom and phone use, otherwise members will either use the bathroom as an excuse to go call a friend or smoke a cigarette, or they will accept personal calls on their cell phones during the session. The best rule of thumb is to have all members visibly turn their cell phones off at the start of the session, where the therapist monitors to ensure that the phones are actually being turned off. The therapist can emphasize that in doing this the group is creating a "safe space" where they can let go of outside pressures and focus on their own therapeutic goals. Most teens are in therapy because they have problems with interpersonal issues. Group leaders should remind members that scapegoating, name-calling, and rudeness will not be tolerated.

When new members are present, group leaders will want to remind members of the purpose of the group. "This is an expressive art therapy group for teens that are having problems with depression. Sometimes it is hard to talk about our feelings. Creating art is a form of communication that allows you to express your feelings. If you are having a hard time communicating your problems to others, art is a real way to express what is going on inside you. Even if you feel your art doesn't mean anything in particular, the act of making something helps to quiet the mind and allows you to get in tune with your inner self and what is going on inside you. Remember that in art there is no right or wrong, nor good or bad. You don't have to have any special art ability. Just feel free to create and see what happens."

During the activity, members should be totally engaged in the process of creating art. Often teens will open up and begin talking about personal problems while they are creating. This is good, especially if the members are talking about therapeutic issues. On the other hand, if members are socializing rather than working, the leader must intervene and redirect. Members should be aware from the start how much time they have to work on the activity. As they are nearing the end of the activity time, it is helpful for the group leader to point out "10 minutes left", "five minutes left", "one minute left" and "stop". Following the activity is the group discussion. This is a time where members share their artwork. Each member should have adequate time to discuss his or her piece. If time is running out, the leader can choose to continue the discussion during the next session. A round-robin turn taking approach works best with teens. Adolescents are often reluctant to share their artwork, so this approach ensures that all members will speak. Each member should discuss for at least five minutes, this encourages quieter members to have equal share time. Teens may be superficial in their discussion of their artwork. Leaders may want to point out deeper meanings they see in the art and encourage individual and group contemplation.

Activities

The sky is the limit in terms of art activities for teens. With a little imagination group leaders can invent a wide range of wonderful art therapy activities. These activities have been used successfully with teens in a variety of settings.

Mask Making

In the mask making activity, teens are asked to create two masks. One mask represents the self they show to society and the other mask represents their inner self. These masks can be created out of papier mache or cardstock. Additional materials to have on hand are feathers, sequins, glitter, paint, glue, scissors, etc. The leader can explain how we act a certain way in society in order to fit in, but really feel differently on the inside. This statement can open discussion where members (1) describe how they feel when they wear each mask, (2) discuss reasons they have to wear a different mask in society, (3) ponder if they are being true to themselves if they act differently in one mask as opposed to the other.

Bag Self-Portraits

In the self-portrait activity, members are asked to make a self-portrait on the side of a brown paper bag. The portrait can be created with crayons, markers, colored pencils, or paint. Teens can glue on hair, fabric for outfits, etc. The group leader should instruct the members to put things that "make them who they are" inside the bag. Members might put in pictures of their family, a favorite book, a CD, a picture of a pet or best friend. On one side of the bag, they can list their fears, on the other side their greatest hopes. On the back of the bag, they can create a tombstone with a eulogy describing qualities for which they want to be remembered.

There are many other group art activities that are excellent for teens. The following books can help therapists in planning expressive art therapy groups:

Liebmann, M. *Art therapy for groups.* Cambridge, MA: Brookline Books, 1986.
Malchiodi, C. *The art therapy sourcebook.* New York: McGraw Hill, 1998.
Malchiodi, C. *Handbook of art therapy.* New York: Guilford Press, 2002.

Although teen groups may take a little extra work, they are deeply fulfilling in a personal way. A counselor who patiently helps adolescents through this difficult and chaotic part of their lives will be remembered by the teen as someone who believed and supported them when they needed it the most.

References

Amatruda, K., and P. Simpson. *Sandplay the Sacred Healing.* Novato, CA: Trance Sand Dance. 1997.
American Psychiatric Association. *Diagnostic and Statistical Manual of*

Mental Disorders (Fourth ed.). Washington: American Psychiatric Association, 2000.

Author. "Sand play therapy with U.S. soldiers diagnosed with PTSD and their families." In G. Walz & R. Yep (Eds.), *VISTAS: Compelling perspectives on counseling 2006*. Alexandria, VA: American Counseling Association, 2006.

Bandura, A. " Social cognitive theory." In V. R. Greenwitch (Ed.), *Annals of child development* Greenwich, CT: Jai Press. 1989:1-60.

Bentley, S. *A short history of PTSD*. Retrieved July 18, 2005, from http://www.vva.org/TheVeteran/2005_03/feature_HistoryPTSD.htm. 2005

Department of Veterans Affairs. (n.d.). Treatment of PTSD. Retrieved July 21, 2005, from http://www.ncptsd.va.gov/facts/treatment/fs_treatment.html

Epstein, J, & Miller, J. *U.S. Wars and Post-traumatic Stress Disorder*. San Francisco Chronicle, (A11.) 2005, June 22

Foa, E. B., T., M. Keane, and M. J. Friedman, *Effective Treatments for PTSD: Practice Guidelines from the International Society for Traumatic Stress Studies*. New York: Guilford, 2000.

Foa, E. B., and B. O. Rothbaum, *Treating the Trauma of Rape: Cognitive-behavioral Therapy for PTSD*. New York: Guilford, 1998.

Hoge, C., C. Castro,,S. Messer, ,D. McGurk, D.,Cotting, and R. Koffman, "Combat Duty in Iraq and Afghanistan, Mental Health Problems." *New England Journal of Medicine,* 351. (2004) 13-22.

Kerr, M., and M. Bowen, *Family Evaluation* (1st ed.). New York: W.W. Norton & Company, 1988.

Kymissis, P. "Developmental Approach to Socialization and Group Formation," In P. K. D. A. Halperin (Ed.), *Group Therapy with Children and Adolescents*, Washington, DC: American Psychiatric Press, 1996,: 21-33.

Leader, E. "Why Adolescent Group Therapy." *Journal of Child and Adolescent Group Therapy*, 1, 1991:81-93.

Liebmann, M. *Art Therapy for Groups*. Cambridge, MA: Brookline Books, 1986.

National Center for Post-Traumatic Stress Disorder. *Iraq war clinician's guide* (2nd ed.). Washington, DC: Author. 2004.

Riley, S. *Contemporary Art Therapy with Adolescents*. London, England: Jessica Ingsley Publishers, 1997.

Rothbaum, B. & A. Schwartz. " Exposure Therapy for Post Traumatic Stress Disorder." *American Journal of Psychotherapy*, 56(1), 2002.

Sandplay Therapists of America. (n.d.). *Sandplay Therapy*. Retrieved July

22, 2005, from http://www.sandplay.org/index.htm
Tyre. "Battling the Effects of War when Combat Veterans Return Home." Newsweek. Retrieved September 14, 2007, from *Veterans for Common Sense* website:
http://www.veteransforcommonsense.org/ArticleID/2468 (2004, December).

Reference Books

Amatruda, K., and P. Simpson, *Sandplay the Sacred Healing.* Novato, CA: Trance Sand Dance, 1997.
Boik, B. and E. Goodwin, *Sandplay Therapy.* New York. W.W. Norton and Company, 1999.
Friedman, H. and R. Mitchell, *Sandplay*: *Past, Present, Future.* San Francisco: Routledge, 1994.
Turner, B. *The handbook of Sandplay Therapy.* Cloverdale, CA: Temenos Press, 2005.

Informational Websites

Sand Play Therapists of America: www.sandplay.org
Information on how to set up a sand tray room:
www.siteceu.com/tools.html

Websites for Sandtray Miniatures
http://www.childtherapytoys.com/store/sandtoys.html
http://www.selfhelpwarehouse.com/sandtray-sandtray-miniatures.html

SPARKING A MIGHTY BLAZE: PLIANT PATIENCE RECALLED

CAROL HENRY

Through the years, I have used what I see as pliant, flexible, patience with my students, both individually and in groups, as we use aesthetics, mostly music and dance, to elicit wellness. The language I choose to use with the students is also an important part of the process, and reflects who I am with them. Writing this biographical material about what has happened between me and these students has been a purge of consciousness for me, at a time when I can take an honest look at my many-layered existence. Perhaps my reader will gain some sense of how I fit into the development of this field, since it grew up alongside my career.

Igniting an Enlivening Spark

It wasn't until inadvertently stumbling upon E. Paul Torrence's *Guiding Creative Talent* that I understood who, what, and why I am. The most relevant thing I learned was that I wasn't alone. (Presently, I'm aware of *sharing* a dream with a *worldwide community!* That affords me a feeling that is very idyllic!) I wrote Paul thanking him for his work. His gracious reply included clippings and pictures from a *Look* magazine of at least ten years prior, and his action commenced a mutually bonding, thirty-year mentoring relationship of unrelenting support. He was at the University of Georgia for many years, and established the Center for Creative Studies there, which is now operated by Dr. Bonnie Crammond. My relationship with Paul was a lifelong anchor for me. I vividly recall my dismal first college teaching job at segregated Southern University in Scotlandville, LA., a bepebbled, unpaved, sandy, foul-scented, and slaughterhouse-rendering plant-fumed, shanty town, shared by poor blacks and whites. Mid-spring 1953, I wrote home feeling like a round peg trying desperately to fit into an extremely tight square hole. I wrote about 23 letters my first week; only D'Mate, a name I gave my mother, replied.

The sly, cunning, octogenarian department head *graced* me with 21 band majors as private piano students, two half hours a week! From that number only one avid soul, the most comely of the lot, passed a performance exam well enough *not* to have to retake piano. He had a smile on his face as he called, "You got me out, Ms. Henry!" Enough thanks for all those who *never* practiced! The director then assigned me to teach a theory class *and* play in a four-hand arrangement of Brahms *Waltzes*, for his wife's choral concert. I had been *royally* had! A week after the choral concert, I went to his office to practice on the piano he'd had moved there from the chapel so I *could* practice; the piano had vanished!

Utterly miserable after three and a half years, dreading a pending revolution, I knew my returning to New York was best! I wrote my father advising the South was befouling my Spirit. His reply pleaded I remain, implying I was not bright enough to be employable in the North. I went anyway.

Spring 1963, I wanted to assuage the distress of dancer Merce Cunningham and Company, who were leaving on an extended international tour. Merce and composer/pianist John Cage were allied for many years and were ranking members of the Avant Garde in music, dance, and painting. Merce and company are now located again in New York. I had gone back to New York to play for dance classes for his Company. I loved playing for them—what pleasure! They were also delighted to have me play, but I wanted most to take the dance classes myself. For over a year, I was happy doing that, until they needed to go on tour. I did not want to play for classes any more.

I answered a notice in the Local 802 AF of M publication, seeking musicians for six month Music Therapy internships at Essex County Overbrook Hospital, Cedar Grove, NJ. I had applied a year before graduating Juilliard; I met and was interviewed by the director when she visited. Questions she asked, and her statements, confirmed our views with regard to arts as healing agents — totally antithetical. Not wishing to either perform or entertain, I refused to believe the mentally ill ought to be perfunctorily presumed insensate, as the director seemed wont to deem patients in her program.

This time she hired me; New Dance Group Studio in the city where I had played before going south discovered my whereabouts, and called to ask me to come for four hours a week. I would begin taking dance classes there to keep me happy, and when the Company returned I would be ready to take classes with Merce again. Things were going my way, after all.

Beautiful, Warming Southern Summer Hour

In summer 1971, with MFA in Performance Arts, as Visiting Professor in dance, University of Georgia, Valdosta, I taught in Project Radius, a program geared for public school teachers. The teachers had three art experience courses per five-day week. One morning, before class, the project director asked me, "Would you be willing to work an hour with children of migrant workers after your afternoon class?" With no hesitation, I replied, "I'd love to!" Working with children was definitely my preference. I adored seeing bored, indignant, glum faces metamorphosized by the mystical magic of time-disciplined freedom, generate the most broad, beaming smiles imaginable! I experienced too much joy to not immediately acquiesce to any such invitation *whenever/wherever* proffered.

My "Miracle watching" started several years earlier in East Harlem/El Barrio, with children in *my* neighborhood; then a Jersey K-12 school program and finally, Children's Center for Creative Arts at Adelphi University, a lively intergenerational program! In the 50's I'd lived in boring, rural, dull, flat, agrarian, soil-depleting, cotton and rice producing Pine Bluff Arkansas, where I witnessed firsthand the distressingly typical plight of migrant workers. Evenings, trucks passed campus, bringing workers back into town from the fields. That plight *could not* match the indignity *I* felt seeing chain gang labor on FAMU's campus, but observing human beings riding as livestock in open slat-sided, flatbed, pick-up trucks was painfully close. *Inhumane treatment,* certainly not civilized conduct; I was observing America's Twentieth Century slaves! On Little Rock's sidewalk curbs, migrant Mexican laborers perching, squatting like indigenous birds of prey, were the norm. "What about the families?" I thought, noting the dehumanizing travail; imagining children's lives in particular. Visions stirred instant compassion and empathy. I knew of no group with whom I'd ever work where sharing *my* time would have more merit. As my day's last scheduled class left the auditorium, approximately fifteen apprehensive, ethnically diverse, somber, lugubriously silent elementary school children filed into the auditorium's orchestra section and walked down the aisle as if attending a funeral mass (I could hear Chopin's Funeral March,) the aftermath of some catastrophic area disaster. Dispersing nametags had occurred to no one. They didn't smell too good, but were quite cordial toward one another and me; I was impressed.

We sat in a circle on the stage floor. I talked; they listened attentively; soon they answered questions promptly, laughed fittingly, smiled often, raptly heeded directions, executed them similarly, and displayed the most courteous behavior. In less than fifteen minutes, the dour, solemn little band that entered so timidly was transmuted to a joyfully engrossed, buoyant troupe! Conferring freely with one another, they facilitated each other's grasping of vital demands for satisfying tasks. I was speaking "New Yorkese"—not Georgian; they were deciphering my accent along with unfamiliar directions and additional tasks! Many migrant workers' children are unable to attend school nine straight months a year. This was an unusually special day for each of us!

Watching their diligent, generous caring about each other thrilled me. In twenty years work with children's classes, not once had I seen any that so exemplified confirming the intrinsic dignity of each human spirit. Their initiative effected a striking, remarkably fluid, disciplined transition. I was enormously honored to have contributed to and observed such an easily achieved metamorphosis. Inwardly sensing, responding to their own transmutations, each exuded awareness of having experienced unique personal accomplishment; their Selves had been properly acclaimed. My reward for freeing spirits was watching them soar!

The hour, too brief, ended too soon. Leaving the auditorium, quietly exchanging comments through a glistening stream of perspiration, the largest boy, perhaps of Mexican descent, radiated an utterly content glowing countenance of deep aliveness. Jose Limon came to mind. I, positively beaming at the group's response, eagerly asked the Project Director, "When shall I see them again?"

Shaking her head, she replied blandly, "Only a one shot deal." That nearly reduced me to tears. Summer's most gloriously gratifying teaching/ learning hour was tossed to the wind... Perhaps, not entirely... Each of us could savor the memory of living through an extra-ordinarily unusual hour... Thirty odd years later, *I* can yet recall! The art of living one's art, the act of fully sharing—both were unforgettable... Salutary memories and good dreams seem synonymous: they remain forever clear... We were together only sixty minutes but no one could/would forget our conversion... experienced en mass... I'd say we were singularly privileged. We had initiated, witnessed, and shared the mystical joy of full-blown, total self-discovery.

Amazingly Abundant Spring Harvest

In 1973, the final Spring of government funding for my first position after Grad School, which was Title III, innovative education; focus on the arts as curriculum adjuncts. It was time for assessment. I was to reintroduce music/movement to about ten, uncommunicative, "lower track" seventh graders with whom I met and worked in their classroom. All rooms had windows in the doors. Intimidated by the idea that 'the other kids' passing in the hall would see what the "dummies" were doing, prior to each class, I'd been requested from last Fall to draw the door's window shade. They group had retained adamant reticence toward the personal, intrusive nature of both acting and dance. Feet dragged the floor to the beat in my sessions. I had played, one session at a time, triangle, claves, and maracas. Since September, they had barely tolerated my presence, had never made any view known—just refused to even *fake* participation. I felt sorry for them; they had no idea what fun they were missing! I had learned dance fortuitously but have not once regretted my decision to study it! Dance is absolutely the best thing that *ever* happened to me!

This day *I would* go for broke! During all eight counts of each phrase, chairs, chosen as partners, must also be kept moving, I told them. Tasks and movements were based on three qualities of *instruments*: triangle; any direction, smooth movement; *maraca*; jagged/ jittery movement, *small slow-motion leaps; claves* acute angles; *body* isolations, arms, head, or *entire body and chair*.

Never ceasing to murmur counts, I played instruments—one at a time in rotation. In a while, all were adhering to directions as told consequently, in less than half an hour, jamming in a jam-packed steam room! Pausing a moment, I offered, "Getting pretty warm in here..." which prompted an instant choral response, "Open the door!" Their call was sent echoing through the open door and down the hall. One boy called to another for help extricating himself from the rungs of his chair. It was the first time all year! Radiant, glistening smiles of sheer delight shone in faces drenched with perspiration. Even as "other kids" watched at the open doorway, the 'dummies' experienced a glorious epiphany! They felt the exhilaration, satisfaction, and excitement of being *involved, plus* the joy of a major win. I thought, "See what being so stubbornly prideful had made them miss all year!" Ignominious epitaph dispelled forthwith. They had prevailed, freed themselves, by themselves. (I had not appeared too bright either, sitting there, playing three instruments, muttering numbers. Not exactly genius caliber class labor, but not *forced* labor either; I was at one with them!) *That* day, for better or for worse, we were a group. The last triumphant hour had been *ours*. Each person could rest *assured* that he or she was absolutely capable of functioning *with self-initiated discipline*.

In June, some of those students were scheduled to enter mainstream classes. Having been *once* self-assured, *making the daring to fail acceptable*, abandoning self-effacement would serve them well. Come fall, they could/ would assume a proud place, squarely, smack dab in the middle of a level playing field.

Abby's Sparkling Exfoliation

Early Spring 1992, prior to starting my first afternoon as volunteer music/movement therapist at the YWCA, I sat in the cafeteria/ lunchroom among a host of predominately disadvantaged, dysfunctional, elementary school African American boys and girls, few of whom I knew. Earlier, the director introduced me to TJ and Dee, smaller boys who had spoken with me briefly; the director had made that selection for me. Suddenly, I noticed an "odd" little girl sitting to my right on the curved, built-in plastic covered seat, steadily jostling me as if to clear a lodged door. Answering a tablemate's question, she gasped, "She reminds me of my grandmother." She turned and asked my name. Passing us, the YWCA director idly remarked, "That's a good one!"

I had volunteered to work specifically with youth "living troubled." Serendipitously, Abby had picked me! Only the director knew my mission. With a body tight and rigid with the tension of a metal robot, forbidding, nine-year-old, fitfully coordinated Abby, readily as possible, sought the attention she knew was needed. Hence, she tried curling up, unobtrusively snuggling, and in a light, polite puppy manner, nudging. I was a door she wished open. Bereft of basic physical agility, her limbs, head, neck and torso moved spastically. She was a small person with a strange disability; as if teased by a fly, she reacted with a facial tic. Frankenstein's child, she plodded like a wounded little bear. To laugh, she would have been asphyxiated; speaking, whispering, for her were onerous—*living,* precarious! *Nothing* about her body flowed or was attached; her breathing was sheer labor.

As children dispersed to individually chosen group activities, she and I wandered onto the empty floor. Stroking her back, offering soft suggestions—"bend knees, touch finger tips on toes or floor," I, simultaneously seeking small sections of her back to physically ease, was manipulating, massaging. We made little to no progress toward normal humanization that day! She had no idea, no conception of bending or bowing. I was trying to knead her back into a flexibility enough to bow; only her irregular pants and gasps verified her live being. In its fitfully unsynchronized way, every centimeter of her misshapen, misaligned, spastic little error-ridden form fought desperately to comply, but she was totally unable to manage *any* ordinary feat!

How, without excessive force, to detach, to usurp her body's crude processes of motion? The solution would involve multiple precise manipulations by experts—rare in urban ghettoes. I was not one. Easy, noninvasive isolations were a start, I hoped. Prudent, patient improvisation was our/*my* sole hope!

Our meeting had been by chance, so staff members detailed pertinent details of her home and history in bits. It was a dysfunctional home that included a newborn. Neither parent evinced undue emotional, nor mental, stability or exhibited much caring. Daily, during the two short block walk between school and "the Y," fights with classmates erupted. Indubitably, she was a peer-taunted victim; tangled in snarled roots, a lone, delicate bud, a fragile flower fighting to survive. In seconds, left unsupervised, the best of "the Y's" group metamorphosized into beasts; they coalesced into frightful boorish packs! Though appearing as a *Frankenstein*, she was mightily outmatched by a grimmer, shifty pack of miniature Mr. Hydes!

TJ and Dee were smaller, more lithe, hyperactive boys about Abby's age who preceded her session. Once, combining two hops and two skips, they burst through the open door, bounded down the hall—a pair of ebullient kangaroos! Abby watched in tortured awe, overwhelmed by her desire to do likewise. She followed them to the door, bent one knee, picked up her foot, stood unsteadily trying to gain balance, and tenuously picked up the other foot. Frozen in mute horror, I watched each disjointed leg's agonized sashay to shift her weight, tax her breathing, and alter her hands into eagle claws clutching golf balls. She forced herself to explore; validate herself, even to her own detriment. It was dreadful to watch. As if a hunter in hip high muddy boots stalking deer, I inhaled deeply, silently easing nearer her. Catching my tack intensified her anxiety. Walking slow motion behind her, I laid my hands on her marble shoulders, lulling repeatedly, as if to a wild pony, "Easy—relax—breathe," I sighed huskily, until, her body softening, she calmed and finally was still. She stood nearly motionless, gasping from the exertion. Placing my crossed arms against her shoulder blades, I felt her release, heard her gasping cease. Tension- ridden, rigid robot had mutated into malfunctioning machine. Any attempts at physical restraint I might have made would have had the potential of provoking either or both of us, and serious injury. Out-of-whack machines cannot *sense their* power!

JR and Dee's personal problems were less blatantly discernable. JR's chronically truant mother abandoned him for *her* mother to raise. Neither a rare occurrence or unique to him, but for him, abidingly traumatic!

Loquacious, he was first of the group to loudly voice loving me, which, enlightening me, and also delighted. Sharing quarters with uncles, who were his "big brothers," he took it upon himself to share what he'd learned of sex education. Nearly non-verbal, Dee had a lone metamorphosis session. Doing a movement exercise designed to "free spirits," he slipped, fell, came up laughing with an enormous burst of spontaneous glee and, in a second, prepared to repeat the "trip." A few weeks later, he advised he didn't want to come anymore. "Don't need me anymore?" I asked eagerly. He shook his head. "That's grand!" I cheered. "Feel free to stop in whenever you feel you do! OK?" He nodded again and left. Before term's end, the family moved away. (Historically, having been a stop on the Underground Railroad is part of the city's heritage. Seems the phenomenon is self-perpetuating for/with troubled youth.)

Agreeing to conduct a *double* session with another teacher's group, proved a frightful error! Dee, Abby and JR seized instant power—"my anointed disciples," "assisted," disciplined, corrected, bossed, and interpreted for others. It was dreadfully frightening/flattering, and most unfair to all involved. A startling revelation! It changed my perception of our relationship. I, in their strange fantasy, became a neutered demon; *not a human personality*. Their *transposition* of reality was truly bizarre!

February through June, Abby and I met twice weekly. At an early session, alternately gasping, puffing, staring blankly out a window, she improvised a gurgling, seemingly endless song, "my mother taught me." Often she would prate long, halting original stories, never owning authorship nor involving either of us. Rambling—perhaps to draw attention away from herself—she related countless, halting, barely coherent, original tales. One day she burst into the room during Dee and JR's session. After I explained that interrupting sessions was impolite, rude, she never repeated the action. Warming up to me as best she could, she wanted me to know of her appreciation. To release back tension, I massaged her back; soon, she would work *with* me, helping to straighten her back.

One day, requesting we exchange roles, she directed holding hands. Her countermanding order at once was, *"first,"* I had to ascertain her ability to merely hold—not clutch—a human hand! She was standing still, arms dangling loosely from shoulders; I requested she slowly, gently, lift my arm, move it in different directions, drop it when I told her. Hearing my relaxed hand slap my thigh, was totally flabbergasting to her; but it became a ritual. We did that for each other at the beginning of each meeting henceforth; we would "test" each other's *relaxed* arms before strolling "easily around the room, swinging arms, singing our song." A tune I had written had exactly the right quality needed; it was free enough to aptly yield to simple, improvised, descriptive words. Often, she offered phrase suggestions which, when incorporated, fit well and quite naturally.

She merely smiled coyly, when her images were accepted; it was clear she was inordinately pleased having *her* ideas listened to, acted upon. It was clearly a totally new and beneficent event. (She taught me empathy I had never known existed!) Shortly thereafter, while singing our song, I noticed her breathing and speaking were unequivocally less labored! Now, I *also* noted that whenever I explained something, questioned, or addressed her directly, she peered at me, listening as if contemplating, perhaps, wondering how I spoke so easily. Clearly, it was a magical new, easily interpreted and readily understood (most of all) *welcome* tongue.

I witnessed her father arriving to drive her home one day. Entering the building as if being pursued by hounds closing in on him, he greeted no one, shot dull glances at Abby, signed a form on the office counter, fled down the stairs. Abby stared at me intensely, quixotically; I wondered if she were wishing me to make her life easier. She seemed then so pitiably alone, a love-starved puppy who hesitantly hurried down the steps toward the door. Whether or not she safely crossed the narrow, fairly busy street to enter her father's car was solely *her* responsibility.

Our sessions were moved into the "auditorium," the largest open space after the gym. As spring arrived, the staff reported not only had fights on route to "the Y" ended for Abby; but she had also begun visiting staff in their offices, stopping them in the hall to exchange hugs. Assuming a leadership role in the new room, Abby ambled about the room listening, testing avidly for sound variations of my drumstick on wood, metal, and furniture. Singing, we roamed the room. At random intervals, I would loosely swing/jiggle her arm. Soon, feeling her arm free, she would look up smiling. In a few weeks, she insisted the director be invited in to see our song/dance piece.

Nearing term's end, she entered the room with most tension redirected, transformed into energy and first informed me she'd have to leave our session promptly; group leaders needing assistance expected her at rehearsal for "the Y's" end of the year special!

Entering easily, calmly, completely poised for our final meeting, she laid a notebook on a chair; calmly, easily, silently. She then walked to the room's center, stood straight, legs together, bent over, consciously setting her fingertips swinging—petting the floor. *Good show*! I cried with delight. At session's end, she jotted on a notebook page, tore it out, laid it on a sofa cushion, *dashed* to rehearsal. She'd written, "I love you."

The door had been opened. Work succeeded beyond my wildest expectation; she now had eased, soothed, conscious, deep breathing. She'll express herself with freedom of breathing; she *never* knew any type of speech before, but now any idea she had, she had won the freedom to say. She had gained access to total easy movement, in breathing, speaking, singing, and walking. Abby could/would relish an entirely new world! She had discovered; savored with dignity, the freedom and joy of *being alive*; liberated her own whole new *Self.*

Thus had Abby's sparkling exfoliation evolved! By September, Abby's family had left town. Unlikely I'll ever see her again, but I'll *never* forget Spring/Summer 1992 when one fortuitous meeting and arts experiments led to sheer love of life and joy of sharing in an exceptionally needy nine year old.

Out of Ashes – What?

Some children are daily offered only deadly, bitter fruit. I met with one middle school's at-risk students far less fortunate than any I had known, and possibly would remain so. Sad fates of the children I met in fall 2001, result from the glob — as in rob — *globalization* of the world's economies!

NAFTA robbed satellite towns collaborating with Detroit, the former world auto industry capitol, to manufacture for less, facilitated moving outfitting first to Mexico*,* which enjoyed a boom about two years before that bubble burst! World Bank, gleefully cooperating, trounced cheap labor in countries around the world!

In the wake of Gulf Wars, a horrified world watched victims/ witnesses of 9/11 in New York City — vicious attack on World Trade Center (arrogant, ugly, *vain* examples of architecture.) — as Michigan's economy, formerly mostly structured by and for the auto industry, plummeted, collapsed, traumatizing the entire "FREE WORLD" including the United States of America! Foul political, diplomatic, chicanery promptly auguring catastrophic educational misery probably lasting at least two generations.

Solving a puzzling route to one devastated, downtown Michigan area, I arrived midst an appalling, nightmarish gloom evoking recollections of Central Harlem's 1960's destruction. However, *this* time external and internal intensity has mounted in schools. Havoc has returned to strike harder! I felt it quite unlikely that any rational concerned thinking had ensued regarding the pitiable plight of *unborn* children ever *needing* decent education! The Power people were too absorbed in checking real/expected gross capital interest earnings from *international* deals.

Hence, the students in my charge were paying for parents' elected officials' vile lusts; apathy accomplishes absolutely nothing! Alien to the Kennedy/Johnson era, or the relevancy of trial and error, once explained corrections were ended. Progressive, innovative modes of teaching/learning were brazenly aborted; negated until non-existent; this would take a toll on *victims* of present virtually abandoned schools

I was asked to help improve reading scores in one school, one hour a week. Returning from the East to arrange moving, I did not care about being paid immediately. My primary wish was to *banish* student *boredom* with intellectual challenge! The students were obviously discontent with themselves, in fact, although they had a "brand new school." It resembled more an air raid shelter, which was an obvious design for disaster! Just before Christmas, waiting in the school office, I lost count of students filing in, asking to call home to report suspensions!

Discovering their imaginations needed a swift boot, for openers, to at least snare attention, I was anxious to work on creating rhyming word puzzles. The pair of group leaders offered no help whatsoever! During the session, he read a newspaper, she, *Malcolm X*, both glancing up occasionally to threaten calling home in a way that forced my quelling hysteria. Vigorous home tutelage had not voided the students' dismal at-risk classification.

Second session with them was amazingly successful. The first stir of images awakened the entire group and enlivened beautiful, spontaneous zeal. Attesting to the rapt attention they gave the project until session's end, an abundant steady stream of fresh, individually written ideas flowed from every student. Rhyming word exercises allowed fountains of ideas to flood from revitalized brains!

At the hour's end, deeming the exhilaration "rude," the group leader, *Malcolm X* reader, apologized to me for them. I wish she had apologized for her own dull-witted attitude! Why apologize for the first sign of life she had seen in the room? Had *planned* insentience trapped yet another ill-fated group? Probably.

There remain too many regularly victimized students, wards of failing schools who are not given opportunity to meet the love, joy, and freedom they could learn through the arts. If asked why I do such work, I *recall almost* euphorically awakening life through art and creativity. But my working years are winding down; at times, I wonder what of the future's students? This had also been one of my mentor Paul's deepest concerns; time has come to do *whatever* I can *whenever* I am asked.

Through flexible, pliant, patience, I have met my students where they were, sometimes at very low times in their lives, and helped them to find a spark *within* themselves. Many times, through my caring, I was able to kindle the gentle flame of genuine aliveness into a *mighty* blaze within them. In combination with my tools of music and dance, it was my caring that helped them to come alive. It does my heart good to recall my small part in sparking such aliveness, but it also causes me to wonder about the future. When I am no longer able to kindle sparks of life for the discontented, will someone *be* taking my place in this good work or will only ashes remain?

Developing a Language for Trauma: Children Communicating Through the Arts

Vicki J. Morgan

Love is the thing with feathers
that perches in the soul
and sings the tunes without the word
and never stops
at all.
—Emily Dickenson

Gross motor and language skills

When a baby is born, parents are excited by the first movements and sounds of their newborn child. If prepared, the parents may have a nursery ready with mobiles to stimulate their child's vision and crib toys to stimulate motor development. They coo and talk to their baby, not expecting much in the way of real words for the first eleven months. What parents do expect is that their baby will learn to lift his/her head within the first few weeks, eventually roll from stomach to back, sit up at six months, perhaps a little wobbly, then crawl, and by the first year try to walk.

The baby is so busy developing gross motor skills that language skills take a back seat during this time. Of course, the fine motor movements of the tongue and the brain's ability to put sounds together into words are complex skills. Yet, once a child learns to talk, he/she seems to take off into the world of vocabulary. While movement is often subject to the laws of nature, speech is not. Take, for example, a child that falls out of a tree. Gravity will dictate that the child fall, yet the child may or may not yell out. A child on a hill will roll down it, but may or may not giggle in delight.

Considering the early development of motor skills over language and the natural response the body has to the forces outside of it, it is easy to understand that trauma would automatically be stored in the body regardless of the ability to verbalize it.

As a special education teacher, I have worked with children diagnosed with learning disabilities and children with behavioral/emotional disabilities. What these children had in common was their ability to be on target in their physical development and motor skills while struggling with the educational curriculums involving reading and/or math. Even though I recognized that some of these children had either witnessed trauma or were trauma survivors themselves, I did not realize the role that language played in their ability to process and express trauma.

Language and PTSD in children

While obtaining my graduate degree at the University of South Florida, I had the privilege of studying under Doctor Michael Rank an expert in the field of Post Traumatic Stress Disorder (PTSD.) It was interesting to note that most of the recognition around PTSD has focused on service members who have been to war. Yet, large majorities of clients diagnosed with PTSD are women who have been sexually abused. The number of children with PTSD may be much lower due to the fact that it is often unreported in childhood. Children who experience PTSD may not be aware that they have the symptoms as research indicates they are at times labeled as having behavior problems. My research focused on how childhood trauma is processed including age-specific features, how it affects memory, verbal abilities, attachment, behavior, and how various forms of expressing through the arts are used successfully with children.

Puppetry

Early in my career I learned how the power of puppetry combined with song was able to reach an introverted child where a verbal invitation to join us could not. I was working as a behavioral modification specialist in southwest Florida using a program called Developing Understanding of Self and Others (DUSO.) The DUSO kit provided the perfect set of puppets using sea animals, the main character being Duso the Dolphin. Since we were located in Florida, the children were familiar with most of the animals portrayed by the puppets we presented.

My group consisted of children ages five to eight with emotional ranges on a spectrum from very withdrawn to outwardly angry. When Duso was introduced to the children, all but one child gathered around me, eager to meet the characters. As we sat in a circle on the floor, a young girl peeked out from behind the couch, observing the show from a distance. This particular child was the youngest of her siblings and had become extremely shy and withdrawn. A large part of her behavioral response had developed as a result of members in her family making the decisions for her. She had not developed the confidence necessary to make decisions for herself or speak up for herself against her siblings.

Aware that she was watching us and trying to access the emotional safety of the group, I continued conducting it without calling attention to her. Behavior modification meant not reinforcing unwanted behavior. I gave my attention to the children in the circle and the puppets, making it as much fun for them as possible. As we modeled an atmosphere which encouraged the children to express themselves to the puppets, this young girl drew physically closer to the group. It was half way through the second group that she joined us and began participating. By the end of the summer, she was very verbal and was "sticking up for herself at home." She had used the puppets to express herself and through reinforcement was able to transfer the skills to her home.

Puppetry, especially with young children, is powerful. In Dayton, Ohio, the Suicide Prevention Center provides elementary schools with a package that includes scripts and instructions on how to make puppets and stages, and how to put on a performance. The center also provides puppeteers who go to classes and answer questions about life and death.

As stated by Ayyash-abdo, "In puppet therapy, it is easy to act out expressions as if they belong to the puppet ...children recovering from trauma can act it out over and over, leading to catharsis" (2001.)

Confiding in Adults

Hamblen states that a label of "PTSD requires that an individual experience an event that involves a threat to one's own or another's life or physical integrity and that they respond with intense fear, helplessness, or horror" (2006.) Lieberman explains that if the parent was the trauma survivor and the child witnessed the trauma, the parent may have been so involved by his or her own traumatic process that he or she was unaware that the child also experienced the trauma. If the parent sexually abused the child, he or she is caught between approach and avoidance. Aspects of the parent's behavior are likely to become traumatic reminders for the child, resulting in attachment disorganization "fear without solution" (2004.) Fear without solution or the ability to verbalize the trauma, or to get the help of someone to process the trauma, triggers a greater than normal physiological response. This exaggerated physiological response is a main factor in the development of PTSD.

Graffiti

In an effort to express the trauma of witnessing the horrific events of September 11, 2001, children turned to art. A forward in Goodman explains the birth of such graffiti. There was an "immediate outpouring of art created by children affected by the tragedy. The work sprung up spontaneously, adorning building facades, storefronts, fire and police stations...we knew that the children felt most comfortable revealing in their art what they had witnessed and experienced" (2002.) Upon seeing the graffiti that began to cover the city, the Museum of the City of New York and the New York University Child Study Center collaborated to exhibit and publish the artwork of children ages five to eighteen that were affected by this tragedy. Children drew self-portraits, people falling from buildings, rescue workers, before and after scenes, tragedy as well as peace. Each one was an opportunity for expression, an open door for discussion and healing. It is easy to understand how words could not express the intense emotions of this trauma.

At a Loss for Words

Van Der Kolk found that the nature of traumatic memories is very different from that of ordinary events. Whereas memory for ordinary events is always constructive, can be verbally articulated or expressed symbolically, is conscious and uninterrupted, and loses accuracy over time, memory for traumatic events leaves sensory imprints which remain accurate over time, are vivid and may occur without the ability to articulate what the individual is feeling or thinking. This inability to be articulated verbally may occur even though the memories are detailed, accurate and persistent. Dissociation at the time of trauma is "the most important long-term predictor for the ultimate development of PTSD." Van Der Kolk describes dissociation as memory stored as sensory fragments that have no linguistic components (1998.)

Knowing how difficult it is for children to express themselves verbally, I created a small storybook. I was working with a group of children who were living with relatives as their primary caregivers. Most of the children's parents were incarcerated. One of the younger boys acted out a lot in school, but he loved art class. According to his grandmother, he was often angry and aggressive towards others.

I wrote an open-ended story for the children about a frog that lived with its parents, but one day had to go and live with relatives who cared very much for him. I printed it in black and white and provided each child a copy and a set of crayons. They were invited to color the book and draw pictures on the last few pages as an ending to the story. This little boy drew two shapes at the end of the story. The first shape was a head with triangles pointing down and circles for eyes. The first picture, he stated was "a very angry frog with sharp teeth." The second picture was a single square with an "x" drawn across it. I wrote his words "the mother has been X'd out." The frog was his angry self and as a powerless child who felt abandoned, he was able to take back some power by crossing her out.

Correlation of Trauma to Language and Behavior

Alexander, et al. tell us that trauma in children results in a reduced forgetting of trauma-related words…and that survivors develop semantic networks ("fear networks") within which trauma- related information becomes stored. The words surrounding the event, although not consciously remembered by the child may trigger a traumatic response (2005.) Given the changes in physiology, unconscious triggers, and repression of verbal abilities, it is not unreasonable to expect changes in a child's behavior.

Mennen found an inverse correlation between the PTSD Inventory and scores on the Verbal scale of the WISC-R. The correlation indicated that higher PTSD scores were related to lower performance on the verbal measure of intelligence. It was interesting to note that the same correlation did not exist for the Full Scale or Performance dimensions of the WISC-R. The tests indicate that trauma is not directly related to IQ but only to the verbal dimension. This finding supports Van Der Kolk's work on linguistics and PTSD. Both verbal and behavioral difficulties have a positive correlation to PTSD indicating problems in verbal learning could lead to an increased number of behavioral problems. The PTSD Inventory also had related scores on measures of anxiety, behavior problems, and dissociation indicating a substantial overlap and correlation between the Child Behavior Checklist (CBCL) and PTSD symptoms. Results showed that "one quarter of the score on the Total Problems dimension of the CBCL can be predicted by the score on the PTSD Inventory". For clinicians, Mennen suggests a possible need to target verbal learning in traumatized children (2004.)

Filial Play Therapy

Lieberman explains that children have limited introspective and articulation abilities. Therefore, a child who responds to traumatic reminders but is unable to express the trauma to the parent will be misunderstood. Since the parents are unable to link a stimulus to the child's behavior, they may respond by scolding or punishing the child and aggravating the traumatic response (2004.)

Rye explains that Filial Play Therapy is different from traditional Non-Directive Play Therapy because parents are trained by the therapist and normally conduct the sessions themselves. It is best suited for children three to eleven years old and specific toys are chosen for play therapy based on the situation being addressed (2005.)

I had the opportunity to attend a workshop presented by Jennifer Baggerly at the University of South Florida. She showed a film of a mother and son involved in Filial Play Therapy. The child was running over a toy figure with his truck. The mother simply stated the child's actions "you are running over the man with your truck." This statement allows the child to confirm and expound on his actions. This is far different from the untrained observations of parents who are quicker to advise the child that he should not run over people, but wait for them to move out of the road. In Bagerly's work with homeless children, she found that they had two themes, money and eviction. Children pretended to be rich. They also threw dolls out of the houses as they acted out what had happened in their own lives (2007.)

The true advantage of Filial Play Therapy is that it includes the parents and is designed to teach them the skills used to communicate with their own child in order to continue the therapeutic sessions at home after the professional therapist has terminated with the client.

Warm up and Wait with Poster Board and Crayons

Considering the obstacles children have to overcome when dealing with trauma, it is important that a therapist be able to direct a child but also let the child determine the pace. The program in which I worked with the children in the care of their relatives is a good example of how the process of art making helps traumatic memories unfold in layers.

I brought in a large poster board for each child folded in half like a giant greeting card. As a warm up, we shared our likes and differences. I added that just like each of them I did not live with my parents. The objective of the statement was to have it expressed as a conscious thought in order to create an environment that would encourage the children to express their feelings about being separated from their parents.

Each child was given a box of crayons and instructed to draw whatever he or she was feeling at the present time. Two of the girls drew a rainbow with flowers beneath it. After a specified time, I announced that it was time to finish their pictures and put the crayons away. One of the girls continued to draw on the inside and back of her card. She had become comfortable with the activity and learned that it was safe to draw without judgment or criticism. The initial drawing of the rainbow and flowers had provided time for her unconsciousness to open up to the art experience and allow her emotions to come closer to the surface. This was not a cognitive decision, but an artful expression of what was happening inside of her. With a crayon in her hand, she was able to draw a picture that she had never expressed verbally in our meetings. Her pictures expressed the extreme emotions she was carrying with her about her mother.

Inside the poster board, the girl had drawn an arch that looked like a black and white rendition of the colorful rainbow on the cover. Rather than linear stripes, the black arch had a criss-cross of lines drawn through the arch. Walking beneath the arch was a small girl. When I asked her to tell me about the rainbow, she talked about a trip to Mexico that she had taken with her grandparents. The arch marked the border crossing between the United States and Mexico. She was there to visit her mother. The girl stated that she was very unhappy and frightened by the visit and that she had not wanted to go. Her memory for the event was a vivid sensory imprint. At the age of seven, she was able to draw what she could not accurately describe. She was not able to articulate what had frightened her about the visit, but she knew she was frightened.

Her third picture was drawn on the back of the poster board. It was a self-portrait with a big smile. The lines on her teeth appeared to be braces. She said she had pretty teeth. I learned later that she had visited her mother in prison and had been traumatized by the fact that her mother's teeth were missing. She had never seen her without them or without her hair done. She was frightened by the fact that she did not recognize her own mother. The third picture was another layer peeled back through art.

Implications for Clinicians

Based on the overwhelming evidence and links between PTSD and the linguistic process, the clinician may be wise to consider therapies that deemphasize verbalization of the trauma. Therapies such as play, art, drama, and storytelling provide the traumatized child with a method of communicating the experience without barriers of vocabulary. A skilled clinician can use art to help a child who relates an experience, which may sound similar to the discussion of an ordinary event, but includes phrases such as, "I don't remember," to fill in the gaps in his/her story. When recognizing that a child is actually seeing or reliving the trauma using the words, "I can see...," a therapist can assist the child in recreating the visual through an art form.

References

Alexander, K.W., J.A. Quas,, G.S. Goodman, S. Ghetti, R.S. Edelstein, A.D. Redlich, et al. "Traumatic Impact Predicts Long-term Memory of Documented Child Sexual Abuse." *Psychological Science, 16:*1, (2005) 33-38.

Ayyash-abdo, H. "Childhood Bereavement: What School Psychologists Need to Know." *School Psychology International*, 22:4, (2001) 417-433.

Baggerly, J. USF Collaborative for Children, Families & Communities. Jennifer Baggerly. 2007 Retrieved October 14, 2008 from http://usfcollab.fmhi.usf.edu/expertdetail.cfm?staffid=3

Goodman, R. F., and A. H. Fahnestock, *The Day Our World Changed Children's Art of 9/11*. New York: Harry N. Abrams, Inc., 2002.

Hamblen, J. *PTSD in Children and Adolescents*. (2001) Retrieved March 8, 2006 from www.ncptsd.org/facts/specific/fs_children.html

Lieberman, A. F. "Traumatic Stress and Quality of Attachment: Reality and Internalization in Disorders of Infant Mental Health." *Infant Health Journal, 25*:4 (2004) 336-351.

Mennen, F. E. " PTSD Symptoms in Abused Latino Children," *Child and Adolescent Social Work Journal, 21*:5 (2004) October, 477-487.

Van Der Kolk, B. A. "Trauma and Memory." *Psychiatry and Clinical Neurosciences, 52*:S5 (1998) S97 – S111.

SOLVITUR AMBULANDO
(IT IS SOLVED BY WALKING)

ALISON MORROW

A path painted on canvas, lying under trees, in a secluded grassy space on a sunny late August day. Knowing little about labyrinths except that there was one path leading to the centre, I chose to step in and walk. Birds sang their end of summer chorus. Laughter and talking could be heard in the distance, but otherwise I walked in solitary silence. What happened? No tremendous revelations. But I came out knowing that I had been in the presence of the Sacred, and with a question that has been the basis for my ongoing discernment about the life path I am to travel. That was in 1998 at the University of Guelph in southern Ontario, as part of *Daring Hope – A Celebration of the Ecumenical Decade of Churches in Solidarity With Women*. Since then, my journey has included exploring the uses of the labyrinth, and eventually developing and facilitating workshops for groups to create their own personal finger labyrinths.

Background & History of the Labyrinth

So what is this labyrinth that has been so important to my life? Where did it come from? How was it developed? How is it used? What can it do? First of all, we need some clarification of the frequent confusion concerning the difference between the terms "labyrinth" and "maze." In his book *Unending Mystery,* David Willis McCullough suggests "...the semantic difference between the words *labyrinth* and *maze* is a new one" (2004:3.) Both are patterns to be walked or otherwise followed. The commonly accepted definition today for a labyrinth is that it is unicursal, or has one path which leads to the centre and back out again. We choose to enter, or not, and once having stepped over the threshold simply follow the path. A maze is multicursal, having many paths, dead ends and choices, which may or may not lead us to our goal. In her article "Using a Labyrinth in Spiritual Care," Ingrid Bloos points out that, "The intention of the labyrinth is to clarify, deepen, and connect … The intention of the maze is to tease, confuse, frustrate, obstruct, or trap the walker at each step." Thus, she continues, "...it is only the labyrinth with its emphasis on wholeness rather than fragmentation, and connection rather than separation that emerges as a tool that can be used to promote spiritual growth and healing" (2005:150.)

There are many forms of labyrinths, primarily based on the spiral found everywhere in nature – in seashells, hurricane clouds, cobwebs, whirlpools, the unfolding petals of a rose, galaxies – you can probably think of many other examples. According to Helen Sands in *The Healing Labyrinth,* the earliest known form is the Classical or Cretan labyrinth with its seven-circuit path leading to the centre. She says, "The oldest existing example to date is a labyrinth carved into the rock of a Neolithic chambered tomb in Luzzanas, Sardinia, dating from 2500-2000 B.C." (2001: 27.) This labyrinth design is found in many places throughout the world, "traced on rock, marked out on the ground with stones, carved into turf and decorating ancient artifacts" (2001:26.) Today, the Pima of southern Arizona weave a labyrinth pattern into their baskets and use this design on the license plates of council vehicles driven on the reservation near Phoenix, Arizona (2001:37.)

In the Middle Ages, the labyrinth was claimed as a Christian symbol. Labyrinths were placed in many of the medieval cathedrals, but the majority of them were lost or destroyed in 18th or 19th centuries. The best-known surviving medieval labyrinth is found at Chartres Cathedral in France, and was completed around 1220. Along with the Classical labyrinth, it is the most familiar design used today. It has four quadrants, or quarters, and eleven circuits of winding path that moves back and forth through all four quadrants, towards and away from centre. Often used as a symbolic pilgrimage for those who were for one reason or another unable to complete a pilgrimage to Jerusalem, it is often called "the way of the pilgrim" or "the Jerusalem Road" (Sands, 2001:36.) Lauren Artress describes her journey to Chartres Cathedral in her book *Walking a Sacred Path,* and reveals how she and her group found the labyrinth covered with chairs that they removed so they could walk (1995:5.)

Today both permanent and portable labyrinths are used in many places. Portable labyrinths are often painted on canvas and laid down on church floors, gym floors, grassy fields, sandy beaches—anywhere there is a large enough space to accommodate them. Temporary labyrinths can be created using tape, rocks or a stick, to outline them in sand, earth or grass. There are many permanent labyrinths, both outdoors and inside, painted on floors, inlaid in stone, outlined with rocks, mowed into grass; in retreat centers, healing centers, spiritual centers, churches, and parks. There are locations all over the world, and labyrinths in any area can be found by using the on-line Worldwide Labyrinth Locator. There are also online labyrinths; some websites are listed in this bibliography.

Parts of the Labyrinth

The main parts of all types of labyrinths are the pathway and the centre. The seven-circuit Classical labyrinth has a simpler, less convoluted path than that of the Chartres labyrinth. The centre is smaller, and the shape is womb-like rather than circular. This labyrinth was often perceived as a journey to the womb of the Earth Mother, back to our original home. The Chartres labyrinth, with its eleven circuits, has a longer path, with more twists and turns. The centre is divided into six sections, often called "petals." According to Lauren Artress, these petals may be named as follows: "Starting on the left as you enter the center, the first petal is mineral, then vegetable, animal, human, angelic, and Unknown." Around the outside are 113 half-circles called "lunations." Artress suggests that these may have been used as "a method of keeping track of the lunar cycles of twenty-eight days each" (1995:60.) Other forms of the labyrinth may incorporate some of these elements, such as the Santa Rosa labyrinth designed by Lea Goode-Harris in 1997, which combines the seven circuits of the Classical with the turns of the Chartres labyrinths.

This brief description only touches on the rich history, background and parts of the labyrinth, and there is abundant and expansive information available from many sources. For those who are interested in exploring these areas in more depth, some of these resources are compiled in the bibliography. If "labyrinth" is keyed into *Google,* almost a million references will be found! Therefore, a search that is limited with words like "Chartres," "Cretan," "Classical," or "healing," will deliver as much information as might be wanted.

Using the Labyrinth

Although following a single path sounds like a relatively simple thing to do, walking the labyrinth is not a straightforward process. The curved pathways, the fixed turning points, the backward and forward shifts, the movement toward, away from, and back toward the centre, all create a balance, an experience of harmony. Through focusing on following the path, we are somehow enabled to let go of the multitude of thoughts tangled in our minds. Just as we think we are coming to the centre, a turn of the path takes us back to the outer edge again. The constant turns cause us to slow down, especially on the tighter centre circuits. The long stretches of the outer circuits swoop us halfway around the labyrinth. Our choice is to enter or not, and when we step onto the path we suspend disbelief and allow ourselves to trust that we will reach our goal. And then, we arrive at the centre and enter. We may stay there a while, praying, meditating or resting before retracing our path to re-emerge into our everyday world.

We can also walk as part of a group, or with others whom we do not know in the labyrinth. As we follow the path through the labyrinth, sometimes in the same direction as others, sometimes in the opposite direction, sometimes together with many others in our section, sometimes alone with everyone else somewhere else, we may recognize a metaphor for our life journeys. This is a time outside our usual busy schedules in which we can re-energize and renew our spirits, minds and bodies.

What has happened there for us? Maybe a sense of peace or calm. Maybe clarity in our thinking that wasn't there before. Maybe we are on our way to solving a problem that has been teasing at us. Sometimes it may seem that nothing has happened, but we later realize that our walk has freed our minds to move in a different direction or perceive our lives in a new way. Every experience is different, and each person has her or his own unique encounter with the space of the labyrinth.

There is no "right" way to walk a labyrinth. The most important thing to remember is to go in with openness to whatever may or may not occur. A response is not necessarily immediate, but may need time to percolate and take form. Sometimes when walking, we find ourselves back at the beginning without ever having reached the centre; or we may find ourselves back at the centre after have left it to return to the outside. This is not a time for distress over having walked "incorrectly," but a time to consider why this happened. One time, while walking my finger labyrinth, after spending time in each of the petals and feeling ready to leave my finger inadvertently went into one of the petals near the opening to the centre. I moved it and started back. Within a very few circuits I found myself entering the centre again. This time, recognizing that I was not finished, I stayed there longer, and when I left again I returned to the beginning easily. Allowing myself the freedom to let go of my expectation of immediately returning and to relax and stay was an important learning about my tendency to move on quickly.

Sometimes it is helpful to have quiet, meditative music playing, and at other times, silence seems preferable. I often pray, chant or sing as I walk, repeat a mantra, hold a question, problem or feeling, depending on what is happening in my life at any particular time. I find it helpful at times when I am unable to sleep to sit with my finger labyrinth, and the walking often calms me so that I am able to sleep afterwards. Bloos suggests:

> [that we] walk with intention ... [having] in mind a clear direction or specific purpose to what is being engaged ... Intentions can be powerful because they can focus and direct our physical, intellectual, emotional, and spiritual resources. Intentions call forth the energy within us and around us to clarify our thoughts and support our movements ... An intention can be as simple as walking with openness ...an intention makes the walker more aware of his/her innermost needs and begins to move these needs forward towards complete awareness. Intentions best support the labyrinth walk when they are put into the form of an open-ended question or phrase ... The key, as well as the challenge, of the intention is to simultaneously carry a plan for what is needed and an openness for what comes. (2005:131)

So each of us can find what works for us, recognizing that it will be different each time we walk, and embracing openness to the movement of the spirit.

Moving On

I have walked labyrinths many times, in several different forms, and whatever else might or might not happen, I always come out feeling calmer and with a sense of peace. I found it easy to recognize the significance of walking in prayer and meditation, for bringing peace and clarity, and relieving stress. Walking can help deal with emotions such as grief, fear and anger or as a ritual of celebration and joy. As I discovered the value of the labyrinth, I realized that I would use it more if there were one available. But I don't have a labyrinth in my backyard; I don't even have a backyard. Although there are several in Toronto, Canada where I live, I have to travel to them by transit, and in the cold snowy winters, most of them are not accessible.

While working in a hospital in a program for women, I met with the chaplain there and helped her prepare a workshop to facilitate the making of lightweight finger labyrinths on Plexiglas. Here was a solution for my desire to be able to walk at any time. I had seen some wooden labyrinths, but although they were beautiful to look at and to use, they were expensive. These inexpensive Plexiglas labyrinths were an equally beautiful and affordable alternative. And each person could create their own in colors of their choice and personalize it in a way that was meaningful to her/him.

I then planned a workshop and went to a retreat centre to lead a group in the experience of making finger labyrinths. Watching and helping the participants make their labyrinths was an amazing experience—the energy in the room was palpable and the presence of the Sacred was manifest; in the quiet music playing, in the occasional hushed voices, in the unfolding beauty of their creations. Since then I have led workshops for church groups and in healing facilities, and made several labyrinths that are used by hospital chaplains with their patients. Whether I am working with a faith-based group or a secular group, sacred energy always flows and enfolds us, so that the creating of the labyrinths becomes a prayer or meditation in itself. And when they are completed and each person reveals her/his handiwork, I never cease to be amazed and awed by the beauty and variety and uniqueness displayed.

Labyrinths are frequently used in church or spiritual centre settings, whether they are portable or permanent, and are recognized as being helpful for prayer, meditation, calming, reducing stress, slowing down, or emotional and psycho-spiritual healing. Labyrinths have been installed in and planned for a variety of healing centers and hospitals. After being asked to make several finger labyrinths by a hospital chaplain, I began to wonder about their value for healing.

I prefer the word "healing" rather than "curing." In her book *Exploring the Labyrinth*, Melissa West quotes from Michael Lerner: "a cure is a successful medical treatment ... that removes all evidence of the disease." In other words, we can say that I was well, I am sick now, and with successful treatment, I will be well again. Again using Lerner's words, she says, "[healing] is an inner process through which a person becomes whole" (2000:168.) I use "wholeness" to describe the process of integrating or weaving together of all parts of our selves, body, mind and spirit, embracing all of who we are, accepting and valuing our whole selves, and living peacefully with ourselves. Healing, then, is saying yes to a new definition of normal for ourselves and recognizing our own wholeness.

I talked with the hospital chaplains who had asked me to make the finger labyrinths for them. They led labyrinth spirituality groups with one to six mental health patients, both long and short-term, with conditions such as depression, bipolar disorder or schizophrenia. The patients were engaged with the labyrinths, choosing colors that suited them, and said that they felt relaxed, peaceful and calm. One of the aims of the unit is to offer "self-soothing activities," and the labyrinth seems to be an excellent tool for achieving this goal. The facilitator generally suggests that they might find God or the Sacred at the centre, and one of the patients in the group proposed taking their burdens of anger or sorrow with them into the centre and leaving them there with God. I find this to be an amazing and moving image.

How does healing happen in the labyrinth? Bloos explains:

> The physical movement of walking stimulates biochemical shifts. Merely moving along the labyrinth's path can be calming and help to alleviate stress, by simply offering a change of pace and scenery. It can help the walker shift awareness inward to focus on self in a more compassionate and holistic way. When we are in our thoughts and minds too much, physical movement facilitates the restructuring of the body's energy and can free up stifled resources (2005:160.)

There are many reasons for walking the labyrinth, as many as there are people walking it. Healing takes place subtly, slowly, often without our being conscious of it happening. Walking does not change the events of our lives, but it may help shift the way we feel or think about them, and consequently deal with them. This shift in energy that takes place when we walk a labyrinth, whether we use our feet or our fingers, can help move us towards healing. We will not be as we were, but will move forward to recognize in ourselves a deeper integration of spirit, body and mind.

Both a large walking labyrinth and a small finger one can have similar results, and each has its own particular benefits. Several of the advantages of walking with our feet are that our whole body moves and is involved; we can use different kinds of movement, such as dancing, or we can hold an item such as a stone, a scarf, or a candle as we walk. However, a full-sized labyrinth is not always available. Finger labyrinths are portable and we can use them at any time, day or night, whatever the weather. We can close our eyes or use different fingers and either hand. Those who have a physical disability that prevents them from walking a full-sized labyrinth can often use a finger labyrinth. Regardless of what kind of labyrinth you use, there is a healing power that can lead to wholeness and integrity within ourselves.

I have come a long way in the ten years since my first encounter with the labyrinth. It has been a fascinating journey that is ongoing as I continue to explore the uses and meanings of the labyrinth, especially in relation to healing. The possibilities for its use stretch out, waiting to be uncovered. Whenever I walk, I encounter the Sacred and through that encounter move more intimately into relationship with God and more deeply and closely to wholeness. I continue with joy and gratitude and hope to walk the paths of the labyrinth and of my life, and stay mindful of this quote from T.S. Eliot's "Little Gidding" used by McCullough (2004:7.)

We shall not cease from exploration
And the end of all our exploring
Will be to arrive where we started
And know the place for the first time.

Selected Labyrinth Resources

Artress, Lauren. *Walking a Sacred Path: Rediscovering the Labyrinth as a Spiritual Tool*. New York: Riverhead Books, 1995.
—. *The Sacred Path Companion: a Guide to Walking the Labyrinth to Heal & Transform*. New York: Riverhead Books, 2006.
Baley, Jana. "Walking the Labyrinth: Healing from Suffering and Loss." *Labyrinth Journal*. V. 1, no. 2 (March 2005) 6.
Bloos, Ingrid. "Using a Labyrinth in Spiritual Care." *Spirituality & Health: Multidisciplinary Explorations*. Eds. A. Meier, T. St. James O'Connor, P.L. VanKatwyk. Waterloo, ON: Wilfrid Laurier Press, 2005:149-165.
Curry, Helen. *Way of the Labyrinth: a Powerful Meditation for Everyday Life*. New York: Penguin, 2000.
Eason, Cassandra. *The Complete Guide to Labyrinths: Using the Sacred Spiral for Power, Protection, Transformation, and Healing*. Toronto, ON: Crossing Press, 2004.
Fairbloom, Lauren. *Walking the Labyrinth: Its Impact on Healthcare Professionals in a Hospital Setting*. Thesis (MA). Toronto, ON: OISE/University of Toronto, 2003.
MacQueen, Gailand. *Spirituality of Mazes & Labyrinths*. Kelowna, BC: Northstone, 2005 (pre-publication copy.)
McCullough, David Willis. *The Unending Mystery: a Journey Through Labyrinths and Mazes*. New York: Pantheon Books, 2004.
Sands, Helen. *Healing Labyrinth: Finding Your Path to Inner Peace*. New York: Barrons, 2001.
West, Melissa. *Exploring the Labyrinth: a Guide for Healing & Spiritual Growth*. New York: Doubleday/Dell, 2000.
Wirth, Jane. "The Labyrinth and Healing." *Labyrinth Journal*. Vol. 1, no.2 (March 2005) 3.

Websites

Labyrinth Community Network (Ontario, Canada)
   www.labyrinthnetwork.ca
Labyrinth On-Line
   www.labyrinthonline.com
Labyrinth Society
   www.labyrinthsociety.org
Veriditas
   www.veriditas.org
World-wide Labyrinth Locator
   www.veriditas.labyrinthsociety.org

EXPRESSIVE ARTS AREN'T ALWAYS PRETTY: A PICTURE OF DID

JUNE M. CONBOY

I provide art material and clients also provide their own. Much of the artwork is produced out of session; often the client is stressed, struggling with reality, and besieged with memories. The directive is simple. I ask them to draw or paint and to bring these to our next session.

Betty was 58 years old when she learned she was MPD (Multiple Personality Disorder,) now DID (Dissociative Identity Disorder,) and was in treatment with me. She had provided volumes of journaling and spontaneous writing and her *Writings for Alters* offered histories and comparisons of the many parts of herself. Her artwork was abundant. Feelings and reminiscences were recorded in watercolor, gauche, magic markers, pastels, crayon, pencil, ink and collages. She responded readily to imaging, relaxation techniques, and hypnotherapy. Psychodrama promoted communication among her different alters and me. Because she was in and out of trance states as a way of life, psychodrama was a natural and existential modus operandi.

Because Betty had a long history of 9-1-1 being summoned for her acting out episodes including drug overdoses, alcohol abuse and reckless driving, she had various hospitalizations. She spent as much as fourteen months as an inpatient during her last hospitalization in a psychiatric institution before I met her. From time to time Betty had wreaked havoc on her family. Initially Betty and her family were relieved to learn of her diagnosis. Finally, something seemed to offer to all concerned a respite from the years of the crazies. Her 35 year old daughter read MPD/DID literature and attended meetings with Betty featuring MPD speakers. They met other multiples and sometimes other support persons. Her husband joined the group I ran for partners of multiples.

Betty was from a middle-income family, became retired while in therapy with me and was then on disability for MPD/DID. Apparently, she could no longer maintain her usual composure at her workplace. Her work history included many years as a supervisor in a large insurance company. She was "kicked upstairs" and was relegated to a dull routine after personnel changes were made. She was extremely resentful of this and was feeling invisible and unimportant. This triggered past traumata and resulted in dissociative episodes and questionable behavior. Betty chose the company nurse, with whom she had felt some camaraderie, to be her confidante. However, the community at large does not understand this disorder and medical people are not routinely taught about MPD/DID. (Skepticism is typical and non-acceptance of DID is *derigueur* even in many psychiatric settings.) Betty's nurse friend was unable to be supportive. She seemed, to me, to be respectful of Betty's plight during our phone conversation. However, her responses told me that the ramifications of MPD/DID and child abuse awed and frightened her. Betty has a tendency to assume that if she could survive the abuse surely others can manage to hear about it. This, not being so, devastated Betty who saw herself to be unacceptable, unimportant and damaged goods, as per usual.

Betty, at times, was afraid to speak in my office. I had a figurine of the "see no evil, speak no evil, hear no evil" monkeys. She imitated this with her hands cupped over her eyes, mouth and ears. Yet, she did write and draw in my office and at home. Sometimes she brought to her sessions a crumpled up piece of paper that she claimed she retrieved from her wastebasket. It seemed that the alter who drew a revealing picture was not necessarily the same alter who would bring the art work to a session. There were parts of Betty who were mystified as to content and authorship; but at times, other parts were protecting Betty from knowing her history. Crumpled up paper usually was the work of an authoritative, hostile guardian of those alters deemed incapable of knowing about the abusive childhood.

When I addressed this situation, I was told by one of the all knowing alters, Shadow or The Quiet One or Mary Ellen, that Betty, the host personality, "would not survive" if she knew the facts. "She can't handle it," they said. Frequently, Lizbeth, a six year old alter, got "them" in trouble. Lizbeth was blamed for "talking too much." There was a price to pay for everything said and done, it seemed. Protective alters were not necessarily nurturers. More often, they were rageful and imitated punishers of the past. In their respective rages they acted out against alters who talked and worked in therapy. In addition, they acted out against me, by imitating past punishers who issued many threats and were menacing and obnoxious. In Betty's case, both the biological and foster parents were harshly punitive. Punishments were meted out and various self-abusive incidents were the norm. Fortunately, some degree of homeostasis was restored when nurturers stepped in to console Lizbeth and any other needy little ones. These nurturers and others who prided themselves on their social skills would apologize to me for making me be the recipient of harassing phone calls, letters, insults and threats.

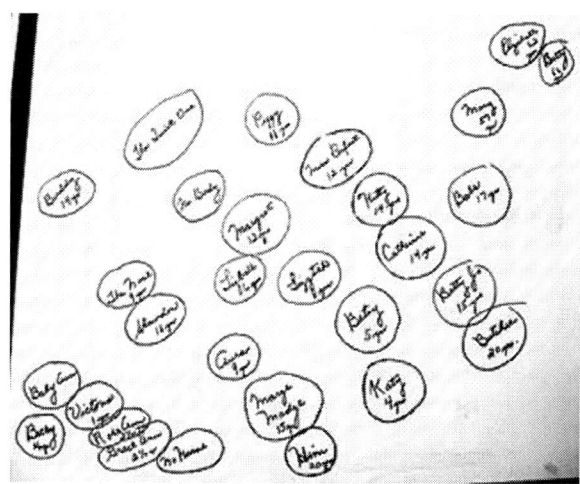

Mapping by Betty

A procedure called mapping can be described as a family tree, road map, diagram, etc. Mapping is a method of defining an internal genealogy. In other words, the names and ages of the alters are listed and they are loosely arranged as to groupings. Betty's map was drawn on 11 x 24 paper. (It has been reduced in size here.) Betty's twenty-nine alters appear to be floating as in a constellation. The babies and toddlers are clustered together at the bottom left. She was 62 years of age when she did this map. There were more alters in her system as you will see in the many reproductions.

Betty and her sidekick, Elizabeth, same age as Betty, are obliquely positioned at the right, upper corner, close together. Elizabeth chooses not to know facts and is modeled on her actual sister Mary, nine years older, who also chose life without knowing. Elizabeth was personable and took on the host role when Betty needed to put on a happy front.

Him, a powerful twenty-year old, who spoke only rarely, was recognized from a deep, basso voice. Most responses were grunts that sounded like they came from his toes. Located at the center, lowest border of the paper, Him is firmly ensconced. His role was to protect all those above.

Butchie was another twenty-year-old male. Also a protector, Butchie had a more benevolent manner and was a watchful guardian. In his self-portrait, he stands tall and straight next to a tree, watching Katy.

Buddy was a sixteen-year-old male who was among the first alters to speak in therapy. The name is derived from fantasizing that he was a drinking buddy with the father. I was told that he had no genitalia. This is not uncommon for persons who have been sexually abused. It follows that if there are no sexual orifices, one would be unsuited to sexual activity. Buddy's role as a house cleaner is legendary. The system especially welcomed this manic side at the conclusion of depressed periods during which nothing was done. Buddy used pastels and applied the pastels with a very heavy hand. These males are noticeably all on the perimeter of the constellation of alters.

Kitty, fourteen years old, was spiritual and aesthetic. She had never been harmed in any way and is a dreamer. Soft pastels in dress and in paintings are her forte and she was oblivious to any of the childhood abuse.

Catherine, age 14, slightly overlaps Kitty as part of the constellation. Catherine was the exact opposite. Her hairdo was a mess when she was forced by the foster father to perform oral sex for him on her confirmation day. He told her, "Now you have something to really celebrate." When Catherine was out, she would shower a few times daily. She disdained religion and spirituality, hated men and was a compulsive over eater, especially ice cream. Her handwriting and artwork were sharp and harsh.

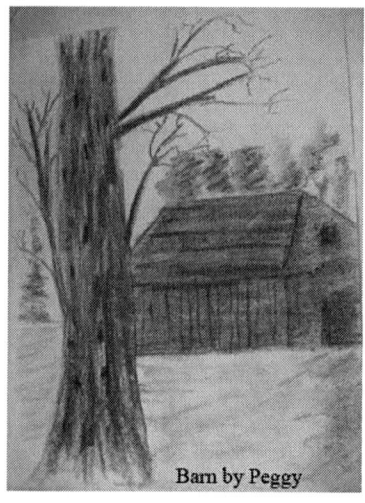

Barn by Peggy

Babs was closest to Catherine on the mapping page. She is 17 and was created by younger alters to appreciate sex. Her seductiveness allowed that part of the system to believe that sex was fun. It was important for Babs to believe she was controlling men. She was flamboyant in her choice of dress and she loved vibrant colored magic markers and colored pencils. Babs had wreaked havoc for vulnerable others though. She did not stay around if the sex got rough. She disappeared and frightened others were left to find themselves being hurt again.

Peggy, 11 years old, was the opposite of Babs. Peggy was always depressed with suicidal impulses. Her handwriting was so small it became microscopic. Her artwork was well done, but it was only in grays and blacks. Twice I convinced her to use at least one color as a watercolor wash over her paintings. Those are the "black and blue" watercolors. Expressing herself in any color was significant because I felt that the potential for more color offered hope for one whose sole outlook was dire hopelessness.

Betty Jo, 15 years old, was unknown to me until a few intense watercolor paintings began turning up. Embryonic forms and infants amidst swirling reds and purples represented one of her abortions. Her foster mother who was a nurse performed this on her. The abortion was done without the benefit of an anesthetic. Betty Jo mourns the death of babies and rages over what was done to them.

Mary, age 57, was named for her birth mother. Mary took the shock treatments during her 14-month hospital stay before she began therapy with me. When Betty was 3 ½ years old, her psychotic mother was institutionalized where she remained until she died.

Once, when Betty was six, she went, accompanied by her siblings, to visit her mother. She remembers her mother hugging her. This seems to have given her something tangible to grasp. Even though her mother was a horrendous abuser, Betty fantasized that her good mom would protect her.

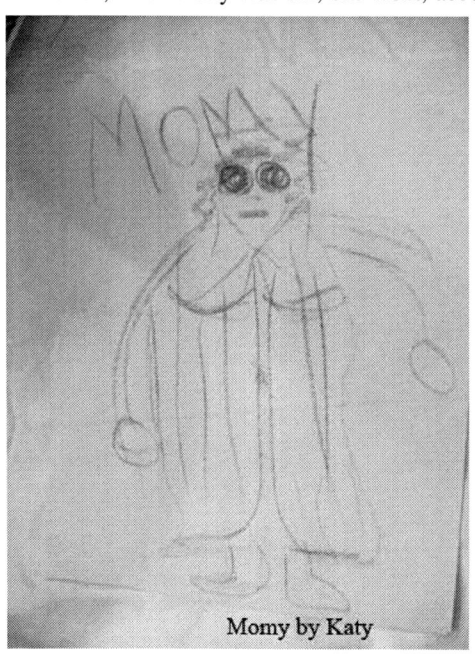

Momy by Katy

Katy, age four, drew self-portraits of a very angry and grim little girl always being humiliated publicly and tortured privately for wetting herself. She painted scenes with yellow puddles under her dangling feet that were not touching the floor. She remembered she was tied up to a hook in the bathroom to teach her a lesson.

Betsy, age five, neither wrote nor drew but other alters did this for her. Her feelings of shame because of masturbatory activity rendered her unable to communicate except through hypnotherapy. Betsy was the target of the foster mother's pedophilic conduct.

The Quiet One, ageless, is the "ish" or inner self helper (Adams, 1989.) Her demeanor was very quiet and gentle. She told detailed stories of particular alters when they are unable to communicate (too young, too frightened, speechless, amnestic.) She had no affect and had suffered no personal abuses. She would tire and disappear when she completed her mission. She wrote very legibly and seldom drew.

Shadow, 16 years old, was the Hidden Observer (Hilgard, 1984.) Shadow had seen it all—the worst of the abuses. She painted all scenes with intense watercolors. Unlike many alters, she always signed her work without being asked. Although she did not speak, she acknowledged, with a nod, her presence at sessions. Shadow held onto everyone's anger.

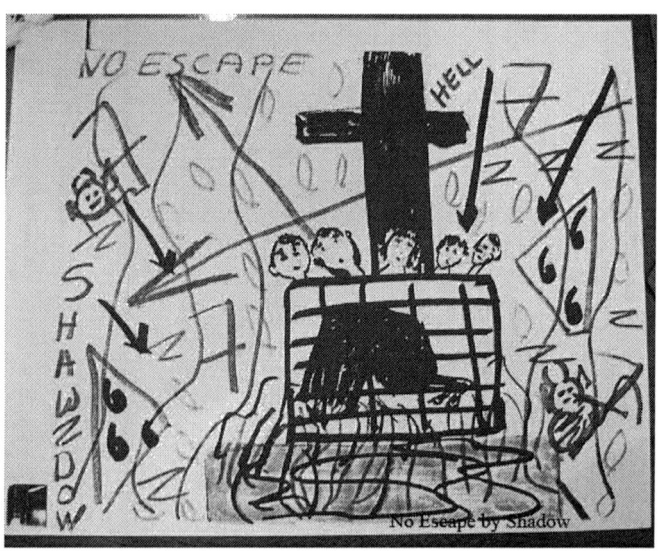

No Body, ageless, was the one who goes into the wall. This way, she was aware that something awful was happening to someone else. Being without a body and from her position in the wall, she observed, without feeling, what was happening to someone else. She was depressed, didn't draw but added her signature to some art that others produced.

The Nose, nine years, will communicate through others. The Nose was extremely sensitive to perfumes and identified trauma with certain fragrances. Certain spices, fires, body odor, etc triggered Odiferous memories. An example of this was a gruesome memory that surfaced from smelling cloves. This was drawn by Shadow. The Nose wrote with a very distinct style of printing and used magic markers with the help of Madge and Shadow.

Aura, nine years old, first met with me when she threatened me. She came across as being incredibly mean. She, like most angry alters, seemed older than she professed to be. I had to remind myself that I was actually dealing with the meanness and rage of a child who wanted to lash out at an adult because of past hurtful experiences. She said that she was subjected to hot wax being dripped on her eyes when she was tied down. She was threatened, she says, with being blinded by the hot wax if she ever told what she saw. In addition, she was told that she "didn't see" what she saw. Her angry written accounts are revelations of the many sadistic events she can now claim she did see. She influences Madge's art.

Lizbeth, six years old, was one of the most prolific writers even though she was limited in her six-year-old ability. She was proud of her precise printing. Misspelled words are phonetically readable. For her artwork, she used crayons and colored pencils. Lizbeth declared her love for me by writing notes in her journal that she expected me to see. She would send greeting cards and would surprise me with small gifts. She desperately hoped to be loved in return. She believed because she was so unlovable that she deserved all the bad stuff that kept happening to her.

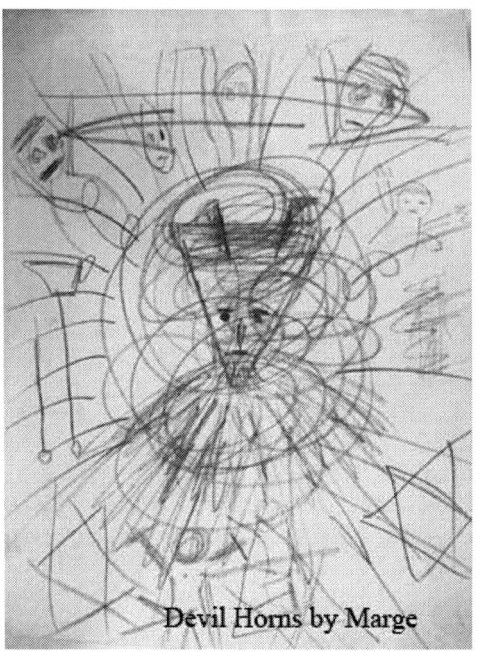

Devil Horns by Marge

Marge and Madge, aged 15, are twins. This

is common in DID. They are among the alters who remember being abused in a cult. Marge, intensely rageful, wrote long narratives of harrowing experiences and could barely control herself when speaking to me. Equally rageful was Madge who never spoke except through her paintings. She chose the largest sheets of paper available and she filled each with horrific details including satanic and cult symbols.

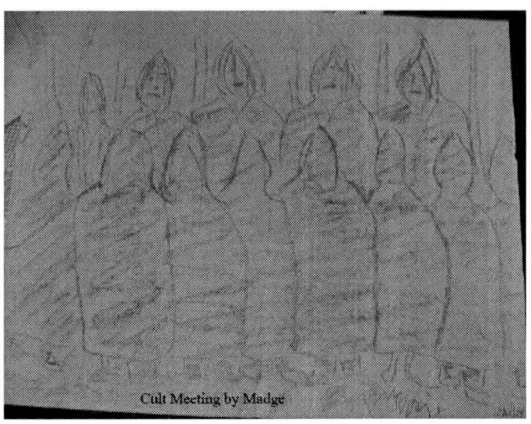
Cult Meeting by Madge

Rose Ann and Grace Ann, also twins, were 1 ½ to 2 ½ years old. Rose Ann abreacted the sensation of slipping down off the birth mother's hip as they (twins) were being carried up a path to a farmhouse and barn. Rose Ann struggled to get away and she screamed while Grace Ann slept. Grace Ann received positive messages and Rose Ann got negative messages. Memories included being placed in boxes and being subjected to unspeakable acts that were triggered by media news, T.V. shows, movies, pictures, books, etc. Certain churches, stairways, caskets, funerals, basements, authority figures including the clergy were among scary reminders that would set Rose Ann and Grace Ann off. Others drew the twins at cult meetings and still others told their story.

Margaret, 12 years old, was said to have pulled Rose Ann from a fire and then they both hid together at a cult meeting. Margaret doesn't know if dolls or babies were thrown into the fire.

Victoria, one year old, believed the birth mother alternated between loving her and torturing her. She shook uncontrollably and her teeth chattered when triggered. Others told her story of surviving a ritualized burial.

Baby Ann, also called the infant, believed both birth parents sexually abused her. She trembled all over, was breathless and stared wide-eyed. Others told her story of being caged and subjected to bestiality.

No Name, ageless, claimed to have no feeling and was just there. She was interchangeable with No Body.

Bethy, four years old, had been declared by the others to be in heaven, where she was safe. Being alive was so awful that she had been assigned a place with the angels. At age four, Bethy was taken from the Angel Guardian Home and placed in foster care for the first time.

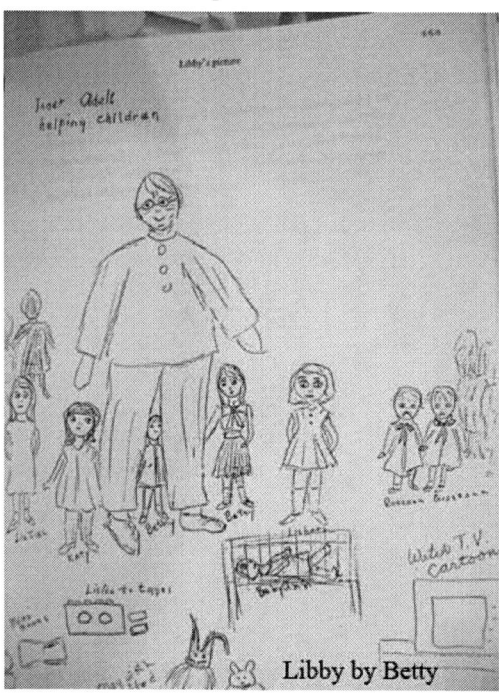

Libby by Betty

Besides the alters in this mapping exercise, there were more alters. Some were holiday alters such as Holly and Holly Beth. Some were fragments such as Cinderella who played handball at school but emptied the foster father's humidor each evening.

Libby was the good mom who never was impatient and never slept because of her constant vigil over the children.

There were other cult alters, such as Lizzy Tish, Bess, Barbara, Barbette, Margarita, Audrey, Pam and Trish. Among alters who dealt with the abusive family were Gail, Polly, Patty, Clover Leaf, Lettie and Nettie.

Sunny was a happy daytime alter, Kay shopped and spent money indiscriminately, Lena was a chronic liar and Mother was a hostile alcoholic, patterned on the birth mother.

Betty's disillusionment with her own mother was the most dreaded moment of truth for her. Betty recalled heinous crimes she believed she witnessed including the killing of her baby brother. Yet, the desire to remember momma as loving and benevolent was so powerful that the alter Mother was created. But Betty's mother gave in to violent alcoholic rages that Betty's alter, Mother, likened to being all-powerful. She equated this with having the ability to control those who seemed less powerful. This was then converted into the role of a guardian who was most powerful and controlled everyone through intimidation, warnings and menacing behavior. Thus, Mother was a protector (as mothers are supposed to be) but she posed a threat to the therapeutic process because she was determined to maintain control. She was convinced that I would be favored over her, just as her birth mother's musician husband was favored because of his talents. Mother's was a thankless job—all work while father played. The alter, Mother, compared me to him. I had been warned that she hated me and was dangerous. She was like a snarling tigress with her cubs.

Mary Ellen or "me" as she calls herself, was out very often because she held the anger toward men. When Betty was very upset and/or mad at her husband, Mary Ellen came out and got nasty. Her namesake for this alter was the foster mother, Mary Ellen Pons, (Pons is a pseudonym) who was indifferent and condescending toward her husband, the foster father. Mary Ellen Pons was also both tough and stoic and/or entirely dissociative. For example, she cooked dinner, as usual, after what was obviously painful dental surgery without complaining. She also, most likely, was anesthetizing herself with alcohol because she was a daily drinker. She was mean and deceitful but clever and cunning as was the alter, me/Mary Ellen. The foster mother, Mary Ellen Pons, apparently never was caught as she indulged in her pedophiliac fantasies and cult participation. She was a paragon of virtue when the foster care caseworker made periodic home visits. Too frightened of the consequences, Betty answered when the caseworker spoke to her but divulged nothing of the sexual and physical abuse that included food and sleep deprivation. Being told she was bad, Betty

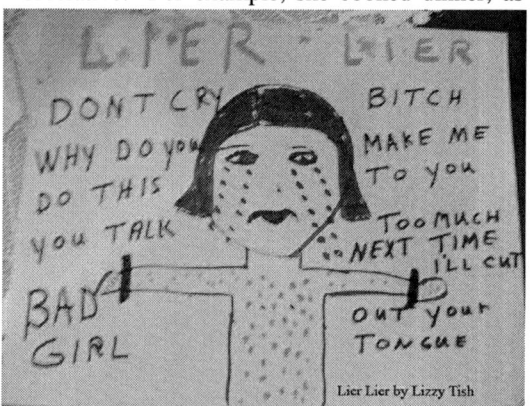

Lier Lier by Lizzy Tish

believed that she was truly bad. The threat of being sent to the "place for bad girls" loomed large and she believed that place would be worse than the place she called home. Besides, Betty was programmed to believe that she was always "asking for it" one way or another. Betty's Mary Ellen was envious of folks who enjoy financial and social security and was quick to put down those who enjoyed prosperity. She was a carbon copy of the foster mother whom she despised. The foster mother was also a fashion plate and had a petite figure. Betty was a larger woman but perceived herself to be whoever was out at the time. This phenomenon can be compared to the 86-pound anorexics that see/perceive themselves as obese. Betty's Mary Ellen could fool most people with her style, good taste and 'duplicitousness.' She eventually apologized to me and admitted that she wanted therapy and would cooperate.

Betty and I learned about her alters as therapy progressed during office sessions, on the telephone and through artwork and her writings. Through abreactions, the reliving of traumatic past experiences, I was privy to introductions and reemergence of different alters. During the early years of therapy, I met many alters by telephone. Not being face to face with me was much less threatening to some alters. Containing her abreactions, at times, seemed impossible. As a result, contingency plans as spontaneous abreactions occurred when Betty was not in my office were necessary for her therapy. Though not always as successful as I wished these plans to be, Betty devoted much of her time at home to projects I suggested. Some of her abreactions caused such chaos in her home life that she and her family were often at their wit's end. During a less chaotic period, Betty did the homework I assigned, *Writings for Alters* that is the questionnaire I developed in 1989. I had accumulated resumes of alters as a result of these biographical and autobiographical responses to twenty questions.

Among the alters who cooperated in this joint venture were Elizabeth, Peggy, "me" (Mary Ellen), Babs and Betty. Babs and "me" always used a red pen. For Babs, red is an attention getter; "me" saw red as a bloody warning to show her potential to inflict pain. Elizabeth, Betty and Peggy chose blue, a more low key and standard color.

Each alter answered on the same sheet of paper but each wrote on separate days. Their uniqueness is manifested in handwriting, style and content. In writing out answers, Betty stated on Question 12 that she was not going to answer any more questions. Therefore, she didn't. (Four years later Betty rewrote her twenty questions. The last two questions on suicide had not yet been included in the earlier Questionnaire.)

Eventually Libby, Catherine and Sunny responded to the questions in *Writings For Alters*. These were all done on separate sheets independent of one another. Catherine's and Sunny's were done months later after the questions on suicide were added. The rest of the writings and artwork are numerous. Much of the contents are disturbing even for seasoned therapists. Some themes are interpreted by more than one alter as are the facts, as Betty's different alters give their versions. The viewer/reader will observe the range of feelings such as anger and rage, sadness and depression, love and hatred, dependence and independence, hopelessness and despair, peace and frustration, serenity, with humor, mischievousness, seductiveness, originality, apathy, empathy, spirituality.

It is my very great pleasure to leave you with this up-beat message. In Betty's own words,

"I at seventy years of age 'celebrate' my life. I am in control. I make all my own decisions. I live with joy and peace. I now can show my love to others and am able to accept their love in return. You might be discouraged that I am free at a relatively old age. That is true. I must point out to you that although being ill for so many years, I wasn't diagnosed until about twelve years ago. I was lucky to be able to find a therapist that understood D.I.D. I had to keep my diagnosis a secret for fear that people would really think I was completely nuts.

I never thought I would ever be a whole person. I now realize how wonderful it is when I get up in the morning just putting on one item of clothing and know that I don't have to change about six or seven times. I now use only one brand of toothpaste. Look at how much money I'm saving. When I go to eat at a restaurant, I know that what I order will not change. That I will not confuse the waitress by ordering a glass of milk, a cup of coffee and a Tom Collins.

Two years ago, I made the decision to move many states away. I didn't ask anyone's permission or advice. I just moved. As my husband's ill health continued to deteriorate, I took matters in my own hands. I now pay all the bills, do all the shopping, cook all the meals, take care of my car, run all the errands. This might not sound like much, but for me it is amazing. I am now able to tell you what I did yesterday. I now know what day it is. I no longer lose time. I am so grateful – Maybe we are not completely integrated, but we have cooperation and except on rare occasions Elizabeth is in control. I tell you this to bring you hope.

Elizabeth"

Bibliography

Adams, M.A. "Internal Self Helpers Of Persons With Multiple Personality Disorder," *Dissociation* II:3 (1989.)
Araoz, D. *The New Hypnosis.* New York: Brunner Mazel, Inc., 1985.
Chu J., *ISSMP&D News* 5700 Old Orchard Road, Skokie, Illinois 1991.
Cohen, B., *The Diagnostic Drawing Series*, (Revised rating guide. available from Barry Cohen, P.O. Box 6091, Alexandria, Virginia 22306. 1986.)
Cohen, B. M., M. Rankin Barnes, and A. B. Rankin, *Managing Traumatic Stress Through Art.* Maryland: Sidian Press, 1995.
Conboy, J. *Hypnosis & Dissociative Identity Disorder* New York: New York Society of Clinical Hypnosis, 1997.
Fraser, G. "Special Treatment Technique To Access The Inner Personality System Of Multiple Personality Disorder Patients." *Dissociation* VI (1993.)."
Fraser, G. A. "The Dissociative Table Technique: A Strategy for working with ego states in dissociative disorders & Ego State Therapy." *Dissociation* IV :4 (1991.)
Hilgard, E. "The Hidden Observer & Multiple Personality." *International Journal of Clinical & Experimental Hypnosis*, 1984
Kluft, E. S. *Expressive & Functional Therapies in the Treatment of Multiple Personality disorder.* Springfield, Illinois: Charles Thomas Publisher, 1992.
Kluft, R. P. and C. A. Fine, *Clinical perspectives on multiple personality disorder.* Washington, D.C. American Psychiatric Press. Inc. 1993
Kluft R. P., "A New Voice For A New Frontier" Editorial *Dissociation* I:2. (1986.)
—. "A New Voice For A New Frontier." Editorial *Dissociation* I (1988.)
Putnam, F. W. *The Psychophysiologic Investigation Of Multiple Personality Disorder.* Psychiatric Clinics of North America 7 (1984.)
—. "Dissociation As A Response To Extreme Trauma." In R.P. Kluft (Ed.) *Childhood Antecedents Of Multiple Personality.* Washington, D.C.: American Psychiatric Press, 1985.
—. *Pieces Of The Mind: Recognizing The Psychological Effects Of Abuse.* Justice for Children, 1985.
Ross, S. Eleventh Annual Expressive Therapy Convention Program, NETA, New York, 1995.
Ryder, *Breaking the Circle of Satanic Ritual Abuse.* Minneapolis, Minnesota: CompCare Publishers, 1992.

Sakheim, D. K. *Out of Darkness: Exploring Satanism & Ritual Abuse.* New York: Lexington Books, 1992.

Torem, M. "Iatrogenic Factors in the Perpetration of Splitting & Multiplicity." *Dissociation* II (2) 1989.

Wasnak, L. *Many Voices Press.* P.O. Box 2639, Cincinnati, Ohio 45201.

YOUR DAILY DOSE OF ART—
A PRESCRIPTION FOR HEALTHY AGING

CATHY DEWITT

> "Art knows no age. The body may change, but the imagination still burns bright."
> —Jane Alexander: Actress and Former Chair of the National Endowment for the Arts
>
> "Every child is an artist. The problem is how to remain an artist once he grows up."
> —Pablo Picasso
>
> "I never feel age…If you have creative work, you don't have age or time."
> —Sculptor Louise Nevelson, age 80

Dr. Gene Cohen was already using visual arts and creative activities in his work, a combination of research and clinical practice, studying the relationship between creativity and aging, but after his own father was diagnosed with Alzheimer's, he took it a step further. Realizing how frustrating it can be for family members to visit with a loved one who has memory deficits, Dr. Cohen found visual arts images to be invaluable memory enhancers, providing a starting point for family conversations.

> "I created the board game, Making Memories Together, and the video biography series—Therapeutic Restorative Bios—to help restore relationships between families and their loved ones with memory impairment,"
> —Dr. Cohen, Director of the Center on Aging, Health & Humanities at Washington University, where he is also a professor of Health Care sciences, Psychiatry and Behavioral Sciences.

A pioneer in research on creativity and aging, Dr. Cohen conducted the first NEA-sponsored longitudinal study of its kind, entitled "The Impact of Professionally Conducted Cultural Programs on Older Adults."

The overall Study planned for 150 in the Intervention Group (programs led by professional artists) plus 150 in the control group for a total of 300 subjects. The median age of subjects in both the intervention group and the control group at the start of the Study was 80. Subjects were selected at three sites:

• Elders Share the Arts (ESTA); Brooklyn, New York
• Center for Elders and Youth in the Arts (CEYA); San Francisco, California
• The Levine School of Music; Washington, DC

Questionnaires were administered in three domains: (1) General Health; (2) Mental Health; (3) Social Functioning. The questions were asked face-to-face during a research assistant visit with the research subjects. The intervention group, in comparison to the control group, experienced:

• Significantly better overall health.
• Significantly fewer falls and less hip damage.
• Significantly fewer doctors' visits.
• Diminished use of medications.
• Diminished vision problems.
• Significantly better scores on the Geriatric Depression Scale and the Loneliness Scale.
• Increased involvement in activities.

"There has been such a transformation of the focus in aging," Dr. Cohen notes. "People are much more serious than they they've ever been about looking at the ways the arts can affect the aging process.'

As the Musician in Residence for Shands Arts in Medicine program in Gainesville, Florida, for over twelve years, I have seen and experienced the healing power of the arts—particularly music—in just about every kind of hospital setting. From the pediatrics waiting room to the geriatric bedside, from the O.R to the E.R., from an auditorium full of caregivers to a small family holding vigil for their loved one, music has proved to be an amazingly effective, accessible and immediate tool for healing. I work with many patient populations, but in the past few years, whether because I am aware of my own aging, or perhaps because Florida is such a Mecca for retired artists and musicians, I've developed a special fascination for the effects of music and art on the aging brain.

Throughout the country, projects studying the effects of the arts on aging have shown interesting results. Alzheimer's patients are looking at art in the Museum of Modern Art in New York, and responding verbally to the pictures when they haven't spoken for months. Dancing is shown to improve circulation, coordination and alertness in elders. Music reduces stress and the need for pain medication. And recent studies in neuroscience reveal that our brains do not age like our bodies. If we keep giving our brains creative activities and challenges, not only do they remain active, but also they may actually increase in size.

In December 2007, the IFACCA (International Federation of Arts Councils and Culture Agencies) published "Above Ground: Information on Artists — Special Focus on New York City Aging Artists." For this project, 213 artists age 62-97 from the five boroughs of NYC were interviewed in English, Chinese and Spanish. The study found these aging artists to be passionate and enthusiastic about their work, and supportive of each other within their creative community. They rank their lives high in satisfaction and self-esteem, and 91% would choose to be artists again. These artists remain engaged with their art and each other, and 77% communicate with each other on a daily or weekly basis. Analyzing data from the interviews, the 210-page report "Above Ground" creates a strong case for artist communities as a positive model for our aging society. (Available through the Research Center for Arts and Culture at Teachers College at Columbia University—http://www.tc.edu/rcac/)

According to Dr. Cohen,

"Becoming involved in group arts activities can even boost the immune system. I'm studying the role of creativity in relationship to both health and illness."

One such activity that has gotten some national attention lately is the formation of New Horizons musical programs. This program, started in 1991, was initially offered to give aging adults an opportunity to make music in a group setting such as many had not experienced since their school days. Now there are over 100 New Horizons bands and orchestras all over the country.

Says director Roy Ernst,

"Many adults want to make lifestyle changes to improve and sustain a positive lifestyle. Evidence shows that music making supports good mental and physical health, and gerontologists have long known that socialization is an important factor for good health. This combines both.

The evidence is also strong that the 'use it or lose it' principle applies to mental abilities as well as physical abilities. The constant mental challenge of learning music is an ideal form of exercise for our brains."

Another study, The Music Making and Wellness research project, was funded by the National Association of Music Merchants (NAMM), the International Music Products Association, retailers and manufacturers, and The National Academy of Recording Arts & Sciences, to investigate the link between active music making and wellness. This program studied the effects of group keyboard lessons on 150 active aging adults, as compared with 150 controls. It found significant quality of life changes in the participating group, including a decrease in anxiety and depression, improvement in stress management skills, and even an increase in Human Growth Hormone (hGH), a hormone which positively affects aging factors like energy level, sexual performance, wrinkles, muscle aches and pains.

Frederick Tims, Ph.D., MT-BC, Chair of Music Therapy at Michigan State University, who was also principal investigator for a University of Miami Alzheimer's project on music therapy, assembled a highly respected multi-disciplinary team of researchers to conduct the project: specialists from the Aging Institute at the University of South Florida; the Department of Psychiatry and Behavioral Sciences at the University of Miami School of Medicine; Karolinska Medical Institute, Stockholm, Sweden; University of Miami; and Western Michigan University.

Speaking for the research team, Dr. Tims said,

"We feel very strongly that the work we are doing here suggests that abundant health benefits can be achieved by older people learning to play music in a supportive, socially enjoyable setting."

Comedian George Burns, who lived to be nearly 100, had no doubt that continuing to perform comedy was what kept him going.

"Age to me means nothing," he said. "When I'm in front of an audience, all that love and vitality sweeps over me and I forget my age. I'm going to stay in show business until I'm the last one left!"

With the advent of medical discoveries and the emphasis on healthy lifestyles, especially for the aging baby boomer population, people are living longer, and the scary specters of dementia and Alzheimer's disease loom ever closer. Soon seniors will outnumber children for the first time in our history. Alzheimer's strikes nearly half of those 85 or over. However, the good news is that active participation in the arts has been clearly shown not only to enhance good mental health in an aging population, but to improve the quality of life for those who are already struggling with some form of dementia.

With that goal in mind, Sean Caulfield and Dr. John Zeisel started ARTZ: Artists for Alzheimer's™, a 501I 3 non-profit initiative of the Hearthstone Alzheimer's Foundation. ARTZ is an organization of artists throughout the country who volunteer to do interactive art with Alzheimer's populations in their area.

> "Art has the ability to transcend the limitations of conventional communication and language," said Caulfield, "leading to rich emotional connections and in many cases enabling people with Alzheimer's to break out of their shells, to become awakened, if you will."

In a partnership with the Museum of Modern Art (MOMA) in New York, clients with Alzheimer's, along with their family members and caregivers were brought to the Museum for special interactive tours and discussion led by specially trained Museum educators focusing in depth on iconic art from MOMA's collection. It was discovered that even just looking at these works by such modern masters as Henri Matisse, Pablo Picasso, Jackson Pollock, and Andy Warhol could trigger a verbal response in a patient who had been non-verbal for a long period of time.

Music brings dramatic results to patients who have Alzheimer's, dementia, and other memory disorders. Patients who, according to the staff, have not spoken a coherent sentence in weeks may be able to sing along with entire songs. Patients who have a flat affect and sit slumped in their wheelchairs become animated and start moving. Moreover, sometimes singing these songs actually triggers something in the mind that makes it suddenly possible for the patient to remember and speak of an experience.

Oliver Sacks, noted author and expert neurologist, explains:

> "... a stroke or dementia can cause aphasia, the inability to use or comprehend words. But the ability to sing words is rarely affected, even if an aphasic cannot speak them. Being reminded in this way of words and grammatical constructions they have forgotten...may help them start to regain old neural pathways for accessing language...Music then becomes a crucial first step in a sequence followed by spontaneous improvement and speech therapy."

Although I generally see patients only for the time that they are in the hospital, there have been cases where I followed them through the later stages of their process, continuing to visit them in a rehab center or hospice. One such patient was M., who had suffered severe brain injury from an accident. After being in a coma for nearly a year, she had recovered enough to be placed in various hospital rehabilitation settings, but still had problems with memory and with speaking coherently. She would insert nonsense words into sentences that otherwise made sense. Previously, she had been a successful professional psychologist. The hospital speech therapist was interested in how music might affect her. When I asked M. what her favorite song was, she said "Jingle Bells." So, I started singing with her—first Jingle Bells, then Elvis, the Beatles, and Motown, as she began to remember other songs she liked. She seemed to get more coherent every time I saw her, and soon all of the staff was singing with her as much as possible. Eventually she was well enough to be sent to off-site Rehab. I went there to visit her and she seemed to be completely recovered—she knew everybody's name, remembered me, remembered the accident, her family, everything. She was getting ready to go home, and said she was nervous and scared, which certainly seemed appropriate to me.

Dr. Bruce Miller, Professor of Neurology at University of California, San Francisco, is the Clinical Director of Aging and Dementia and the Medical Director for the John Douglas French Foundation for Alzheimer's disease. In his work there during the past decade he has seen people with Alzheimer's develop extraordinary abilities to draw, paint, sculpt or play music.

"Working with an exceptional patient made me realize how much creativity is actually left in our dementia patients," he said. This led him into detailed research of the brain and its creative connections. "I think we're increasingly going to have to think about the fact that these dementias...don't wipe out all of the aspects of creativity and cognition."

The National Center for Creative Aging (NCCA) is the overseeing organization for most research projects, organizations and programs that involve the arts and aging. In 2007, NCCA implemented a strategic move, in partnership with George Washington University: Center on Aging, Health & Humanities, to reposition the organization in Washington D.C. This new partnership with George Washington University combined with the strategic positioning in Washington D.C. alongside its D.C. partners provides the NCCA the opportunity to be at the center of growing public awareness and education. In his role as a valued member of the

NCCA staff and board, Dr. Cohen is even more active in the field of creativity and aging. In his recent book, "The Creative Age: Awakening the Potential in the Second Half of Life", Dr. Cohen states that as people age, they begin to use both sides of their brain more—rather than remaining mostly "left-brained" or "right-brained" in their approach to life. This may explain the onset of late-life creativity in some people. There is even some evidence that creative challenge keeps our brains flexible and active in ways that actually increase their mass and weight.

In their book, "Secrets of Becoming a Late Bloomer" Connie Goldman and Richard Mahler seek to redefine the concept of aging, exploring its many gifts, including the opportunity to reinvent ourselves. While we are all aware of the most famous "late-bloomers"—Grandma Moses, Groucho Marx, Norman Vincent Peale—the book introduces the reader to many ordinary people who have found extraordinary excitement, productivity and creativity during the so-called "retirement years."

Dr. Cohen takes this idea even further, noting in his research on aging a pattern of "practical intelligence" and "pragmatic creativity," resulting in what he calls the "liberation phase" –that period when one has developed the freedom and the confidence to try new endeavors, find more creative ways to solve problems, and discover a new "limitless inventive potential."

> "Age allows our brains to develop a repertoire of strategies developed from a lifetime of experience," says Dr. Cohen, "and the liberation from social restraints gives us the courage to pursue new paths."

To join the journey down this healthier road to aging, instead of making excuses like, "I can't draw a straight line" or "I couldn't carry a tune in a bucket," maybe it's time to sign up for that painting class you've often wondered about, or finally realize that lifelong dream to play the piano, or even take dance lessons. Dr. Cohen would say that now is the time to ask those three vital questions that can help you make the leap into the next creative stage of your life:

First, "Why not?" Then, "If not now, when?" And finally, "What are they gonna do to me?"

***

Here are some ideas for ways to bring creative arts into your life:

1) Make a collage, using photos and images from your own life, to create your visual history. This is a great project to do with a family member or friend.

2) Take a class in silk or fabric painting and create curtains or pillows for your home or a community home for those in need.

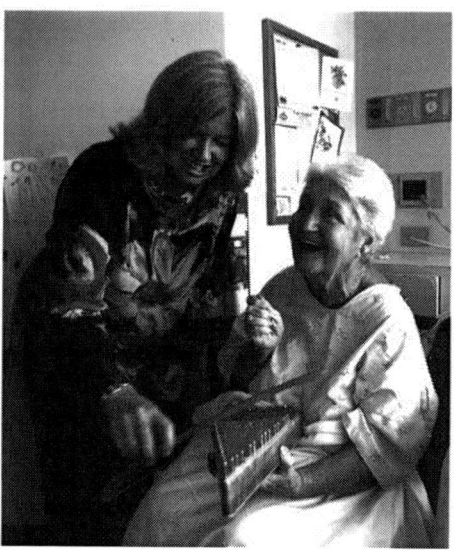

3) Learn to play an instrument—or if you already play, take up a new instrument like the bowed psaltery or banjo!

4) Join a community choir. Then volunteer to sing at your local hospice or hospital.

5) Take up journaling. You can even make your own journal, or create your own paper.

6) Take a watercolor class. You can paint your own postcards to send to friends!

7) Sign up for a dance class—it's a great way to stay fit.

Sidebars

Many cities have senior centers that offer programs in dance, art or music. University towns and community colleges often have Learning in Retirement classes or creative programs for people over 55.

For more information about Dr. Cohen's work, visit http://www.gwumc.edu/cahh.

For more information about user-friendly art projects and products, visit www.healingartsource.com.

Other websites of interest:
www.thehearth.org/artistsforalzheimers,
www.kairosdance.org,
www.theSAH.org,
www.creativeaging.org

Bibliography

Goldman, Connie, and Richard Mahler. *Secrets of Becoming a Late Bloomer*, New Hampshire: Stillpoint Publishing, Hazelden Foundation, 1995.

Additional Resources

Personal conversations and notes taken during the *Aging Well* conference in Florida the winter of 2008, with Dr. Gene Cohen, MD, PhD, in a session entitled "Vintage Voices: The New Senior Moment," have been used.

BIBLIOTHERAPY FOR OLDER ADULTS

ROBERT M. BELAND

Introduction

Long before books, magazines, radio, televisions, modems and cell phones, people told stories to each other to entertain, educate, pass on cultural values and heritage, and even to motivate soldiers for battle. Stories are the beginnings of traditions and shape our lives and communities (Rosen 1986:227.) The value of reading books aloud may be understood when one observes the interaction and subsequent compassion that occurs when parents read a bedtime story to their children. Without a doubt, some of our earliest and fondest memories of childhood are focused around storytelling and the reading of books by our parents and caregivers.

What is Bibliotherapy?

Bibliotherapy is the guided use of selected books as an adjunct to treatment and in some cases a primary method of treatment (Cohen 1993:70.) In recent years, bibliotherapy has expanded beyond the use of self-help books to include many forms of literature (Beland 1995:18; Cohen 1993:70.) Researchers have demonstrated the effectiveness of bibliotherapy in psychiatric (Katz and Watt 1992:175,) geriatric (Landreville and Bissonnette 1997:37,) and pediatric settings (Amer 1999:92.) Bibliotherapy has also been used with children in foster care (Pardeck 1990:64) and persons with cancer (Pardeck 1992:225.)

This chapter will explain how bibliotherapy can be used as a treatment procedure and as a recreational activity for older adults. Specifically, using children's books that portray older adults in positive ways can be an effective method to treat older adults in nursing homes, retirement communities, senior centers, assisted living and adult daycare facilities.

Rationale

The need for this type of program can be based on several factors. First, all the books used for this program are short in duration (may be read in 5-10 minutes.) This appeals to the short attention span experienced by some older adults, especially those with dementia. On the other hand, many other older adults view these books as just shorter versions of short stories. Secondly, all the books used for this program include an older adult who is a major character in the story. In addition, the older adult character is depicted in a very positive manner (Beland and Mills 2001:639.) Consequently, older adults are able to identify with the story very easily. They enjoy seeing an older adult character depicted, not only in positive ways, but in heroic and inspirational ways, too. They sometimes see themselves in the stories or see how they would like to be in real life. Sometimes they see how they would like the world and society to treat them.

Thirdly, conducting bibliotherapy programs such as this one can provide an enjoyable outlet for older adults. They feel like they are being catered to, because another adult is reading the book to them. In general, there is the stereotypical "happy ending" in the stories, which provides a pleasant experience for the listeners. Many of the stories provide humorous experiences. Older adults have reported that one of the few times they may laugh during the day is when these stories are read to them. Moreover, many older adult listeners also enjoy seeing the colorful and interesting illustrations in the books.

Fourth, when these stories are read in small group situations, social interaction usually occurs. Many times older adult listeners may comment about something that is read or how something in the story may relate to them or to someone else in the group. Lastly, another important feature of using these books is that they stimulate memory, reminiscence, and life review. For example, in many of these books the older adult characters tell stories about their past. The listeners can relate to stories about vaudeville, working on the farm, immigration, wartime and family histories. The stories also remind them of a time when there was no television.

Selecting Appropriate Books

As much as possible, the therapist should let the listeners select the books to be read. This can be done by selecting a small sample of 5-9 books and putting them on a table for the listeners to view. The therapist should carefully observe the participants for any signs of interest when the listeners look at these books. When selecting books for a group activity, the selection should have a combination of humorous and serious books, since this usually provides a balance for the emotions that may be expressed within the group. It is also good to select books which may have seasonal interest like *The Day Before Christmas* (Bunting 1992,) *Kwanzaa* (Chocolate 1990) or *The Tie Man's Miracle* (Schnur 1995.) It is also helpful to encourage the listeners to suggest categories of books as well as specific books. A comprehensive annotated bibliography concludes this chapter.

When selecting books for an individual activity, the therapist should attempt to pick some books that are meaningful to the person. For example, if the person has military or aviation background, then books such as *Grandpa is a Flyer* (Baker 1995) or *My Grandma Is a Pilot* (Yong 1995) would be useful. Knowing the person's ethnic or family background may also aid in selecting books.

Functional Intervention

For functional intervention, this program can be used to address such specific emotional functional goals as improving self-esteem, by making older adult listeners feel good about themselves. This can be accomplished by reading books that may make them feel good because there is a happy ending. Books that have been especially useful in promoting self-esteem are those books in which the older adult character is not only a positive role model in the story but may be considered a "hero or heroine." These heroes are older adult characters who fix things in the story. They usually solve problems, like the grandfather who is a tailor and usually makes a navy blue coat for his granddaughter in *The Purple Coat* (Hest 1986.) The mother does not like her daughter's idea of wanting a purple coat, but grandpa saves the day by making a reversible coat – navy on one side and purple on the other. These books have also been useful in working with older adults who have depression. For example, books such as *Love You Forever* (Munsch 1986) and *Come Back, Grandma* (Limb 1983) have provided older adults who have depression with very positive feelings and an opportunity to feel better about themselves.

A number of books could be used to help older adults become more aware of family leisure activities. A large percentage of these books depict older adult grandparents who are actively involved with their grandchildren (Beland and Mills 2001:643.) For example, in *When I Go*

Camping with Grandma (Bauer 1995) the grandmother not only fishes and has fun with her granddaughter, but also camps out overnight with her. A grandfather teaches his granddaughter to fish in *Fishing at Long Pond* (George 1991.) A grandfather acts in a local community theater to the delight of his granddaughter in *Grandpa's Face* (Greenfield 1988.)

The books can also be used in conjunction with music and art programs. For example, several of the books include music as a major theme in the book, so these books could be used in conjunction with the music program. Some of these books are *The Jukebox Man* (Ogburn 1998,) *Grandpa's Song* (Johnston 1991,) *Georgia Music* (Griffith 1986) and *The Song and Dance Man* (Ackerman 1988.) Since almost all of the books include colorful illustrations, older adults could draw pictures of what occurred in the stories that were read to them. They could also make sculptures, decoupages, collages or ceramics of persons or objects in the books. In the story, *Emma* (Kesselman 1980,) this 72 year-old woman receives a painting of her village from her children and grandchildren. She is delighted with the gift, but does not think the village is exactly how she remembered it. So, she decides to paint her own picture of the village and she is transformed by the experience.

Specific Concerns

Alzheimer's disease is a major cause of senility among the older adult population. Memory problems tend to be troublesome for both the older adult who experiences this phenomena, as well as family and friends. There are books used in this program that address the issue of memory loss. These books can be appropriately used with older adults, and in many cases, families have appreciated them also. This is possible because the authors have presented these problems in a very positive manner. For example, for those persons who are in the beginning stages of the disease, the story *The Memory Box* (Bahr, 1992) describes how one family prepares for the disease. Grandfather and grandson put items in a box to keep the memories of all the times they had shared. At one point, the grandfather tells his grandson, "Your Mom's going to hurt.... When it gets bad, bring out our Memory Box. Show her what I remember." In *Grandpa's Song* (Johnston, 1991) the grandchildren help grandfather to remember his favorite song.

In the story, *A Window of Time* (Leighton 1995,) the grandson and grandfather enjoy their times together even though grandfather is starting to forget things. He even points out that it is easier to remember things from his youth rather than his old age. Consequently, the grandson uses this to his advantage – that he can see what life was like before he was born through grandpa's "window of time." In the story *Great-Uncle Alfred Forgets* (Shecter 1996,) a young girl takes her great-uncle, who has Alzheimer's, for a walk and patiently answers all his questions.

There are several books that discuss illness and disability in very positive ways. In *Gramma's Walk* (Hines, 1993,) a young boy enjoys traveling with his grandmother who uses a wheelchair. Actually, they never leave her house, but they travel because the grandmother tells such vivid and detailed stories about taking a walk to different places like the beach. In *Can You Hear Me, Granddad?* (Thompson 1986,) granddad has a hearing impairment. The granddaughter keeps trying to tell him about the things she is going to do, but grandfather keeps twisting them around. Grandfather says, "We're going to the zoo. What's that? Glue? You've fallen in glue?" The story continues like this and there is no question that the story is humorous and that the grandfather and granddaughter enjoy each other's company.

In the story, *Now One Foot, Now the Other* (dePaola 1980,) the grandfather teaches his grandson how to walk and talk, tells the grandson stories, and plays games with him. After the grandfather has a stroke, it is the grandson who teaches him how to walk and talk again based on the stories the grandson heard of his own upbringing from his grandfather.

Several of these books deal with death and dying in a very realistic but positive way. In *Granddad Bill's Song* (Yolen 1994,) the grandson approaches various family members as to what they were doing the day granddad Bill died. The responses are pleasant memories that each person had of the grandfather. The grandson, Jon, eventually realizes that by talking to family and friends about their recollections, he is in a sense communicating with his grandfather. In *Great-Grandmother's Treasure* (Hickcox 1998,) it is the death of the great-grandmother that finally reveals the treasures she had kept secret for so long. She was wearing an old apron when she died and the pockets with stuffed with the symbolic treasures. "There they were, all the special treasures! And no wonder nobody could see them. They were the things she had given away. There were the smiles of course, and peanut butter cookies, ghost stories and Mud Puddle Soup…"

In *Come Back, Grandma* (Limb 1983,) Bessie loses her grandmother (her best friend,) when she is a young child and misses her very much. Eventually, Bessie gets married and has a little girl. As her daughter grows, she realizes that she is just like grandma in terms of looks and personality traits, and feels like Grandma has come back.

Conclusion

One type of bibliotherapy for older adults involves the use of children's books that positively portray older adults as major characters. It may be used as a functional intervention, leisure education or recreational participation program. It can be used with small and large groups as well as on an individual basis. The availability and diversity of current children's books allows the therapeutic recreation specialist to select stories that may reach a large number of clients. Moreover, there are many variations and modifications that can enhance this program.

References

Amer, K. "Bibliotherapy: Using Fiction to Help Children in Two Populations Discuss Feelings." *Pediatric Nursing.* 25:1(1999) 91-95.

Beland, Robert. "Bibliotherapy and Aging." In *Proceedings of the ICHPER-SD 1995 World Congress,* ed. Jill Varnes, 1995:18.

Beland, Robert and Terry Mills. "Positive Portrayal of Grandparents in Current Children's Literature." *Journal of Family Issues.* 22:5 (2001) 639-651.

Cohen, L. "Discover the Healing Power of Books." *American Journal of Nursing.* 93:10 (1993) 70.

Katz, G., and J. Watt. "Bibliotherapy: The Use of Books in Psychiatric Treatment." *Canadian Journal of Psychiatry* 37 (1992) 173-178.

Landreville, P. and L. Bissonnette. "Effects of Cognitive Bibliotherapy for Depressed Older Adults with a Disability." *Clinical Gerontologist,* 17:4 (1997) 35-55.

Pardeck, J. "Bibliotherapy and Cancer Patients." *Family Therapy.* 19:3 (1992) 223-232.

—. "Children's Literature and Foster Care." *Family Therapy.* 17:1 (1990) 61-65.

Rosen, H. " The Importance of Story." *Language Arts* 63:3 (1980) 226-237.

Annotated Bibliography of Children's Books

Ackerman, K. *Song and dance man.* New York: Dragonfly Books, 1988. Grandpa takes his grandchildren up to the attic, opens an old trunk and becomes a vaudeville actor again.

Bahr, M. *The memory box.* Morton Grove, IL: Albert Whitman & Company, 1992.
When grandfather realizes he has Alzheimer's disease, he starts a memory box with his grandson to keep memories of all the times they have shared.

Baker, S. *Grandpa is a flyer.* Morton Grove, IL: Albert Whitman & Company, 1995.
Anne's grandfather tells how he became interested in flying in the early days of flight, when barnstorming was popular.

Bauer, M. *When I go camping with grandma.* Mahwah, NJ: Bridge Water Books, 1995.
A child enjoys a camping trip with grandmother that includes hiking, canoeing, fishing, and cooking out.

Bunting, E. *The day before Christmas.* New York: Clarion Books, 1992.
Four years after her mother's death, Allie goes with her grandfather to a performance of "the Nutcracker" and hears about the special day he had with her mother.

Chocolate, D. *Kwanzaa.* Chicago: Children's Press, 1990. The story of the African American holiday and its roots and heritage.

dePaola, T. *Now one foot, now the other.* New York: Putnam, 1980.
Grandfather and grandson develop a close relationship in the boy's early developmental years but switch roles after granddad has a stroke.

George, W. *Fishing at Long Pond.* New York: Greenwillow Books, 1991. This beautifully illustrated book tells the timeless story of a grandfather teaching Katie to fish.

Greenfield, E. *Grandpa's face.* New York: Philomel, 1988. Tamika learns about family love and grandfather, the actor.

Griffith, H. *Georgia music.* New York: Greenwillow Books, 1986. Grandfather did not like leaving his rural home and became depressed. His granddaughter played music for him and made him feel better.

Hest, A. *The purple coat.* New York: Four Winds Press, 1986. Grandpa provides the perfect solution his young granddaughter's wish for a new coat.

Hickcox, R. *Great-grandmother's treasure.* New York: Dial Books, 1998. Great grandmother puts all the treasures of her life into her apron.

Hines, A. G. *Gramma's walk.* New York: Greenwillow Books, 1993. Donnie and Gramma, who is in a wheelchair, take an imagined walk to the seashore and smell the salty breeze, walk barefoot on the warm sand, observe animals and build a sandcastle.

Johnston, T. *Grandpa's song.* New York: Puffin Pied Piper Muffins, 1991. Grandpa, who loves singing, forgets the words to his favorite tune and it's up to his grandchildren to find a way to help him remember.

Kesselman, W. *Emma.* New York: Doubleday, 1980. A grandmother decides to paint the village as she remembers it instead of the way it is depicted in a painting she received as a gift.

Leighton, A. O. *A window of time.* Lake Forest, CA: NADJA Publishing, 1995. Shawn and his grandfather enjoy wonderful times together, even when grandpa forgets things and calls him by the wrong name.

Limb, S. *Come back, grandma.* New York: Knopf, 1983. Grandma love Bessie and always has time for her but one day Grandma dies. Bessie misses her and keeps looking for her and eventually does find her.

Munsch, R. *Love you forever.* Willowdale, Ontario: Firefly Books, 1986. This story of parental love has caused a cascade of human tears.

Ogburn, J. *The jukebox man.* New York: Dial Books, 1998. After watching her grandfather repair broken jukeboxes and change records at work, Donna dances with him to her favorite tune.

Schnur, S. *The tie man's miracle.* New York: William Morrow and Company, 1995. On the last night of Chanukah, after hearing how an old man lost his family in the Holocaust, a young boy makes a wish that is carried to God as the menorah candles burn down.

Shecter, B. *Great-uncle Alfred forgets.* New York: Harper Collins Publishers, 1996. A young girl takes her great-uncle, who has Alzheimer's disease, for a walk and gently and patiently answers all his questions.

Thompson, P. *Can you hear me, granddad?* New York: Delacorte Press, 1986. A humorous look at hearing and comprehension problems.

Yolen, J. *Granddad Bill's song.* New York: Philomel, 1994. A young boy learns about his dead grandfather from different relatives.

Yong, C. *My grandma is a pilot.* Woodbury, MN: Chandelle Publications, 1995. Andy discovers that Grandma Liz flew during WW II

A GATHERING OF ANGELS: ARTS AND MEDICINE SHORT STORIES

JOAN ABRAHAMSON VOYLES

The following is a collection of journal entries and stories about my experiences as a volunteer in an arts in medicine program at a local hospital, and then concludes with two Hospice patient stories. I am using the title, "A Gathering of Angels," as the larger umbrella over this collection. The *Angels* appear in many forms, groups and activities. There has been a special heightened sense of being part of something bigger than just myself and the other person in each encounter.

"We need to emphasize that art is about finding meaning...It is not about recreation."
— Dr. Paul Jacobsen

I begin in "Artist Rounds:"

My Question: How do we, the artists, "fine tune" and become better and more effective in working with patients one on one?

A: As a new volunteer, I need help. Let's talk about how do you do the transitioning from gathering supplies and the group energy in the office to changing focus and being totally present for the patient. How are you able to respond to the patient in a more intimate setting at the bedside in a hospital room? The logistics of getting a cart ready is frustrating, but I can learn this. How do others get themselves mentally ready?

B: When I work "one on one," I am conscious of a 3rd Presence. I become grounded...I do not go with any agenda or expectations. ..I see what happens and what the person needs. There is that quality of "being present"... and then going where the patient is... and this takes time. I always receive from the patient.

C: I do Reiki. I am not looking at my own way of judging if the encounter was good or bad. I cannot judge where just one word may have helped someone.

B: We do not understand the importance of just going from room to room or saying there are options in our arts in medicine program. Just our presence with them has a value. Someone thinks, "I am important enough for you to take the time to talk to me or appreciate that I am here...It helps me feel important and valued."

D: Being the witness is empowering. Sometimes just holding a hand makes such a difference. I try to leave my beeper off so that I can be present and focus on the people in the waiting room. Going around with the pamphlets lets people know that "we are here for you." There is a releasing of personal ties...and just an offering of oneself.

C: In the art process, you have to get out of self to go to what you are doing. A work of art is "the space." It is a type of entrainment. This is where the meaning comes...it is not something I can tell you. I invite you to participate. Eye contact is important. Honor the process.

Someone: The line, "This is a loaded brush," is often an invitation that works. The process is like a prayer...a marker of moving into another space.

C: This is living on another level.

'D' passed around a rock wrapped with raffia and a feather.

"The feather and the stone...bound together...bone to feather
Thankful hearts...the burden and the transformation."

I.

Pat knocked on the door of the room of the patient whose name was on the referral slip. The referral note from the nurse noted, "The patient had a question about an angel."

She was modeling protocols for me in the hospital's bone marrow transplant floor. In contrast to many areas where patients stay for only two or three days or the outpatient clinics, patients in the bone marrow unit stay for extended periods of time.

I am now, after several years of study of Expressive Arts at the University, an intern in this arts in medicine program. Most of my previous clinical experience has been in hospital waiting rooms or other places where patients and families were at the hospital only for the day. My other experience working with patients in the intimacy of a hospital room had been with an alert patient in a short stay floor.

We checked on the large patient assignment board at the nursing station and confirmed that a patient with the same last name as on the referral slip in the room, but there was a different first name on the board.

Checking with the patient's nurse, we learned Jane went by a different name (Michaelina) and we were told the patient *could* be difficult. I realized this would probably be someone with great stress and pain. I was glad that Pat was with me.

Though we were just responding to the request as a step in making a determination about my assignment that afternoon, we stopped by the sink and washed our hands with specially pumped foaming soap for two minutes before approaching the room. Bone marrow transplant patients have compromised immune systems, so we have a responsibility to be sensitive to the appropriateness of art materials we bring into their rooms, in addition to personal precautions regarding spreading of bacteria and viruses, which could be life threatening.

We came by the room two times and repeated the washing of hands. The first time the room was dark and no one responded to our gentle knock. The patient was probably sleeping. Later in the morning when Pat knocked, someone responded. As Pat carefully opened the door, the hall light angled across the face of a patient in the darkened room. Her bed was unusually close to the door. The room appeared crowded. There was a cot angled along the opposite wall. A man was reclining in the shadows.

Our director had explained to the patient and family member that we were representing the arts in medicine program and Pat now asked the patient if there was any way we could help her.

A young woman with a slender face, large dark eyes, slender hands with carefully manicured nails, and a baldhead tried to talk, but tears welled in her eyes as she struggled for composure. With emotion she asked, "Who painted the angel?" Her hands weakly fluttered as she pointed to the sidewall beside her pillowed head.

As we leaned into the room, we could see a paper pinned on the wall depicting a loosely painted but beautiful angel below which was a message: "An Angel for Michaelina."

Jane had been floating between drugged sleep and consciousness for some time. Several days before, when she had opened her eyes, she had been surprised to see this angel and the message greeting her with her more personal name. This had been an unexpected and positive image for her... a bright contrast to the blur of the routine and plainness of her hospital life.

We knew that one of the hospital artists had stopped by. Because the patient was sleeping, she left the painting on an impulse - a "calling card." Apparently, there had been "medicine" in this angel image.

I was asked to come back after lunch.

So, after lunch, with my small clipboard, I brought watercolors and pens, two papers and one of our plastic recycled water cups. On one of the papers I had drawn a "mandala" circle and on the other, more rectangular, paper a "double mandala," the "mandorla."

I stopped at the nurse's station for validation about the materials I had prepared. With the nurse's eyes, I also saw the color stained plastic water cup. We agreed it should be replaced with a fresh cup I obtained from the nurses' station. Again, I washed my hands and went to the room.

Stopping outside, I paused. I felt somewhat anxious. I knew getting myself calm inside was important. I was in the process of going from theory to application.

I took several deep breaths and slowly released the air. This helped. I said a prayer of affirmation. I declared to myself my intention. "I know the *artistic process* can be stress releasing at the most basic level. My intention is to develop that ability to support artistic processes, and reach to a deeper level of healing... more than Herbert Benson's 'Remembered Wellness.'" I had read and heard of the phenomenon of the healing power of the unspoken body knowledge bringing up internal images that could contribute to the opening of the body's immune system for self-healing, a goal of many arts in medicine programs.

Now the lights were on in the room. Because of the crowded arrangement, I sat on a closed commode seat adjacent to the bed facing the patient. Her husband sat on his cot and watched me passively. I sensed he had spent many days in the confined room.

One of the special hospital features here is that a family member can move in and live in the room giving continuous emotional support for the patient.

I had hoped that the patient and I would be able to paint together on a "mandala," as I had done with another patient the preceding week, but very quickly I decided that her arms remained under the covers due to weakness. I remembered her struggle to gesture toward the benevolent angel. Switching expectations, I asked Jane, "What would you like me to paint?"

"A horse."

I am a landscape and abstract painter, but have never had much interest, skill or experience in painting horses. Well, this would be a challenge!

"You're asking for a horse. Tell me about your interest in horses. Do you have one?"

"Yes. Star. Reddish brown. A white blaze on her forehead. Her colt looks just like her but without the blaze."

Two horses.

There followed a short discussion with Jane's husband, who corrected her memory of some aspects of the present status of the horses. She then asked me also to put in two other horses, "More brown than the first."

A four-horse challenge for my artistic response!

I began with a forward view centered in the circle. Using the water to block in shape, I dropped color and let the horse paint itself. This was expressive art. I began without planning and just intuitively painted.

A nurse came in to change the chemotherapy treatment. She had difficulty getting the lines to flow correctly. (A metaphor for what was happening to me with the art?) Time passed. Jane fell asleep.

There was only the bubbling sound of the machines and the quiet of the room. I painted the four horses. One to the right was the colt. A third became a frontal view peaking around "Star." The fourth was a silhouetted profile in the distance. For some reason this became the arrangement that had painted itself in a circle.

I changed paper and asked her husband if he would be willing to paint with me. My instinct was that *this* was the person who could be helped by a change in focus to relieve *his* stress.

He demurred and was hesitant. I encouraged him with the comment that I would be honored if he would do a "painting dance" with me.

Hesitantly he picked up a brush and looked at the paper with its two overlapping circles. Reaching into the black watercolor, he carefully drew the lines and curves of an apparently remembered oriental symbol. He looked at me to see how I was going to respond. *This seemed to be a tired but politely quiet challenge.*

I selected red, as this color is often used in the limited palette of oriental brushwork. With my brush, I danced echo lines around portions of his image, leaving a clean white island between, then extended a line and added a few brushy dots. The intent was an affirmation of the mood and quality he had begun.

I supported him in the risk he had taken into an artistic process.

He appeared surprised but intrigued. He became more alert.

He selected blue, turned the paper and carefully painted another figure. He then explained that for ten years he had done karate and had achieved a black belt.

This was our only conversation.

I put in my mind the intent to have this painting process help him remember some of the feeling of power and control he had felt in the past.

I chose orange to complement his blue and did a similar mirroring, but with extension to the previous patterns and placed an orange dot next to one of his red dashes.

The man was now into the process. The dance pattern was unspoken but known. He initiated and chose the placement of the oriental pattern and I responded with complementary colors, variations and connections to each stroke of his artwork.

We were both in deep concentration and focus of artistic process. The monitor gave a gently bubbling background sound. Jane was sleeping.

Finally, after making six or seven figures, he carefully rinsed his brush and set it down. He took a deep breath and gave a long sigh of relief. I took the cue that he was finished.

He held up and turned the painting around. He was smiling. "This is pretty good!" he said. I echoed and affirmed his opinion.

"Now you have your own painting to hang up and decorate the room. She has the angel and the horses. You made something special for you."

I thanked him for sharing with me. Jane was still sleeping. I picked up the paints and brushes and left.

I had experienced a gift of being part of the story of this couple's very private and painful time. I had seen the rising of a symbol that had in some way created a change in the body and mind of, not the patient, Jane, but of her husband.

That day my gift was to him. The other artist's gift had been the "Angel for Michaelina."

Addendum...

I read the rough draft of this story to my expressive art class as an illustration of my experience of seeing images arise while working in clinical settings. Much of the class application had been in a "wellness setting." We talked about the application to humans in higher stress and illness.

There is an incredible amount of stress for a caregiver of someone ill, especially when the person spends so much time in the hospital room. My understanding was that the spontaneous selection of the very personal karate images by the husband gave him memories, feelings and a change of body chemistry. His deep breath and long exhaled sigh was a significant indicator of physical release.

No one else could have known what to select for him. He did not make this selection consciously. It arose from his unconscious.

Without that image, the painting process would have validity on the surface level of the stress distraction. When he was painting his power symbols, his mind and body worked together in a process of change. Maybe it served as a way of "re-charging his batteries" to give himself "reserve power." Most likely whenever he looks at the images of his very personal process, he will re-experience an echo of the same sense of well being. The picture value is not as a painting or a work of art. It is the symbol of a healing process uniquely for him alone.

This experience gave me a great respect for such applications of "artistic process." This was my first experience of seeing the power of arts in medicine in such a powerful process.

One of the Expressive Art class fellow students who works with grief and children for Hospice very quietly said, "Yes. I saw the angel, too, and wondered who had made this special gift for the gir ." She had been at the hospital to consult with the mother about her directives for caring for the children the previous week.

We were in awe about the coincidence of our mutual caring for this family in different but complementary ways.

II.

In a third floor room, the dark haired man had an irregular haircut that was the result of some type of head surgery a few weeks before. When presented with several arts in medicine options, he expressed interest in having an artist visit, but thought it would not work out as he was going to be dismissed the next day.

This was my first day back after the Christmas holiday and Bee and I were visiting rooms. I volunteered to come back today as it was 3:30 and there was time before I had planned to leave. Working more often one on one with patients was the goal I had stated earlier in the monthly staff meeting and this opportunity presented itself.

I selected watercolors and pastels, two brushes, a 12" x 18" paper on which I drew a circle and clipped this onto a Masonite board. Pausing in the privacy of the landing between the two flights of stairs between the third and fourth floor, I stopped to center myself, focus and say a short prayer.

Alex was given the option of material choice and selected pastels. "I have never done anything in art before," he said "and I think you do not have to be so accurate with chalk…. we did not have art where I went to school."

"I thought about this when you left to get supplies. I decided I would make a sponge boat."

The board was propped on his knees and he sat up higher in the bed. He looked at the chalk and started to draw. There was not a hesitancy to get started.

My instinct was that he was going to work alone and now I wished I had another paper for myself or for a backup. And for some reason I felt that he would be more comfortable working alone. I left to get another paper.

When I returned he had drawn a solid, simple boat. He explained to me that these boats are white. To help him stay involved in process, I offered him a way of helping the boat become whiter by coloring in the background so the boat would be a contrast. I offered him a blue or aqua color for the sky. He selected the aqua and I broke it in half so it could be used on the side.

This rubbing process and toning the sky seemed to be very satisfying to him. He began to talk about riding the boats several times a day as a boy. His father had a store near the docks and he was often able to ride these boats as a child. Then he described the dangers of being a diver that came especially from the propellers of other boats. The divers wore helmets, weighted suits and had lines for oxygen pumped to them. Sometimes they hid sponges in their suits so those could be produced to please the tourists.

He continued to block in the chalk background and the conversation continued. I listened attentively and did not paint.

Alex talked about his pride in his heritage now, but he did not have that as a boy. When he met his wife, whose father was a fisherman, somehow this became a time of growth in his pride. His young boys do not have this pride that he wished they would gain sometimes.

I asked about the boat's name that looked like it might have been Sylvia or Sybil. He said it was a name from Turkey, from which many of the early settlers from his town immigrated. As he spoke about these simple, but honest, hardworking people, he became choked up with emotion and tears.

"For some reason since my surgery, I find myself in tears often."

I stated that that was not a problem. I felt touched and offered the possibility that perhaps he was honoring them with such honest emotions of respect and sensitivity.

He continued his conversation and rubbing the chalk on the paper.

He decided to embellish the boat by adding a flag. He closed his eyes and said he wanted to visualize the scale of the flag. He needed to make a white flag now and was pleased that the white chalk blended and produced a white area. Selecting blue, he blocked in a cross and added blue stripes. "I do not remember how many there are of these."

Then he built a series of layers of stokes on a basket on the end of the boom which I learned was used to cover the propeller of the boat as the engine had to be running while the divers were down in order to pump the oxygen. Oxygen lines as well as divers needed to be protected from the blades.

We had also discussed the possibility of making a visit to his homeland as a goal for the family. He said that being ill had made him put a number of things into a different perspective. In his youth, he had turned down several opportunities to go there because it was not of value to him then. Now he had a different perspective.

He decided to make a higher water line and was starting on this when an attendant came to take him down for a procedure. Our process was concluded. Half an hour or more had passed so quickly.

I brought him a soapy paper towel and a dry one for cleaning his fingers as I hung his picture on the bulletin board next to his bed to inspire him.

As he was wiping his fingers and looking at his displayed picture, he volunteered, "I feel so much better now. I do not like to be here with only the TV to watch. Thank you for coming and giving me this opportunity in art and thinking."

I shared that I was honored to have experienced his sincere sharing of memories and had learned about his heritage. I offered that sometimes taking risks in personal expression, trying something new such as doing this art work, has special healing power, too.

Another memorable encounter in arts in medicine.

III.

The social worker stopped by the studio area and filled out a request slip for an artist to paint an angel for Mario. She also said, but did not put this into writing, that "he was a bit slow." This gave the impression to be sensitive to his more special needs.

This was shortly after Christmas. At an earlier meeting after the holiday break, I had said I was looking forward to having more experience working with patients in their rooms. This request seemed to an answer to my earlier statement.

Now I wished I had saved some Christmas cards for a reference of how to make a simple, delicate angel. I took some of the paints and with paper scraps searched for my concept of "an angel." I remembered the simple but effect quality of the whimsical one my fellow artist had left with the other patient, which had resulted in my encounter with that family. I felt an obligation to continue the power of the "artistic gift of angels" the other artist had started. Apparently, the social worker had seen them, and thus the request.

What is my image of an angel?

Angels have blond hair...a soft pink face....a little red and more yellow for flesh color... some gold paint for a halo and sprinkles elsewhere for good luck dust and effect... probably blue eyes for color and contrast. Then the white dress or gown.... a gold cord crossing over the chest and around the waist, dangling down for a soft, waving gold pattern....

I experimented with negative painting washes to pop out a white, long, flowing dress.

How do wings look? ... Do they have gold on them?

How will I make the wings relate to the shoulders ...

Do they show out on the sides of the arms and dresses?

Mmm, add some lavender shadows for folds and color contrast.

These were details I had not seriously thought about until I was to "perform" the task, as an artist, fulfilling this request to paint an angel.

After several minutes of experimenting, I didn't have a "formula," but I was more confident and ready to be spontaneous.

Today, just being here and resuming my arts in medicine intern role has special significance for me. This would be the first day away from eleven days in a caretaker and patient family member role. There had been the recent trauma of watching my husband knocked off a ladder by a large limb, falling onto a brick patio, calling 911 for help and transporting him to the hospital. After surgery, I spent days and evenings anxiously at the hospital in a nearby town. He had progressed to a week in the "rehab" hospital. With the schedule of rehabilitation classes, today I feel confident enough to leave him and to resume a more normal pattern of life.

After gathering materials, I did some introspective analysis and caught myself operating still in that "wary, on guard mode" that sustained me at the Memorial Hospital. However, I was conscious that I had a responsibility to drop that mode of operation. My usual personal stress-relieving behavior was "just being busy." Neither of these was appropriate now. I had to melt into a sensitive state of absorbing clues and focus to support a patient in a room here.

I took the stairs down to the third floor patient area. Mid-landing, I paused to center and focus in the privacy of the back stairway. My body was still dealing with unexpressed personal trauma. I wasn't back to a normal or an ideal mental stage, following two or three minutes of meditation, but felt "I could fake it until I could make it," to quote an old adage.

With the Masonite clipboard, paints, brush and paper, I approached the room. The door was ajar. I knocked and looked inside just as the phone rang.

I experienced a profound sense of shock.

There my eyes rested on a young man around 19 or 20 half sitting in bed. Grateful that I could defer to the phone call as a higher priority, I said I would return in a few minutes. I left.

I had just experienced both a personal shock and personal revelation.

Now I had the gift of ability to totally focus on my role and my upcoming encounter with this patient.

What I saw was an African American boy with large, wary eyes talking on the phone. I expected to see an older man.

The "planning" of "my" angel was glaringly incongruent. I had "stereo typed" a blond haired, blue eyed Caucasian angel. I chastised myself and was thankful for the gift of some extra time to think.

I was instantly aware of a great lesson for myself. As I walked away, my mind raced with surprise by the implications, and my change in attitude. I chuckled at myself.

I slowly climbed the same back stairs to the fourth floor so I would be alone and have time to think.

Back in the studio, two of the artists were concluding a deep, serious conversation and said they were late for a meeting. The others had gone to other areas of patient contact. So, I had to solve this problem by myself.

I examined the validity of my "cultural sensitivity." I did not know if I presumed to paint a brown -skinned angel if that would be experienced by the patient as patronizing or appropriate. I was still in the shock of having my confidence sensitized. I didn't have a clue about the best way to respond.

Then I thought that the most logical action was to ask for the patient's verbal description of what an angel looked like. In anticipation of how he might answer, I offered the scenario that perhaps a young person like him would relate more to a humorous angel, perhaps a dog or cat angel. Humor is always good in a hospital room. Then again, I could create a brown-faced angel. That would be easier to paint and actually be a

nice contrast to the "white robes". *Would the wings be white or brown?* This was getting stressful. I realized my mind was playing games. *What would his response be? And what would mine be?*
I went back to the room. He was still deep in conversation. This gave me more time to think.

I was looking for a "gut instinct" to arrive and it had not.

By now, I had evolved to dropping the presumption of the "assignment of painting an angel." How likely was it that any young male patient would ask for an angel painting? Maybe the social worker knew about the other artist's angels and asked for one to surprise him.

Instead, I would just begin by talking with him. Based on this, I would evolve into an art process. That seemed to be safest. Let him take the lead.

When I returned to the room for the third time, I was greeted by a smiling young man, quite a change from the wary look when I first peered into the room.

After my introduction, he first wanted to know if I knew how to work the large VCR and separate TV that was on a cart at the foot of the bed of the large room. Without my glasses and in the darkened room, that would be difficult for me, even if I had been home with my own equipment.

With my lack of VCR skill acknowledged, I had difficulty moving into a conversation flow. I also had difficulty understanding him because his English appeared to be a cultural variation, with different emphasis and patterns, so that I had to really concentrate. Sometimes I would paraphrase what I thought he said rather than make incorrect assumptions.

I asked how long he had been here in the hospital. He responded with, "Too long."

I commented about his smile and that his mood seemed to have changed from when I first looked in at him. "Was that an important phone call?" I asked. This opened the floodgates of conversation.

I learned there had been an added dimension to the expected trauma of dealing with cancer and with the necessity of having to be hospitalized. This was a very lonely boy, who apparently had not seen or talked to anyone from his family on the East Coast since he left there to come to this hospital. No matter the real length of time, it was a very long period for him. He wanted so badly to go home.

This telephone call was his first contact from his family since arriving. They were telling him how important it was to them that he stays here where he could get the best care. In addition, they were going to arrange getting off from work so they could visit him within the next week.

He felt relieved, assured that they wanted him to be here, and apparently, he felt less isolated.

I asked if he ever painted or did any art projects. He shook his head. He seemed dubious about participating. I asked if he would be willing to paint with me - if we would take turns.

Since he was sitting up in bed, I placed the Masonite board on his lap. I offered him a choice of brushes and invited him to bring the paints to life by pinching drops of water from the brush onto the paint pans. "Just let the brush show you what it can do."

He made the first mark using a slow hesitant line. I responded with the same deliberation and some wiggles and dots. He selected another color and made some more spontaneous lines. Then I responded by dancing with thin lines and around his work and said the lines were dancing and sharing the space. The rest of the time there was not talk, just the taking of turns. The patterns seemed to take on risks.

When he sighed and put down the brush, I knew the painting was finished. I started to ask him if he thought the painting said anything to him but then the hospital chaplain, a tall African American with great warmth and style, walked in. He made very supportive comments about our painting and said he would return later.

Mario asked him if he knew how to run the VCR, but he got the same declining response from the chaplain. (I felt a little vindicated.)

I volunteered the synopsis of the story I had been told and said I thought Mario would like to talk about this further, and that I would be leaving shortly.

I asked Mario if he wanted to paint by himself. I had more paper.

"No, I want to find someone who can run the VCR," he said.

"Would you like to have the painting pinned on the bulletin board to decorate your room?"

That was fine.

While I was putting up the painting, another person arrived, a hospital attendant.

"Do *you* know how to run the VRC?"

Mario finally got a positive response to the VCR question. His attention was now focused on this with anticipation.

I shook his hand and thanked him for sharing his story and time with me. I also suggested that if he wanted something else or someone to come with art materials again, all he would need to do ask the nurse to make a request.

I left as a much wiser facilitator - but I still do not know how to run that VCR.

Now I regret that I had not inquired about what video was waiting to be played.

Later Thoughts:
I still smile to myself when I recall how physical my response had been to my awakening. At that time, I had become quite conscious of the lessons, the humor in the situation and *I learned so much about my personal expectations or assumptions.* This was a valuable lesson and experience!

I thought about the social worker's comment regarding Mario "being slow." My sense was that there was a lack of broad cultural experience. His speech indicated an immersion in a black culture with little influence of the larger popular culture. The "white" atmosphere of the hospital and most of the people in his interface had no doubt created an additional layer of unease and stress.

I hoped the chaplain would return to talk with him. My sense was that he could add a unique role of support for Mario.

My contribution was greatest as a listener and being there after he hung up the phone. Talking about something good and "telling his story" was a stress reliever for him and a part of the good medicine of the phone call. The sigh after painting, which seems to occur regularly after an art process, is also an indicator of the release of stress as well.

The heroine of the story, however, is the social worker. The social working was "Gathering all of the Angels" to help this young man.

As I reflect now, I believe she observed a very unhappy patient who had been assigned to her. She gathered all the resources she could to help him: a VCR with movies, an artist and chaplain visit and a call from home. I happened to be part of those responses of support for a *lonely young man.*

I also thought that perhaps, dropping color on a wet paper as a painting beginning might have been more spontaneous and fun that what we did – but who knows?

Each experience working with a patient in a room has been special and different.

I learned the most about myself. Mario was the angel who taught me.

IV.

The woman I was talking with was the most stressed patient I had encountered. She was sitting in a waiting area for patients, anticipating chemotherapy treatment. People usually are sitting in clusters about the room. Some are reading or sleeping, a few may be working on the puzzles available at a side table and others just stare into space. There is a mixture of patients and family members or friends of patients. There is a core reason for being here. Someone is involved in a process of treatment requiring a series of returns and waiting in this large room. The arts in medicine activities are brought into the area on certain afternoons, usually one of the busiest days, to help relieve the stress levels.

I realized from a new perspective, that unless I observed the obvious wig or camouflaging of the head, often I was unable to discern which the patient was and which was the family member.

There are a variety of responses as people are invited to participate in the painting activities. Part of the learning for me is to be sensitive about appropriate ways to engage people in a waiting room. I continue to be amazed with the number of people who feel wounded about their potential to do anything with art. Others, I often sense, just need that little bit of encouragement. With a simple comment like, "This brush has your name on it," they will join in the artistic processes.

The woman that caught my attention was bending over her lap, in what seemed to be an uncomfortable stance, working on tracing a fan shape pattern onto the back of a cloth strip. As I expressed interest in her process and looked more closely, I could see that her hands were not steady.

"Perhaps you would have an interest in the silk painting process. It could have implications for future quilt projects," I posed to her.

She declined and said in a low voice:

"I am having difficulty coping with 'this.' The first two times I was here, I could not do anything except keep from being hysterical. I cannot think straight. I am working really hard to just focus on this task."

I was not certain whether to continue the conversation or not. Perhaps talking to a stranger will help ease the bottled tension. However, I immediately knew that her line of control was fragile.

I shared that I had limited experience in quilting myself, but that had taught me about how important it was to be precise in all of the steps of the process. That understanding and acknowledgement seemed to have some comforting aspect to her. I did not feel closed off.

Something led me to ask if she would mind showing me how the fan shape related with the larger quilt pattern. There was a large bag of supplies under her cardboard pattern tracing area. She did not raise her eyes to look at me but fumbled until she found a segment of a larger pattern to show me. I saw how lovely and unusual the colors were. I made some affirming comment. She proceeded to take her pencil and sketch out the overall relationship of how the blocks interfaced in the finished quilt, but now in a relaxed manner. I nodded in understanding and thanked her for sharing with me.

I said I hoped her choice of the working on the quilting process would continue to help her. "Your own instincts are probably also good medicine for you."

I smiled and went on.

This encounter has left me concerned and more sensitive about the hidden stress. I know it exists intellectually. This was the most "raw" and acknowledged encounter I have experienced. *It also reminded me of myself at a time of great personal stress about fifteen years ago.*

About eight or nine months after we moved from Illinois to Florida, I got around to scheduling my annual PAPS smear test with a new OB-GYN doctor. He told me I had fibrous tumors in my ovaries and endometrioses, I likely had had years of pre-menstrual pain. That was so true. For years, no doctor had been of much help to me. Those periods of pain were something I just endured. The comments were comforting and gave me greater confidence in him. However, there was also the concern why that had not been explained to me before. I had gotten my share of inferences that my pain was largely mental.

The conclusion of this examination was the announcement that I should have a hysterectomy. This was a great shock. I became somewhat skeptical, as I knew that some doctors "make money" reportedly with this particular unnecessary surgery. I asked for a second opinion. Because I was new in the community, I asked for a referral doctor. (We knew so few people and I went to this doctor as a referral from one of my few new friends.) That second doctor confirmed the first diagnosis.

Timing was important. My insurance from a prior job lasted for one year. Soon we would be getting a new policy that would not cover a pre-existing condition such as this. It seemed to be wise to do this surgery while the policy was still in coverage and have some time for coverage in event of any complications. We had to move quickly to have this financial help of insurance and fit in with the doctor's vacation plans.

My husband was very matter of fact about this. There was no emotional support. I did not have any female friends to talk about this surgery. I felt trapped by the necessity of a logical financial decision, the nagging thought that this was not really necessary and still the shock of my personal "vulnerability." I was not sick! I was only forty-five and this was not supposed to happen!

When I attempted to talk to the doctor on a return trip, we were in his consultative room and he was sitting behind a very large, formidable desk. When I became emotional as I struggled to bring to words my anxiety, he seemed to withdraw. This "turndown" of any emotional support only made me more anxious. I had a history of really stuffing my feelings and had good control. However, now I had a further feeling of abandonment and falling into a terrible unavoidable trap. There was a whirling vortex closing in on me.

I was scheduled to visit the hospital unit to help me feel "comfortable." This confronted me with the greater reality of what I feared. However, the introduction of the first sensitive and caring people penetrated my amour. I started to cry hysterically in my conversation with a nurse. She took me to the office of the nurse manager and left me to cry and unwind.

Later I discussed with her my ambivalence and feelings. The part that I could least handle however, was being told that I could stay at my home that "*last night*" and come to the hospital at five the next morning for the surgery.

That assumption was the final straw. I knew I could not sleep the night before this dreaded surgery. I was not sleeping now. In addition, I felt great tension with the stress of making those early morning connections. My (former) husband was usually in such a grouchy mood in the mornings. I was not sure if I could cope with both him and me.

She asked if coming that evening, rather than the morning would be better. Now that I had talked aloud about a number of the concerns and cried, this solution seemed to offer additional relief. No one could have anticipated how much this would relieve my stress.

I returned later that day to the hospital. Once I was "in the process," I began to feel relatively relaxed even before they gave me a sedative. I was alone in the room and enjoyed feeling in control of my time to do nothing but be there and read and relax.

The angel of the whole thing was the gentleness and concern of the anesthesiologist who visited me that evening. His demeanor and concern gave me the first confidence I had for anyone in the whole process. That evening I told my husband in great raves about how this person, who is usually an invisible part of surgery, really helped me.

Rather than cancel a previously scheduled speaking engagement, in an earlier discussion I had encouraged my husband not to cancel the talk. It would be perfectly acceptable to me for him to be away the day after the surgery. I would be too medicated to need company.

Later I leaned he used the personal story of his wife's emotional response to the anesthesiologist as part of his presentation. Now such visits are typical of pre-surgery procedures.

That is the story and remembrance of my terror that came to me because of the anxiety I picked up from the patient in the waiting room. *I find that the word "terror" applies more to how I felt than the word "stress."*

I began to think more acutely about the terror of each of the other people waiting for the chemotherapy treatment.

Would I be able to be so calm? My surgery was curative, not hinging on life and death decisions!

Or, would I be like this patient, just on the edge of hysterical terror?

How do these people manage to act so calm and in control?

These are life and death steps. Many people get violently ill as a direct result of the treatment. They usually lose their hair.

I had come with a friend last summer to this very room and went with her as she received her treatment. I had planned ahead and had contacted one of the arts in medicine artists. She came to the chemotherapy unit and sat with us for a block of time. As my friend received her treatment, the artist talked about her work and showed us pictures as she read poems. This helped us pass the waiting time.

The others I saw in the many chemotherapy stations seemed to be accepting and stable emotionally or, at least, in control. I wonder now about this and the illusions.

I would like to learn more of how I might appropriately help others such as this woman who was in an extreme state of denial and non-acceptance. She had intuitively sought her own "art process" as her personal therapy.

Was my conversation with her good or bad?

Would ignoring her have been better?

Could I have taken a different approach and offered more support?

I wonder how much does this degree of anxiety and stress impact the patients' reactions to the chemicals.

How much does this affect the immune system?

Sometimes some resistance is healthy; the person does not give up.

Later I thought through my experience, and contrasting my mental attitude about reoccurring menstrual cramps with those of the patients who keep returning for chemotherapy treatments. Maybe the way I continued in life with the knowledge of the re-occurring monthly pain, is a metaphor for attitudes that develop in acceptance of the treatment. Once the pain was over, I forgot about it. In both instances, the pain and after effects of treatment can create a wide range of differences. I'll have to think more about this perspective.

I write this without conclusion, only stating my memories, identification with the suppressed emotion, my empathy, my concern and desire to be of help as a member of the arts in medicine team.

V.

Anne, a new arts in medicine volunteer intern, was shadowing me in her introduction to working with a patient on the third floor.

As we washed our hands at the sink just outside this room, we could see through the blinds that the patient was again sleeping, but her nurse said, *"I don't think she'd mind being awakened; probably she only appears to be asleep."*

So we knocked and entered after hearing a response from inside. The patient rolled from her *fetal position*. As typical in this cancer hospital setting with long-term patients in the bone marrow unit, her head was bald. She looked at us with dark circled and dull eyes.

I introduced us and asked if she would be interested in an art visit that afternoon. She hesitated, *"I am depressed and would not do anything."*

I said *we* were just seeking her permission to visit. Her face brightened. *"I am lonely. I would love a visit!"*

Our opportunity and mission seemed to be clear and welcome.

We returned to our base and packed a cart with art options, including a hand-painted silk scarf done by patients earlier for the stimulus of touch and color. To create an atmosphere of sound, I added a CD player with a flute disc. For art materials, I chose the most basic: large papers with circles drawn on black and white backgrounds, watercolor paints, brushes, chalk, oil crayons, colored pencils and gel pens.

Our next step required us to provide calm, healing energy. Anne and I sat and gazed out the windows as we prepared the energy of body and mind. In soft voices, we affirmed our intention to provide companionship and creative play. We would support and help her make her own discoveries. We took several deep slow breaths and had a few moments of personal meditation.

Giving deliberate patient choices are important components of arts in medicine processes. We had first asked permission to visit. Now we asked for permission to play music and clear the table for the three of us to sit around. Anne respectfully moved items to a nearby shelf. *An untouched lunch tray was one item.*

The paper choices were offered and Fay, the patient, did not hesitate: white paper. I made the decision to use transparent watercolors. Fay was instructed to use the largest brush to move water, as magic, to activate the dry watercolors in the paint tray. Three water containers and paper towels were available for rinsing and cleaning. There was symbolic sharing of the same tray of paints.

Quiet music began. The three of us moved to sit around the table with the white paper with the large circle. Calmness seemed to radiate from this center. With a sense of ceremony I handed the scarf to Fay to bring a focus on the hand-painted art object. She stroked the softness as we discussed the beauty of patterns and blended colors. The scarf was swirled around then placed as the "fourth" at the table setting.

Fay began to relax with the companionship and conversation.

Taking a deep breath, and then exhaling, I presented the process.

*"This can be a different way of becoming acquainted... through 'non-verbal' conversation. Fay, let a **color chose you** and then begin by making the first marks on the paper. Then it is Anne's turn and mine, and we keep going around and around.*

We will know when it is finished."

She took her brush and selected the color red-violet. Filling the brush with color, she hesitantly began with a curved line with a little wiggle on the upward end. Anne reached for the orange and made a mark in the same quadrant with a few dots and dashes nearby. I took blue, stayed in the same range of energy and carefully extended the line into a more distant section of the space. Fay chose another color and made a series of six or seven curving lines. Anne added more marks, but this time she echoed Fay's painted lines as an unspoken affirmation.

Fay broke the silence, *"There is no right or wrong way...we are just having fun!"*

We smiled and nodded agreement. The magic was working. We lost track of time, taking turns repeating and changing colors. Fay continued to paint different patterns of curving lines when she had a turn. Anne and I sometimes moved into new places, sometimes we paralleled existing lines or danced dots or stars in open places. Colors and dashes became paths linking patterns, connecting and becoming secondary networks.

There was an easy creative flow embracing our trio, an acceptance that each addition was perfect and unique. Most of the time there was silence. Decisions came spontaneously from somewhere deep inside our bodies.

Fay carefully brushed three daintily drawn hearts. Anne mixed a light pink and drew lines around these hearts with loving stokes. I used the same pink to draw other hearts outside the circle. Fay's hearts were the brightest and most important. The symbolism was obvious. The communication, unspoken, was a special type of knowing.

The silence was broken by occasional comments from Fay such as,
"I love making curving patterns."

She sighed and laid down her brush. We knew the process ... and the art ...was complete.

Then, most significant and rewarding, were her somewhat astonished statements:

"I have forgotten about being here in the hospital! I got away from thinking about it!
I was just thinking about what is happening here in this room. I am feeling better!"

To this I responded:

"Thank you. Because this happened and you told us, you also have given us a gift. We hoped to bring you the magic of a different type of hospital experience."

As we thanked her again for allowing us to come into her space and spend time with us, she asked, *"Would it be OK to share hugs?"*

We laughed and each embraced and held her warmly. I consciously gave her a back rub of extra touching. Anne did the same. These hugs were also exchanged with great warmth, ceremony and caring. *"We will be among your new friends here. Would you like us to request that our resident musician come to play some guitar, too? "*

She thought that would be fun as well.

Fay appeared now to be an entirely different patient than when we had arrived.

Neither Anne nor I saw her again. Perhaps she was discharged from the hospital. Perhaps she did not need us. That is not important. The value in our role was to give a gift of the different hospital experience for those moments.

VI.

There are "gifts" that come to us at unexpected times and from unexpected people. These moments are some of the rewards of volunteering in the arts in medicine.

Amy, Anne and I are in the large waiting room of the hospital. It is Wednesday. We set up our activity table in a new place as the furniture had been rearranged. The only clear space is right in the middle of the room.

Today's new setting feels comfortable. We notice that because of the silk display in the lobby of the main building, people have a heightened appreciative attitude towards our activities. A large percentage of the silk painting had been done in this waiting room in earlier months by patients and family members. This is part of the story we take care to acknowledge as we walk around to introduce ourselves and invite people to participate in the art processes.

Today silk painting and marbleizing on paper are the two activities offered. It is a busy day with many participants who come to the table and experience one or both processes. Others watch quietly and participate with comments or just by walking by to look. We hear stories of patients and families as they interact with us.

I notice a man with a maintenance uniform and an employee badge who comes by to watch for a moment; he is here on an errand. These activities are for the staff as well as the patients and families. We are always pleased when employees, especially the doctors, stop and participate. I invite this man to take the coffee stirring stick and involve himself in the Japanese Suminagashi marbling process of dropping ink onto the surface of the water.

He hesitates for a moment, smiles, takes the stick and quietly starts the process.

He breaks the blank presence of the water in the shallow pan by touching the surface in a progression of changing sticks in the eight colors and types of inks. Colors appear and disappear as the surface tension changes. There are a few quiet intakes of breath from him and someone else watching as unexpected dancing of patterns occurs. He repeats the touching of the centers of existing circles and also adds new circles. The progressions and variations of ink create changing tensions, relationships and movements that skim across the surface in fragile and delicate patterns.

Next, he is offered the "magic wand."

This long thin stick is used to slowly draw lines into the surface to create even more surprises of unexpected, more complex and beautiful patterns. When he lays the stick down on the table, I know he is finished.

As a final step, a piece of white paper is dropped onto the water surface. As we watch, the paper becomes moistened and we can see a pattern appear that gives clues as to what might be on the side facing the water. He carefully picks up the corner of the paper and I hold a piece of newspaper for him to place the dripping patterned paper to drain.

He looks approvingly at the beauty of the colors and patterns. Others watching give quiet appreciative non-verbal "Ohhs."

I look at him, smile, and say, "You have something to keep that you created!"

Then he speaks his wisdom:

> "You know I see in this what we are about here in our arts and medicine. In my job in receiving... few people know what I am doing. Just like some of the colors here that do not show up...yet you can see they make a difference by the way the other colors change...there is a chemistry... a connection. It is like... if I did not do my job, many people would soon notice. There are many people like me here at the hospital. We do not have the visibility of the doctors and the nurses...and even you artists.
>
> But there is a connection and a support with each other. We all work together for the patients. It is like when you take the stick and move the colors...when we all work together we create something beautiful. We help many people. Working together, we create a special place. It is beautiful, too."

Here speaks a true angel!

VII.

Each time the Improvisation troop enters a waiting room there is a sense of suspense. What will happen today? Will the people be receptive? Will we be able to offer for them an aspect of healing? This can come most simply with losing, for a short time, their anxiety and sense of isolation that is typically part of the waiting room scene. Other times there are moments with greater gifts.

In the many waiting rooms throughout the hospital, each day there are several people sitting with the privacy of their own thoughts and fears. *How can I deal with this pressure and fear? What will the report be on the blood test? Will I have to wait long? Will this hurt? Will I get sick? Will I die with this disease? Will the operation be a success?*

Some people are here alone. Others have a spouse or friend that offers a quiet supportive presence and shares the same anxiety and stress. They all sit in the hospital's waiting rooms. Though the chairs are comfortable, the colors soft, and the staff warm and very aware of their supportive role to each vulnerable individual, the mental stress is a growing private pressure for each individual. Some can disguise this with vacant looks in space or down turned heads. Others read, pick at fingers or attempted conversations.

There is a strong sense of isolation and strangeness as they sit and wonder about each other and most of all, their problems or that of the family member they are accompanying.

On this Wednesday morning, we had a centering warm up session that began with a stimulus from nature. Helen had brought several long green leaves fresh with moisture from the early morning rain. One was nestled inside the other, as they were unfurling. The six of us brought ourselves into a circle and began to improvise movement. The classical guitar became part of the process as the Certified Music Practitioner Terry's fingers also began an improvisation. We were all moving and exploring the experience of being a leaf ourselves.

I moved arms upward with a slow twist, moving as I revolved around and lost myself in the focus. This process of silence and turning inward gave its peaceful gift. After several minutes of "leafing" there was an unspoken sense of group closure, coupled with a quieting of several shared deep breaths.

Amy, our leader, held a plastic bowl containing strips of folder papers with ideas for movement. We took turns selecting one and then creating, in movement, the written concept. I chose one with the idea "opening an umbrella." Others were things like "painting a wall," "playing a big drum," "planting a garden and waiting for the flowers to emerge." We took turns in silently focusing upon, then exaggerating the movements of each idea. There was the energy of suspense as each quietly took movement turns and the rest searched the visual clues in order to know the portrayed idea.

I suggested, after using some ideas, that we add more of them to the "bowl" in order to maintain, in the waiting room, the same interest and freshness we seemed to have.

Thus centered and quiet, we gathered the sign and the pole with hooks for hanging hat props, and we went to the new waiting room on the third floor. It was about 10:30 AM on the busiest day of the week for outpatient procedures.

We had a good improvisation morning, beginning with some new ideas as we centered ourselves.

We entered the third floor waiting room. Terry had preceded us and was playing live acoustic music. One tall blonde woman said something I overheard; she had been stressed out, and the music helped her begin to relax. We shifted the focus in this room with two sections separated by a coffee shop. As a hat introduction, I did something about being cold with a heavy hat and then going skating. We evolved to drawing ideas from the fish bowl.

On an impulse, Amy asked people to draw the topic from the bowl, and then choose who would act it out. This moved us into more audience interaction immediately. Meanwhile, we shifted the action focus to the more crowded part of the room. A tall blonde woman deliberately moved to be able to see what was going on. She seated herself at an empty chair next to another attractive woman, a brunette with a yellow-green dress. When it came time for the woman in yellow-green to choose someone after drawing her piece of paper, the first woman asked if she could do it, too. That was such a surprise and a breakthrough! I do not now remember what the other woman drew or what subject matter we improvised. I had my focus on the woman who had volunteered.

Then the woman who held my focus drew her paper and asked if she could act out hers out as well. We were all feeling so good. There was the intense focus and feeling of camaraderie developing in the waiting room.

Amy did something else that was new. She took a purse from the rack and asked if anyone had a story about a purse. She was using the idea of an object to trigger a memory. This time our same tall blonde responded and shared a change she had made. With her illness, she had begun to look at places to go for a trip. They talked about Hawaii, Paris, etc. Then she realized that they were already living here, which is one of the top destination vacation spots in the world. She decided that every day after work, the purse symbolically meant taking this into the car, that she was going to start acting and living like she was on vacation. This was every day as well as every weekend.

Her story offered such a positive and uplifting message for everyone.

The troop acted out the story with Helen as the woman, and I was the husband who was driving while she was talked about her ideas for a vacation and the change in her thinking. The others were a chorus that acted out the Hawaiian idea and others. This was part of the brief planning. My tall blonde woman beamed.

Then we moved to the other side of the waiting area and continued the same kind of process. I loved having the new ideas and watching the unexpected occur!

When we were leaving, several of us took the brochures, went to each person in the waiting room, shook their hand, and thanked them for being so supportive. The tension level had changed so much. We were feeling very rewarded.

In the afternoon, later, with the painting set up in another lobby, I saw the tall blond woman arrive with her husband. I went to them and told them about the silk painting. Next the brunette and her husband came as well. They sat next to each other, and soon explained to me that after our improv troop left that morning, they had started to talk and ended up enjoying each other's company so much they exchanged names and phone numbers. The women hugged each other as one learned of a positive test result. There was satisfaction for me in knowing that two couples, who started sitting on opposite sides of the waiting room, had become friends and even later were continuing to support each other.

Our improvisation troop shared many magic moments in the waiting rooms. There are memories that fade as other great times occurred. I wish I had journaled them more carefully. I had no idea these experiences would become so rewarding.

Angels can arrive in varying forms and with varying processes.

VIII.

This gathering of angels is in a different setting: Hospice.

"Usually I shift in my bed constantly to get comfortable. But when I am painting, I seem comfortable. I do not think of the discomfort of my bed. I am not numb either - sometimes when I sit in the same place for an hour I get numb...When you are here and I am busy painting, I have an hour or so when I do not think of my cancer or that I am sick."

"Now I can paint!"... My fingers seem more flexible."
—A Hospice patient I will call Peggy

After working at the hospital, I expanded to working in a different setting. I was one of the first to work with a Hospice patient in their home in this area of the country. I gave a verbal report, but then was asked to document and give supporting comments back to the coordinator of this new program. He wanted a written report to share with others as part of advocacy for further development of a program using the arts in Hospice.

July
Dear William,

You asked me to share this quote with you in writing. In this letter, I have elaborated to document and clarify, for myself as well as you, the response of this Hospice patient to an expressive arts experience while bed bound.

Upon hearing Peggy make the above statements I asked her to say it again while I wrote down her comments. Her spontaneous statements also included, *"My pain stopped while you and I worked together. "*

Peggy was sharing with me, saying that I see her only as a relaxed woman lying in bed. However, she usually had to keep moving and modifying things with the bed controls, her angles and position. In contrast, she has been able to feel more relaxed and experience less pain during the time I am supporting her in artistic process. For a period of time she gets relief from her bedridden patterns...she forgets she is ill.

I thanked Peggy for sharing this. These statements were a gift to me - confirming that the processes have benefits she is able to articulate clearly.

Then I repeated them to her and had her repeat, again, her statement that working with art helped eliminate her sense of pain for a period of time. I suggested, as a gift to herself, that when she was feeling particularly uncomfortable, she could experiment by asking her companion to set out the paints and deliberately paint as another way of possibly controlling pain.

I would be delighted to learn from Peggy that she could modify some of her pain symptoms by painting by herself. *I would also be surprised.* That would require a big leap of personal confidence to move so quickly into working by herself. For that reason, I had her repeat and reinforce her new beliefs.

The unfortunate reality is that many people are intimidated about their abilities in artistic processes and have unhelpful beliefs that are deeply ingrained. To ask, or tell, anyone, especially a Hospice patient, to paint by his or herself *could* be adding stress.

At this time, upon reflection, I would not want to promote to a patient that working in an art process might eliminate some pain because that could potentially set higher expectations than could be achieved. The surprise, the discovery, if this happens, is the magic of the gift in the experience. If you predict "magic" or promote directly "magic," I think some of the power can be lost. There is so much disappointment in Hospice patient's lives; I would not want to add to that.

However, this testimony is of value for us to share professionally. I am pleased that you called me and there has been opportunity to do testing of artistic process for this Hospice client. As we all know, people experience pain in personal and unpredictable ways. For her, the artistic process works. We are doing our own informal research.

You and I have not formally discussed our goals for me coming to work with the patients. The unspoken assumption is that we believe that participation in art processes can improve the present quality of life for some Hospice patients. If there is less depression or less pain, those are secondary or spin off values. I am bringing training in the expressive arts and the "Arts in Medicine" approach that is different from what a traditional artist might bring to the bedside. I am comfortable and respectful of the sacredness of this person's space and time.

For your understanding in how the expressive arts approach is different, I will share more of my understanding that may explain what is happening for Peggy.

In the expressive arts way of working there is a core premise of the value of having someone attending... just being there... our term is being a "witness," while the individual or client is experiencing the *risk* and the *discovery* of the artistic process. The quiet and supportive witnessing, not just watching, which could make a person feel uncomfortable, is unique and something I had to learn. It is not passive; it is being very attentive and is also near to being suspended in time.

Perhaps this witnessing, sharing an experience that is happening "now," has an aspect of personal validation—countering the feeling patients may have of becoming "invisible" or non-existing. There is also the possible explanation that the patient becomes so focused on a new experience that brings pleasure that the brain disregards the pain stimulus, the dominant pattern, and follows the new stimulus.

A small part of it may be similar to feeling better after simply talking to someone who is a good listener. Talking aloud helps one hear oneself "safely." Just the "talking," and having someone consider *you* as important enough to give time to listen to, has a healing component.

The most basic part of this, the pure power of the artistic process, can occur in all creative expression. It taps into a core part of being human and connects with the mystery of the life force itself. There can be that element of creative surprise, discovery and excitement. There is a type of relief that comes from the flow of spontaneous action as one follows small impulses to put color here and there...*to move without conscious direction.*

I am aware that I enter that home setting differently than I would have done before. As a master's prepared art teacher of twenty-two years, my prior approach would have been to be directive and informative. I would see myself feeling responsible to share some technical knowledge.

With the expressive arts training, I have learned an entirely different approach – nearly an opposite approach. I come in with a clear mind and little expectation. I take my clues from the patient. I am not directive, but "go under" and support individuals to take risks. I support them in whatever direction they go, and build upon the spontaneous happenings of each moment. This is part of the expressive arts training and understanding. It is very subtle, but very important.

I appreciate your giving me the opportunity to apply my expressive arts training, and the experiences of working with people as inpatients in a large hospital, applied now to the home setting. The interaction with Peggy is a gift to me as well.

The time spent traveling to and from the patient in addition to the time spent on site and the gathering of materials makes the money minimal. There are about four hours spent of my time with each visit to Peggy. I have a greater understanding of the time and logistics in other Hospice programming and service with the number of people who work continuously in many home settings!

Sincerely,
Joan Voyles

(Note: I wrote this before I went to see the patient Arthur.)

After that first visit, I received a card from Peggy. Inside was a message thanking me for coming. She had painted a lovely border on the card. I was touched by the effort and planning that went into the card.

My visit with her concluded with some time listening as she talked about not being ready to die. She was looking for some personal goal or challenge that would keep her going. Because she was on morphine, and not taking formal allopathic medical treatment, she was helped by Hospice. However, she had not given up. About nine years ago, she was given first about four months to live. Several other times doctors had given her short time frames. She has proven them wrong. She has done many alternative therapies.

I began to document my experiences with Peggy more closely.

A week later:
I talked to Peggy about her painting on Friday without me. She spoke of beginning a painting of a blue bird and putting on a beak and a twig in its mouth. She was focused on the product and the way it looked. She would show it to me when I came.

I told her I was so proud of her that she painted by herself, that the product was not nearly as important the process. We would talk about this on my next visit.

Ten Days Later:
Each time I came, there was a period of assessment of the *present* physical and emotional status of the Hospice patient. I brought the silk paints, and anticipated finishing our first project, then embarking on painting spontaneously on another piece of silk stretched on a 14-inch embroidery hoop. In addition, I have other materials for flexibility to change direction if appropriate. Maintaining flexibility was my watchword.

I saw Peggy's pretty oval face framed by the combination of the natural light and graying of her faded red colored hair that had been growing out. She seemed slightly more fragile looking, but her demeanor and appearance had been consistent in the five times over the two months we had been sharing art experiences. She had a morphine IV drip in one of her arms continuously for pain management, and she was unable to move her legs and get out of bed.

When I arrived that morning, parking by the mobile home was more difficult as there were two other cars. In addition to her companion, Peggy had two other visitors who were just leaving. One was introduced as a caseworker from Hospice and the other was a man in his early thirties. Their visits overlapped and they apparently had a shared conversation.

On most days that I had seen her, Peggy had been upbeat and ready for the day's adventure in art processes. But her conversation was more somber on that day.

"When I get depressed, the social worker comes and talks to me and I feel better," Peggy told me.

That day the conversation had been a little different and the essence was shared with me. Peggy relayed that she had been close to death many times with her illness of nine years and it had happened more often lately. She had been planning Bible verses and other parts of her funeral service with her friend and companion. They formed a unique supportive team as they attend the same church.

Recently a new thought had become a priority. The Hospice counselor had suggested that Peggy think of something she would make in her art activities that could be a gift from her to friends. This art would be given to them at her funeral service. It should be something symbolic of things she loved and valued.

This idea was a change in plans and most important to support. I had a different role. I became very still inside. I wanted to listen for inner guidance. This was a new path for me to facilitate. I became the student.

We reviewed options, beginning by looking at the blue bird she started using the gauche paints. She had used blue and white and was experimenting with brush strokes, the gouache paints, and monochromatic color schemes, as contrasted with the earlier watercolor experiences. The soft brush stroke's emerging patterns began to suggest feathers. Peggy saw the potential for this to be a blue bird and painted then to develop that image. There had not been time to complete the painting.

When I had to cancel the previous Friday's session, with help, Peggy had painted. This painting, without me, was important. Two weeks before, Peggy had shared with me that statement again:

"When you are here, and we are doing art, the pain is gone. I am able to lie in bed without the turning and moving that is the usual pattern during my days."

I had had her repeat her discovery that when she was painting she did not feel pain. Then I had suggested she experiment with painting on her own. This could be a gift to herself. It would be very powerful if she *could* help modify pain by painting without my presence. I felt that the unexpected need for me to cancel that Friday was actually an opportunity to test this idea without conscious planning.

But last Friday, not much progress was made. The aid that came to give Peggy a bath had arrived just about the time the painting materials had been set up. The painting had stopped. By this time, as Peggy looked at her work, she felt the blue bird did not seem appropriate for this new symbolic piece of art...it had not arisen from the conscious symbols she was seeking. It emerged from another place in her creative expression.

Peggy said she loved trees and loved Bible verses especially. She laughed and remembered when she and her husband first moved to Florida, he told her, "Peg, you have to stop hugging the palm trees...people are looking!"

She also recounted that for years she knew her gift was the ability to reach out and help people by sharing with them her knowledge and love of the Bible. In her religious sect, she found great joy in relationships and the people who thanked her for her help and guidance. However, she was frustrated with being unable to give these "gifts" to people now that she was bedridden.

I assured her that her presence and radiance were clearly gifts to me as to others. The most obvious example of this has been by permitting the newspaper reporters to come to the intimacy of her bedside and allowing them to write the beautiful story of her life journey and the role of Hospice in helping people. She had given a gift of inspiration to far more people that way than she had in all of her years of other outreach. Sharing her story was a courageous act. The newspaper honored her with beautiful touching photos and writing. My truthful response seemed to quiet her distress about not being able to reach out with the typical "gifts" she felt she wanted to give as part of her life's work.

Peggy returned to think of *her symbols*. "She loved her husband, the Bible and trees. Indians love trees. *The trees somewhere are called the 'Standing People' in Indian lore. Their hearts are breaking with the pollution of the earth.*" But traditional Indian symbols were not really symbols for Peggy.

In the creative process, there is a normal sequence of what appears to be chaos, but what is actually just part of progress... Peggy's search moved on, to thinking aloud about how to create something with Bible verses and trees. *"But I do not know how to paint trees well, that is a problem."*

"You have practiced using the brush to dance and make grass blades and growing plants. Painting trees is similar. Do you want to have northern deciduous trees or Florida palms in your 'image' of a tree? Decide this first I think. Or ... just begin and let the tree emerge." These were some of my supportive comments.

She was not sure and decided to work at this from another direction, from the content of a Bible verse. She began calling out verses. Her friend got a Bible with word references and read selected verses carefully. We all listened intently for the words that spoke to this occasion and the new goal.

Job 14-7-8:" There exists even hope for a tree."

Isaiah 65:22: "They will not build...for like the days of a tree, will the days of my people be and the work of their hands, my chosen one will use the fall."

"...Maybe a picture of a man, a family, walking out of the trees of a forest. No, this is getting too complex and not right."

Revelations: *"The leaves of the tree are for curing...Then he showed me a river of the water of life."*

" No, I want to make something lighter for MY funeral."

The friend had an idea and made a sketch of leaf shapes overdrawn with stick lines for a trunk and branches... a beautiful sketch. Still not something that gave Peggy confidence.

I had been sitting quietly, listening with awe, but now I had an inspiration. I got up and went outside.

Searching for leaves, I pulled off hibiscus leaves, bottlebrush and other leaves from foliage around Peggy's home. Bringing them in, I told her of a way to use the same paints she had used on the 'Blue Bird' but in a different way.

"Experiment with painting the back of the leaf with the diluted gouache paint and press it onto the paper."

Hesitantly, she followed my directions. With her graceful hands, she turned over the painted leaf and placed it on the clean paper. A paper towel allowed her to rub the leaf surface and make contact with paint, leaf veins and paper. Then, carefully, she lifted the paper towel and then the leaf. With a look of delight, she saw the bold blue leaf shape printed with a transfer of delicate veins patterned within the larger leaf shape.

Yes, this she could do!

So, carefully choosing different colors for different leaves and experimenting with diluting the paint, she added and arranged six more leaves. She was getting tired. The page was not filled.

I took a mat, blocked out the creation of leaf shapes, and suggested that perhaps the open space was a good thing. Now she had room to print the Bible verses. She also could consider moving the writing around the shapes...it did not have to be printed in a straight line in artwork.

Another verse came to her thoughts:

...And as the days of a tree, so the days of my people will be.

Then, yet another verse came to mind:

"The leaves of the trees are for the healing of the nation." That is it. That would be the verse, the gift she would be leaving.

It was past noon and time for lunch and a nap. Peggy would think about this project during the week and maybe acquire some new insights, she said. This was a good project for her. We would finish it next week on Friday. There was a feeling of satisfaction we three shared. We had made so much progress in helping Peggy create this "gift of art."

I left with reluctance; the spirit of the room was so warm. But I could see heavy eyelids and Peggy had not had lunch. It was 12:50 and I had arrived at 10:00. There was another person for me to see yet that afternoon.

One Week Later:
I called Peggy to thank her for such a lovely visit. I had been inspired by the thoughts and the creative process we were sharing...it had been a gift to me. I wanted to acknowledge this to her. As I wrote this story, I was reminded about that special day of sharing and felt honored to have had a role in her artistic process.

Peggy said there had not been any other verses that had come to mind to replace any of the ones discovered on Friday. However, she was thinking about going back to the idea of drawing trees as another part or an addition to the first prints. *"But sometimes when I think of too many things, I get exhausted."*

I assured her that we were on the path of a good process and we could do whatever she wanted to do. I would facilitate that on Friday. That... or whatever new, creative impulse came to her.

I watch the process with wonder, appreciation, awe and consciousness.

A Week Later:

When I arrived, I saw a beautiful sight. Peggy was lying in bed painting. Her bed table had a piece of watercolor paper and her bedside table held a book propped up with a cookbook wire holder. There was the sound of soft music and a gentle voice talking.

Her friend had brought in a Public Broadcast Tape about the artist Tasha Tudor and this was playing on the TV at the foot of Peggy's bed. This elderly woman, Tasha Tudor, lived a simple, close to nature life. She painted children and her world of forests, flowers, and vegetable gardens with a gentle loving spirit depicting an idealized life of the late 1800's. The friend had put this on to inspire Peggy as an artist that loves nature and especially trees.

Earlier in the morning, they had looked through books to find a picture of a tree that had an image that appealed to Peggy. Then, to surprise me, everything was in place before I arrived.

I complemented them on the beauty and charm of the whole environment. I was genuinely moved by the sight and asked if I could take some pictures. They seemed pleased and several were taken to honor this "painting party."

For convenience, in the past, I had not brought a CD player because in the trailer living room there was not much room. But today I am reminded that the right music does add a background that can be magical. Later the music of the video changed to dialogue and became distracting.

The three of has so much energy together. The rest of the video was turned off for later viewing.

They also showed me several color Xerox copies of last week's painting of leaves. There was concern about taking off the pressure of a "mistake" on the original artwork. Now there was paper to practice the placement of the writing. Peggy would try to do this herself, but we would help if she could not write the Bible verses.

When I first came to see Peggy, I had been told that she could not write. For some reason, with the medication, when she used her hands to write, she would appear to stutter or repeat words or letters. She was uncomfortable using her hands. However, I saw her having good control and dexterity with her hands. She worked with a delicate, sensitive touch as she painted. She had a different level of confidence. And we were not doing things that required the precise sequence and shapes of a Bible verse message.

This time, I had brought the silk piece that Peggy had painted several weeks earlier. I had drawn with resist an image of a happy face design on silk stretched on an embroidery hoop. At home, I had completed the setting of the color with steam and today was the day to unveil it. I saved it until just before I left. I did not want to take any energy away from the tree painting focus.

This was my easiest day. Mostly I sat and supported Peggy as she painted. Before I arrived, she had painted a gently curving brown shaded trunk and was beginning to paint leafs with green and yellow brush taps. This stippling process was going very slowly and made her tired. When she was feeling frustration with the time element required, I showed her options in painting sections of the tree leaves with irregular splotches of paint and then, when this was dry, returning to her stippling of lighter yellow green leaves in scattered places. It was not necessary to do all the leaves in one process. This new understanding seemed to please her.

Actually just sitting and watching is not easy. However, I knew it was important to empower Peggy by not talking or distracting her or telling her what to do. It was important to allow her personal discovery and expression to emerge.

Before the tree painting was totally completed, I could tell by her drooping, heavy eyelids that it was time to stop the painting process ...and show her the silk.

I asked her if she knew about *Rogers and Hammerstein* or *Lerner and Lowe*. We were a new team, *Peggy and Voyles*. I did the drawing and she was the colorist. Then I showed her the silk picture. Both Peggy and her companion were delighted with this new artistic product. It was pinned to the bedside curtains for all to see. Next week we would both sign the silk painting when I brought some fabric markers.

The silk was showy, but for Hospice work, not nearly as important as the products that came in images and sources directly from Peggy. The creativity and images bubbling from her alone were the ones that offered the most healing to her. The other artwork, such as the silk, was fun and had given her confidence. Their greatest value may have been as a topic of conversation about Peggy's world that was beyond illness.

I was looking forward to the next Friday and the further evolution of the art project or projects that would be finished to share with friends at Peggy's funeral. Whenever that would be, these gifts would have been made in an atmosphere filled with love and joy!

August

Peggy told me on the phone that she was hurting; a movement in bed had brought to surface a new pain. On Friday, the companion confirmed her discomfort when I called to check on the best time.

I arrived after lunch, at one o'clock . I brought several art material process options that I kept in the car. These were "back ups" to the simplest activities I carried in my art case. On Thursday and Friday mornings, I had been going over ideas for creating art process options that might help Peggy experience some "flip side" or transformative insights about herself. I had not been bringing this as a conscious activity before. With the open discussion of death coming from Peggy, in contrast to a month or so before, the discussion about wanting to get better, I considered continuing such dialogue if she was so inclined.

We moved from the discussion of feeling pain to art updates. With the help of a friend, the silk painting was hemmed and now going to become a flag or banner. The tree painting was completed but not bold enough or finished looking by the artist's evaluation. On display was the finished leaf print painting with beautiful calligraphy writing of the Bible verse rippling around the prints of the leaves. Again, help given by a supportive friend.

For that day, I brought out a bottle of bubbles. *"Peggy, I sensed you could use some lightness and bounce in your life. Do you have enough energy to blow bubbles?"* Peggy affirmed she had always loved this activity. She could blow the bubbles. All three of us had time to enjoy the color of the reflections and the movement of the bubbles as the fan moved them with the airflow and Peggy blew more.

Then I introduced my second bubble option. "This is for someone who does not have as much breath." Years ago, I had been given a "pen" with its shaft a container for the bubble solution and the "eraser" section, actually a lid with a stem, which had a double circle frame for the bubble solution. This contrasting size scale brought laughter. When Peggy blew into this tiny frame covered with solution, a double row of many bubbles filled the air. That sight was even more delightful.

I offered to lend her the miniature to share with both her grandson and her niece the next week.

Then I brought out the next activity…a jar of Play Dough. I split the contents among the three of us. On her bedside table, I also gave Peggy a fork, a knife and a pair of scissors. *"Sometimes there is pleasure in just poking and pushing, cutting and rolling this material. We do not have to make anything; just let our fingers move and play."*

And we talked, about the art projects, but mostly about the upcoming visits of family and some family problems in the past…

Peggy talked about making a worm. I listened but observed two arches made by a series of rounded shapes that were sitting several inches apart on the bed table. So I made a small rolled "snake" that could go under the "arches" or bridges. When I looked back, the two arches were merged adjacent to each other and Peggy was putting on a head. What I saw as arches was actually to her the body parts of one large worm or caterpillar.

I spoke to her and pointed out how I had misunderstood, until then, her creation…we had talked and looked at the same pieces. We thought we were talking about the same thing, but we were not. My perspective was different.

There was a rush of feeling, a shift in thinking, when I realized we only *thought* we were talking about the same thing. How much this was like life! We experience the same things but see things differently. Maybe there was an analogy for things that happen to people in the same family. This was not something that required an answer, it was only my observation.

Peggy shared with me:

> "When people come in to visit, they first look around to see what is on display in my 'gallery.' There is a value beyond helping me feel better. I think seeing the art helps other people too."

I reminded her that this all began with the friend who brought her some art supplies and suggested Peggy might enjoy them. When she asked Hospice for help in learning how to use the supplies, our relationship and this journey of sharing with "The Three of Us…The Art Triplets" began.

It has been rich for me too! We have this "friend" to thank. Her gesture had grown to an extent beyond her expectations and ours as well!

It was now almost three o'clock and time to leave. I kept watching Peggy for clues about tiredness; her eyes were beginning to look droopy.

"I feel more relaxed now."

Hearing this I felt that my instincts for the low level of activity had been appropriate. I left having experienced a different role. Fewer products and all process. Nothing to show in the gallery, but a time of relaxed conversation and sharing among friends. She acknowledged spontaneously, more to herself, that she was feeling better at this moment.

I looked forward to learning more about the philosophy of interface that could be most appropriate in my role with this Hospice patient.

Ten Days Later:

I called and left a message for Peggy on the answering machine. I was conscious that the recorded message is one made by a happy healthy Peggy of sometime in the past. She called me back shortly apologizing that she had been unable to reach the phone. This was a tired Peggy with a different voice. I was happy to hear the visit with her sister had been good. She gave sighs of happiness about that, and I felt relieved. I confirmed my intention to come on Friday if that was OK. We would continue, and Peggy would create more art.

Three Days Later:

I receive a call at Peggy's directive to suggest we cancel. She was feeling more pain and a team would be coming tomorrow to work with her to help try some new ways for relief. I thanked her husband for calling and sent greetings to her. I would call and maybe visit in a few days unofficially.

I was feeling concern about whether her goals had been met. Perhaps the toll of the cancer was gaining on her now….at the Hospice briefing last Wednesday, they implied amazement at how she had dealt with her pain.

I listened to a tape about meditation with someone who is dying. When I listened, I participated in the last meditation. The person in my focus was Peggy.

Sunday, Two Days Later:

I talked to Peggy's husband and learned that she was failing. The nurses were having difficulty keeping the pain under control. He said people were stopping by. He assured me it was fine to visit and not to worry about any schedule.

When I arrived there were several cars parked around the house.

With a washcloth on her forehead and eyes closed, I could see that Peggy's face was changing. She was not very aware of what was going on. Outside I had an opportunity to talk with a few friends and caregivers to share how honored I was to have known Peggy. They said that she had been a dynamic person in the days of good health. They had nice things to say about the art…how happy the pictures looked.

One of the women had chosen a frame and framed a contour drawing I had made of Peggy the day she painted the tree and I had made time to watch her. I felt pleased and the frame choice with the picture was pleasing to see.

I had a few minutes to hold Peggy's hand and talk to her. I thanked her for sharing her time and creativity with me. I was truly honored and humbled.

I left and felt at peace. I was glad that I had come back for this last time. I wondered then how long the weakened state would continue. I asked one of the women to call me when she died.

I kept checking for messages on the home phone - only personal family messages.

I wrote this and sent prayers of love and peace to Peggy, her husband and friends.

Two More Days Went By:

I received a call from Hospice that Peggy died that morning. I was surprised she maintained that thread so long. On Wednesday, I saw the obituary and learned she was only in her early 50's.

The day before the service, I had a conversation with the friend who had been there in most of my visits. I was mostly listening. The dying process had been lengthy and painful. Friends stayed to give Peggy some sort of a sense of safety. This one needed someone to talk to. It helped me process and have closure, too. She spoke of coming, shortly after I left on Sunday, and with another friend staying all night. A doctor was called to consult about ending the pain. He said she was getting enough narcotics to "kill everyone in the room." He had not seen this resistance in his forty years of practice.

Peggy was alert until the end in spite of much medication. Seemingly, she was in so much pain she could not die. At 4:30 AM the morning of her death, she joked with the family and friends about what flavor of pizza to order for her. Then, on the next shift, a nurse came who helped Peggy to relax and she finally relaxed into death.

The last time I was there, we had discussed options for giving the tree painting some "punch." When I had an opportunity to follow-up, I saw the results. This had been accomplished using a computer. A friend had cut the last painting Peggy was working on, the tree, and pasted it on the blue pattern, the one we first did with dropping colors on a wet blue background. This became the sky. She had then added a drawing of a lamb and a lion sitting under the tree. On the lower left was a photo of Peggy at a healthier time. I did not see the long oval facial lines that I saw when she was in bed.

It is an impressively personal and touching keepsake.

As a memorial to Peggy, there was no emotion or sadness - just a telling of the story of her beliefs and inspiration. We referred to her joy in painting during the last months of her life, and it was pleasing to me to have this process acknowledged.

This had been a sacred experience.

I have a feeling of joy from the experience that I have had in my sharing and enriching the last four months of Peggy's life. That has been a gift to me. I entered into this relationship knowing this was only going to be temporary. I had no idea it would be so intense.

IX.

This next gathering of angels was also in a Hospice setting. There is a short overlap of time with the journal entries for Peggy, as I was seeing both. (I will continue this entry in present tense, as written in my journal.)

I saw Arthur yesterday. He was not able to "play" the first time we worked together. For this encounter, I had to move into more of a role of "teacher" and less of a "facilitator." I am not sure how I feel about this, but I acknowledge that I can do both. I write this to process the experience for myself. I had left his home feeling unsettled.

Perhaps my personal focus was different. I think back and realize I had not stopped to meditate and clear my mind before stepping into this encounter.

Arthur and I had had several conversations on the cell phone as I had to recheck and confirm his directions in the maze of turns in the community of homes that twist around golf courses with different housing themes, dead-end streets and cul-de-sacs. I pulled up in front of an attractive home. I knew he was waiting and my knock would confirm that his directions were accurate.

I want to evaluate my potential for helping this man. I have been an "art teacher" and had twenty-two years of public school teaching experience. But that role is no longer satisfying to me since I became trained as an expressive arts facilitator. I have come to understand and practice art with a completely different philosophy for myself and in my work with others. I come to the Hospice setting with an understanding that artistic process can be healing. That to me is profound and sacred.

Today my role is to facilitate an artistic process experience that I am hopeful will bring a healing experience for this elderly Hospice patient.

I came because he had expressed an interest in portrait painting. I had been called by Hospice and asked if I could help someone with this interest. Portrait painting is something I had done years ago, but that has not been a current interest. However, I draw people frequently and have taught the basics of drawing people and faces. The drawing is necessary before the painting. But there is the possibility that portrait painting was the outward request and there may be something deeper or different that was important to have revealed.

My plan was to assess his abilities and encourage his art interest. My question was how much did Arthur know already and how much could I support his interest? In my art bag, I brought several reference books and had made copies of ten pages of basic instructions for his future reference. I did not know if this would be a "onetime" visit or a series, and I wanted to leave him with support material.

Arthur was friendly and responded to my outstretched hand of greeting. But he did not look up with direct eye contact. He talked "to his lap," head bowed toward his wheel chair. He stayed that way all through most of the 1½ hours that I was there.

I imagined that in earlier years he was a powerfully built man of perhaps six feet and heavy build. He did not stand except to move from the wheel chair to a chair at the table adapted to a studio table. A red oilcloth covered and protected the surface with piles of books and some art supplies. The expanse of tile flooring made moving around with the wheel chair and the sliding of the oxygen hose easy.

Arthur showed me a drawing copied from a magazine picture. It was based on a photo of a smiling Arab chieftain's head covered with a white cloth. I could see that he had acquired some skills that led him to initiate this himself. Making this drawing was a positive sign. I complemented him on this achievement.

There were some other comments I made, as a teacher, such as the value of not pressing so hard on the thick pad of the drawing tablet. Embossing the art surface with outlines, such as the strong teeth pattern, which could make it difficult to soften and blend tones as part of the overall effect.

Then we looked at the box of art supplies sent to him from Hospice. He had not used any of the assortments of watercolors, colored pencils, oil pastels, magic markers, Conte and charcoal sticks. He had some Prismacolor pencils of his own and gestured to a bag of art supplies.

"Before my wife died, I had started taking oil painting lessons and was enjoying this activity. But after she died, it was bad. I just could not do anything....now I have "this." His head hung even lower and he gestured to the length of 50 feet of cord connecting to the pulsing oxygen pump in a back bedroom area.

I learned his only art experience had been with the oil painting of landscapes. The recent pencil drawing of the Arab chief was a new venture. I made a decision to expose him first to the other available media that could be a less involved process than painting with oils. (My sense was that he should not be exposed to any art material fumes.) This would also give me an opportunity to assess his intentions and abilities.

I was also looking for the potential to facilitate his experience in other more *spontaneous art processes*. In these, one does not know what the end product will look like...there is a flow, discovery and creation. *This is the expressive arts approach.*

I had him use each of the art materials in the art box with experiments on a sheet of paper from his sketchbook. This included comparisons of the colored pencils in the box with his Prismacolor pencils in their ability to build layers of color. When he used colored pencils in the Arab portrait, he did not realize he could layer the pencils and create color techniques similar to color mixing of oil paints.

I was heading into a teaching role, not that of expressive arts. I reminded myself that this seemed to be appropriate for his goals.

I showed him how the watercolor could be painted over the oil crayon resist areas to create new effects. The oil crayons had a relationship to the oil paints he used before but did not require the use of brushes and solvents. Layering of colors can be done with these, too.

Then he gestured to large book on fish, both photos and cooking techniques that his daughter-in-law had brought to his attention as a possibility for painting sources. So I decided we could make a fish together. This would be a variation of the "shared dancing brushes" way of developing a picture that has been a good way of warming up and becoming acquainted in the hospital artistic process.

I had him start and we took turns beginning with the oil crayons. His instincts were to be realistic. I would make colorful and playful variations. The sharing of a painting surface was a new experience for him. He was polite and patient, but this was surprising to him I sensed.

Then I introduced him to using the watercolor over the drawing. Wetting the background made it easy and he could quickly block in the space.

He used the white oil crayon to add scales and spoke for the quality of shine on a fish and supposed there was not a color for that. Next, he chose an orange color for the body of the fish and while that was wet, I suggested he experiment with drops of other colors for a softened, changing body color. The white oil crayon marks popped out with the contrast of the colors. There was a contemporary shiny look, though not as realistic as the ones in the fish cook book. Perhaps this experimenting could be of future reference if he was working by himself. Together we had made a totally unique fish!

However, this activity did not bring from him any behavior that clued to me that the play was fun. I suggested to him that sometimes artists work in several different media to discover what they can do, and, to have just "fun" with the materials. Often they may have several things in progress, just as oil painters often do. My intention was to reinforce the idea of play and fun.

Meanwhile, I observed a mountain scene painting hanging in the hallway. I learned Arthur had painted this. For my eye, I could tell the artist was not yet an expert painter, yet some of the effects were well done. I shared my compliments about the shimmering reflections of the water that were a beautiful contrast to meadows suggesting summer flowers blooming. He seemed pleased with this validation.

After seeing this, I asked about his painting kit under the table. Arthur brought out a box filled with paints and many brushes. He obviously had been working at not only painting, but also acquiring equipment. He talked about a variety of people who had TV programs showing how to paint that he had watched over the years. With this information, I encouraged him to return to painting, or some artistic processes, now that he had so much discretionary time each day.

Then I changed my focus to encourage his development of skills and satisfaction with portraiture…to empower him with some knowledge that would increase his personal satisfaction.

"I do not know anything about the rules and ways of drawing faces."

So we moved into drawing …a step leading to painting a portrait.

Taking a pen, I showed him one way of drawing, a contour drawing. *"This is a way training your eyes to really see. It is a process that is scary at first…you draw while you are looking away from the paper. You do not erase. It is an exercise in looking. Learning to really look and see is essential in portraiture."*

In about 5 minutes, I drew him, starting at the top of the glasses that hid much of the left eye and drew around the other features of the bent face. As I started, he raised his head and looked at me, directly, with a touch of surprise. Now I laughed and asked him to tip his head and return to the position and alignment that I had started. As I drew, I eliminated the oxygen cord and the nose clip.

"This is something I do in which I compare what is unique about you that I see; it is a variation of the formula drawing I will now show you. There is a long history of artists developing their drawing skills by looking at themselves in a mirror. That is something you could also do."

I did this drawing to give credibility and balance my sense of playfulness with the paints earlier, as well as to model the idea of practice in looking to see the real shapes. So we began a lesson in drawing. Each of us had a piece of Conte crayon from the big box of supplies and a sheet of paper from a sketchbook.

I have done this exercise so many times...but it had been almost fifteen years since I last did it. The "formula" face that appeared on my paper is one that has looked at me many times over the years.

Arthur created his version of "the formula face." He was attentive and very interested in following the process. After having him draw an eye or a nose on the paper borders to practice, he then added the features on the main drawing. Then I would reference other variations of these same ideas on the pages that I had. They would be something for him to copy and practice as a way of developing skills to simplify and de-mystify drawing faces for portraits.

I began to realize that I had been here for some time and there is only so much one can absorb. Since I did not know if I would be returning, I felt I had presented much. I reviewed with him options for continuing. He was interested in getting some reference books. We talked about perhaps an outing to one of the large bookstores or an art supply store that was near his doctor's office; Arthur did not want a library book that you had to return soon.

I complimented him again on his skill in using his hands and his careful, delicate touch. I had learned he had been a maintenance man in some large facility or manufacturing plant. Then I affirmed to him that using his hands was something that does help him in art as well. I gathered my books and supplies, but left a mat for the shared fish drawing or for anything else he might create in the future. He followed me to the door, still with a bent head, and thanked me for coming. I shook his hand, thanked him for sharing his time with me, and left.

Personal Evaluation

As I looked back, I had several emotions. I mentioned to Arthur several times that one could play with the paints as well as work on some very detailed processes to feel pleasure. I thought he was one who would "get lost" in the details and the laborious steps. That type of artistic process was appropriate and might serve him well. If I returned, I would review what we did and then contrast this with some of the short cuts on drawing faces from the profile and ¾ views. He would enjoy the intellectual knowledge that I would share as "an art teacher."

But I would like to discover something that would help him hold his head higher and something that would bring out laughter. I heard a few reserved laughs as we drew and he looked at his work. *I think he would be helped if there were more times of unexpected, spontaneous fun. That would be my main goal if I returned to work with him.* As I write this, I think that maybe doing cartoons could be an entry to having fun. They are a part of learning the art of painting and drawing faces and even figures.

I left a message on the family answering machine inquiring about how he felt about our time together. I had not heard from him yet.

I wrote this to process the experience and contrast this with my working with a different patient who was bedridden and in pain. These two had different types of depression and illness. These are only two, but my first experiences in working in the home of patients being served by Hospice. I realized with humbleness there are so many other people and stories that Hospice serves each day. I felt honored to have had these experiences of sharing my art knowledge and skills in these new settings.

Mid-July:

Since I did not hear a response from Arthur after leaving two messages, I began to think that perhaps he had been disappointed. If so, I was anxious to encourage having some other individual help him and left a message at Hospice to this effect.

Very shortly, from the Hospice Art Coordinator I learned that Arthur had been pleased with the art lessons. He had shared, *"The only thing I have left is my art."*

Upon hearing this, I melted into an even stronger personal commitment of giving the most I could to Arthur; I felt an even greater sense of responsibility.

I was authorized to go several more times and then we would re-evaluate. I scheduled a visit for the following Friday.

Remembering my resolve to help him experience some laughter, I packed some reference books on cartooning for Friday. In addition, I went to an art supply store and bought a large block of plasticine clay and some clay tools. My instinct was to bring to his large hands the tactile experience of moving the clay. This artistic process would reinforce the two-dimensional drawing concepts with something novel. When I taught school, making clay faces was always a time when minds and hands would be intensely involved. *And, most importantly, there was always laughing* as clay faces would emerge and begin to look back at their creators.

I arrived about two o'clock. Arthur was still in his wheel chair but there was an air of something different. *He talked less "to his lap" and more to me.* We compared numbers and I realized now that I had copied incorrectly the phone number. When I used the number in the notebook, I had been leaving messages on someone else's answering machine. This explained the misunderstanding and the communication problem.

Arthur seemed to be eager to show me a tiger that he had drawn using a picture from a National Geographic's magazine. The tiger was made with a combination of magic marker and paints...*he was experimenting with the new materials.* However, in the face area there were several holes in the paper. Here he had changed to using the paints, attempting to bring in more of the white tiger stripes. In the process, the paper fell apart.

I explained that this tablet paper works for pencil or pen, but something with more body was appropriate when water paints are added. I gave him several sheets of index card stock that I find work surprisingly well for painting. I made a note to myself to get some heavier illustration board pieces for next time.

Again, I complimented him on how pleased I was that he was working on his own. And I reminded him that I knew he had developed some skills when I had admired the oil painting landscape last week.

However, I told him that I had been thinking about the oil painting process and had a concern about encouraging the return to oil paints now with his lung damage and the present oxygen support therapy. Sometimes fumes can trigger a physical reaction. We discussed that in the past he had been using a turpentine substitute and he was not aware of any oil paint odors.

I explained I was bringing less complex materials and encouraging his expanding into new experiences. I asked him if he would like to try my plan to have two parts to our time together, first a return to drawing. We would look at using the same rules but now draw a profile view of a face.

He quickly was into the process and very attentive. We soon finished the day's lesson on drawing faces.

For the second part, I brought out the big block of plasticine clay. I explained that usually in school I had clay that came in butter box sizes. Each person got one stick, a half cup of clay. As adults, we had bigger hands and we were going to play with bigger allotments from this ten-inch clay block. There was a chuckle about this analogy.

I cut off wedges of clay and showed Arthur how to make the clay more plastic by warming it with his hands. We began with an egg shape by rolling the clay between our palms instead of drawing. The half way down eye location began with pushing thumbs into the middle to create eye sockets. And so the process evolved as we reviewed the techniques of both drawing lesson with this new application in form.

And it worked.

I heard some laughs as he periodically held the face at arm's length away and evaluated decisions about ears, noses and hair. His clay head had a good right ear, but the left one was oversized and dropped down to the jaw corner. Using a thumb, the extra ear size was "erased." With the plastic tools and our fingers, both of us were able to model, add and subtract clay, to create a clay face.

On an impulse I took an empty shiny tin can holding some pencils, turned it upside down, and placed his clay head there ceremoniously...a metal formal pedestal base for his creation! It made a good combination. I asked if he would like for me to leave the rest of the block there. He could get more cans, make heads, and create his own "gallery" of faces or portraits!

As we concluded today's session, I thanked him for finding my expensive #7 watercolor brush I left last week and made certain it was now packed in the art bag.

Arthur shared that he had a project of making baklava on this table later yet that day. He observed that using the phyllo dough was similar to working with clay. He had the cinnamon, walnuts and sugar ingredients ready. I learned that the secret to making this pastry, that I love, is to cook the dough and nut mixture and then pour a cold honey mixture over the hot pastry. I thanked him for sharing the process with me and admired this role of contributing cooking for his son and his daughter-in-law.

As a teacher, I was anticipating the next few sessions and the sequence of activities, planning to build on this sculptural experience. On my trip home, I stopped at an art store. I had purchased some of the newer Sculpty Clay and a reference book on making cartoon-like figures that could then be baked into a permanent shape. This would be an evolution into colors and more fun for an artistic process in Arthur's requested theme.

I left feeling good and looked forward to next week.

Arthur had laughed several times. Sometimes, when we were talking, while both working in artistic processes, we were looking at each other. I could then more easily relate to his spirit and there was a comfortable flow of conversation. He had looked confidently at me as I departed.

On Monday, in the morning while I was away, someone from Hospice called and talked to my husband. I was left a message that Arthur had died. The family wanted me to know that he had been very happy about the art encounters and they were appreciative.

I was surprised. I was humbled. It made me realize how fragile the life force was.

On Friday, Arthur had seemed to be so much better than the week before. I was expecting we would be having a much longer time of sharing. He had been an apt and responsive student. That is always a reward to any teacher or a facilitator; our sharing had enriched me.

He had also given me of gift of my beginning to enjoy, once again, being a teacher. I had discovered I could blend my new and old ways of working with art materials, processes and students in a healing environment.

But most of all, I had the additional gift of being rewarded; for I saw the change in his behavior as he participated in the expressive art processes and... the art lessons. He held his head higher. He would look directly at me. He worked on his own initiative for pleasure. But... most rewarding: I heard Arthur laugh spontaneously.

Laughter is good medicine.

Angels love to hear the sound of human laughter.

I reflect on my days of volunteering at the hospital and Hospice as I read and edit these journal entries. The emotions and sacredness of this time in my life flood back. I have a knowing that I helped people at a special moment in both their lives and mine. I received many gifts. I feel so honored to have had that journey with some of the many angels in arts and medicine.

Many of my angels were the patients themselves.

Author Biographies

Olive M. "Hollie" Adkins, MA is an artist/poet-in-residence in an arts in medicine program in FL, with one MA in guidance/counseling and one MA in visual/performing arts from USF. Having retired from a counseling career in the state prison system, she facilitates open art studios, the Poets' Circle, and the Scribes' Hour weekly and directs "Echoes," an improvisational theatre troupe, as well as visiting patients' rooms with the arts. She facilitates workshops and outreach programs. E-mail: holliego@tampabay.rr.com.

Dr. Paula Artac, D.Min, ATR-BC, C.E.A.T. is a professional watercolor artist, business owner, certified expressive arts therapist, registered art therapist and art educator. Her paintings have won both local and national recognition for many years. As an art therapist, she has developed her Colors of Life (R) art and wellness program. She has presented numerous advanced educational courses, workshops and papers on a cosmological approach to creativity, spirituality and creativity at regional and national conferences. Her radical approach to the healing grace of the creative process has been developed into a cosmological theory for the practice of expressive arts therapy. In her consulting work, she specializes in the development of innovative creativity programs for personal and organizational transformation. Paula facilitates spirituality-based art and wellness retreats (Brigid's Garden (R),) as well as creative wellness groups in Arizona and California. She teaches watercolor painting classes at the Shemer Art Center in Phoenix. As a faculty member of San Diego University for Integrative Studies, she teaches online courses in expressive arts therapy. Paula also facilitates a holistic expressive arts therapy group at Sundance, in Scottsdale, Arizona, and at the Sedona Cancer Center at the Verde Valley Medical Center.

Dr. Robert Beland, PhD has been teaching at the University of Florida for over 28 years. He has been involved in the Center for Gerontological Studies and was its Associate Director. In 2007, he received the Distinguished Teaching Honor from the Association for Gerontology in Higher Education. He has consulted for nursing homes, assisted living facilities and community senior centers. He has published and presented extensively on recreation and aging and has received several grants related to older adults. He received his PhD in Therapeutic Recreation from the University of Maryland and MA in Therapeutic Recreation from Columbia University.

Wayne Berman was born in New Jersey. During his teenage years, he was passionate, almost fanatical, about music and the arts. Growing up in N.J. was great for him because he was so near to NYC and had abundant opportunities to see many of the best artists in the world. He was always at a music recital, poetry reading, dance concert, art gallery, museum, or the library. But his interest in the arts developed partly as a result of his mother's illness. Francis DeNoia Berman became ill with Alzheimer's disease long before many had ever heard of it. Wayne was forced to quit High School to watch his mother so his dad could work. In the 4 years of taking care of his mom, he discovered the powerful force music was in keeping her alert and happy. Mr. Berman received a BA in music from Bard College in N.Y., and did his masters work in composition and theory at Bowling Green State University in Ohio. While he was at Bard he had the extraordinary experience of studying with Dr. Benjamin Boretz who shocked him into a whole new way of putting together his musical world, although he had already studied and worked with many of his favorite artists, such as John Cage, William Burroughs, Allen Ginsberg, Jackson McLow, and Gheorghe Costinescu. Wayne currently lives in Pinellas County, Florida. He is a composer, performer, director and teacher in the arts. His approach to teaching and learning in the arts is unique because of his interest in art as therapy. He uses sound as a way to navigate one's life. Contact Wayne at 727-641-0714.

Nancy Cappo. Although the majority of her life has been spent in Florida, trips to the back woods of Minnesota have greatly influenced Nancy's artistic flair, photography, and writing. As a college graduate, along with decades of life's experiences, she has learned that the process of learning is many times more important than the final outcome. By focusing on her own creativity and self-expression, Nancy launched "Photo Meditation/Introspection" to enhance thoughts, discussion, growth and self-understanding. Her current volunteer work with the Palliative Arts program at the Hospice of the Florida Suncoast has allowed Nancy to incorporate this process as an integral form of healing. For further information and to see examples from her personal publications, please visit her website at: cappocustomcreations.com

Author Biographies

Melanie Circle is a painter, printmaker and expressive arts guide. Her mandala-based painting workshops incorporate breath, movement, poetry and sound – a reminder that whatever we do, we do with all of ourselves. She is a graduate of New York State University and the Haliburton School of the Arts Expressive Arts Program. Along with regular workshops in her Vancouver Island studio, she has offered workshops for Hospice, at the Canadian Congress of Gather the Women, and in the Waldorf System. She is an instructor in the Expressive Arts Program at the Haliburton School of Arts. To learn more, visit: www.melaniecircle.com

Dr. June M. Conboy, Ph.D., C.E.A.P., an adjunct professor in the Department of Counseling & Development at Long Island University, is a licensed and certified Mental Health Counselor, a member of the National Expressive Arts Training & Research Association, and an Accredited Certified Expressive Therapist and Diplomate. A member since 1986 and Fellow since 1997, Dr. Conboy was invited to the 25th Anniversary Annual International Society for the Study of Trauma & Dissociation Conference, 2008, as a Fellow honoree. Dr. Conboy has maintained a private practice since 1981 and teaches counseling and psychology to graduate students. For reprints of Writings For Alters and information, contact: June Conboy Ph.D., 631-486-2391/2392, juneconboyphd@aol.com.

Laura JJ Dessauer, MS, ATR-BC, LCAT, the founder of the Creativity Queen, LLC, is a Board Certified Creative Arts Therapist, Certified Parent and Teen Coach, and Doctoral Candidate. Laura brings 20 years of experience working with families, children and teens in over 18 school districts. A national presenter, esteemed clinician, and winner of the 2007 Small Business of the Year Award (SCORE), Laura believes that all individuals have the potential to tap into their creativity to solve problems, make healthier choices, and connect with the important people in their lives. Visit the Creativity Queen website for more information: www.thecreativityqueen.com

Cathy DeWitt. A successful and eclectic career musician, Cathy DeWitt has been the Musician in Residence for Shands Arts in Medicine at the University of Florida (www.shands.org/AIM) since 1994. From piano music in the lobby to elevator singalongs, from hallway concerts to bedside harp in the ICUs, Cathy uses music to transform the hospital environment and the patient experience. While participating in several research projects involving the healing power of music, she became particularly interested in its effects on people with dementia and memory disorders. Her work with creativity and aging began in 2003, at the Florida Center for Creative Aging, where she coordinated events and produced their newsletter. In 2006, and 2008, she helped coordinate and facilitate the NEA/NIH-funded Vital Visionaries Program at the University of Florida. To hear Cathy's recordings, read her writings, and find out more about her work, visit www.cathydewitt.com

Laurie Doyle, drawn to the arts, healing, and social ministries, is intrigued with how these disciplines interplay. After graduating from the University of Florida, she worked in journalism, education and youth ministry. Her most enriching experiences happened while on staff for Young Life with teenage moms and as an adult education teacher in a psychiatric hospital. For the last four years she has worked as a chaplain's volunteer at Bayfront Medical Center and as a member of her Episcopal church's intercessory healing team. She is presently an Intern Chaplain in the CPE program at Tampa General Hospital.

Frances Falk, MFA, REAT, a Franciscan sister, has devoted much of her life to creating art. Her two predominate interests are art as healing and art as spirituality. Born in north Louisiana, she grew up with her identical twin sister in New Orleans. Her first art instruction came as an art major in Boston where she later studied for a degree in education. In the years that followed, she acquired an extensive background as an educator, teaching in colleges and schools in this county, in India, and in Ghana, West Africa. Frances holds a Master of Fine Arts degree from Marywood University in Pennsylvania and is a Registered Expressive Arts Therapist. Coming to Tampa, Florida in 1994, she established the Expressive Arts Center both as a fine arts and as a therapeutic studio. In 1997, she was invited to design and coordinate an arts in medicine program for a prominent regional institution, where she directed the program for 10 years. She presently resides and maintains an art studio in St. Petersburg, FL.

Rev. Dr. Kurt Fondriest, Ph.D. MFA, REAT, CPC, ATR. Reverend Kurt Fondriest is an Expressive Art Therapist in Chicago Illinois at Misericordia Home, a residential facility called home by nearly 600 young to older adults living with various developmental disabilities. He has worked at the Home for over 18 years in an artist studio setting where he implements his philosophy of the expressive arts. He also lives with a physical disability himself called Fibromyalgia. Reverend Kurt has been published in various healthcare journals and metaphysical periodicals. He is an active painter, writer, storyteller and holistic minister.

Susan Patricia Golden, MA, LCPC: Susan Patricia Golden, received her masters degree from the Adler Dreikurs Institute at Bowie State University. She has many professional certificates in various aspects of her profession and 30 years' experience. She is a professional speaker, 'Reconstruction Musician,' writer and teacher. She invites people back to the original way they came into this world, as singers, musicians, artists, dancers and all-around creative people. In this rediscovery process her clients enhance all parts of their lives. Susan authored the ABZ's of Musical Instruments Book 1 and teaches the importance of music-making for all of us from birth to death. Susan believes that there is more to music than only being a passive listener. Music-making creates well-being! She founded UniversalMusicDay.org in 2007 for the second Saturday of October every year. Susan studied with Music for People and Music for Healing and Transition and completed two years with National Speakers Association Academy in Central Florida. Susan lives in Clearwater, Florida. Visit her websites www.UniversalMusicDay.org and www.FamilyMusicNetwork.net, to learn more about the *ABZ's of Musical Instruments* Book 1 and to listen to the sounds of the instruments.

Russell S. Buddy Helm was classically trained since the age of eight. His books, *Drumming the Spirit to Life, Let the Goddess Dance,* and *Way of the Drum* were published by Llewellyn Worldwide about the healing aspects of drumming. Buddy has worked with many greats; Tim Buckley, Frank Zappa, Allman Brothers, Mike Bloomfield, Baba Olatunji, Peter Ivers (New Wave Theater), Big Joe Turner, Wolfman Jack, Bo Diddley, Chuck Berry, Ray Manzarek (Doors,) Billy Burnette (Fleetwood Mac,) Bethlehem Asylum, Kinky Friedman and others. He has done Ron Howard soundtracks, Whitney Museum Art films, Star Wars comic strips for George Lucas, and National Festival of the Arts documentaries. He was postproduction supervisor at Lorimar (Dallas, Knots Landing, Falcon Crest, Hunter) and drum teacher for Guro Dan Inosanto (Bruce Lee's partner.) Buddy has spent twenty years teaching Helmtone Drum Therapy Protocols for healing rhythmic reprogramming of abuse, trauma, delayed stress, grief, anger, cancer, depression, addiction, OCD, ADD, autism, etc. He has taught his protocol at Kaiser, Bayfront Medical, ISEEM, KU, Dominican Nuns, Vanderbilt, NIH, Unity, and healing centers in Malibu, Santa Monica, Cape Cod, Austin, Asheville, USF, New Jersey, others.

Contact: Russell S. Buddy Helm, Seasons-on-Montana, 1021-A Montana Avenue, Santa Monica, CA 90403, 310-650-9438 www.buddyhelm.com, buddy@buddyhelm.com

Dr. Lynn Carol Henderson, Ph.D. is a Feminist, Ritual Leader, Storyteller, Artist, and Adjunct Professor teaching courses in Magic, Myth, and Ritual in Art at Eckerd College, St. Petersburg, FL. She holds a B.A. from the University of Pennsylvania, Philadelphia, and a MFA from Washington University, St. Louis, and an Interdisciplinary Doctorate in Art History and Women's Studies from Union Institute and University, Cincinnati, Ohio. For 30 years she has been a ritual leader in the Women's Spirituality Movement, blending her art installations with Expressive Arts techniques and neo-Pagan traditions, including rituals of seasonal celebration, life passages, healing, and empowerment. Contact: EnigmaArtStudio.com.

Carol Henry, MFA received a BS in Piano from Julliard in 1951, a MFA in Performance Arts - Music, Theatre and Dance from Sarah Lawrence College in 1969. She became a Certified Musical Therapist for Essex County (NJ) Overbrook Hospital, in 1963. Carol wanted to help others obtain and maintain a semblance of coping with life, and to help them perceive how to find a place where they could easily fit. In 1971, while working as a movement specialist in a New Jersey public school system granted by a Title III Federal Government grant, she came upon E. Paul Torrence's, *Guiding Creative Talent*. After reading about herself on most pages, she wrote thanking him for helping her accept her differences. He responded. This resulted in Carol having an avidly attentive mentor for thirty years. His death in 2003 has left an awesome hole that Carol feels absolutely bound to help fill for others.

Dr. Benjamin B. Keyes, ThD, PhD, EdD is the Professor/Program Director for Masters of Counseling Program at Regent University in Virginia. Prior to taking his position at Regent, Dr. Keyes was in private practice, with offices in Clearwater, Florida. His specialties include dissociative disorders, domestic violence, child abuse, addictions, and mood and anxiety disorders. Dr. Keyes received his first Doctorate in Rehabilitation Counseling in 1985, from International College and his most recent in Counseling Psychology from the University of Sarasota in 2004. He also has Doctoral Degrees in Theology and Ministry. Over the years Dr. Keyes has worked extensively with hospitalization programs and private practice, and has established himself as one of the leading program innovators for partial hospitalization programs. He recently returned from the People's Republic of China where he and a colleague were invited to teach on Dissociative Disorders at University of Shanghai and Beijing University. This invitation came at the culmination of a six-year research project which will have the effect of opening treatment for dissociative disorders for their entire country. Currently, he also heads the Center for Trauma Studies and is developing and training graduate students in a First Response Trauma Team. They plan to deploy to Africa over the next few years to teach and work with trauma survivors. Ben is happily married to Kim, has two adult children, Shawn and Jasmin, and a beautiful granddaughter, Amber. He is also known in the Tampa Bay area as a singer-songwriter

Rev. Kathy Luethje, MA, MDiv, LMHC, CEAT, CMP, is a Licensed Mental Health Counselor in the state of Florida. She is a Certified Music Practitioner through the Music for Healing and Transition Program. As a graduate of Ball State University & the Quaker Earlham School of Religion, both in Indiana, she has 35 years experience as a teacher, college instructor, pastor, counselor, and hospital chaplain. Kathy spearheaded an arts in medicine program at Bayfront Medical Center in St. Petersburg, FL. She earned a graduate level certificate in Intermodal Expressive Arts Therapy at University of South Florida, which concluded with an internship at a local arts in medicine program. She is ordained through On the Path Ministries. Kathy founded the Regional Expressive Arts Practitioners (REAP) group, which meets monthly, for support, advocacy, and continuing education in the field. She has spoken internationally about the expressive arts and is currently writing a musical 'dramady' about 12th Century mystic Hildegard of Bingen. She and her husband Jon were a 'Brady Bunch' family when they married, and are expecting their 17th grandchild. You can reach Kathy at godsendink@gmail.com or visit the website of www.FloridaREAP.com

Joan Forest Mage, MA, CMA is the founder & director of Life Force Arts Foundation in Chicago, presenting performances and workshops in shamanism, shamanic healing and shamanic visual, literary, and performing art. Joan received a Master of Arts Degree from School for New Learning, De Paul University, Chicago, with the focus of "creating healing ritual through the arts." She is a member of the Society for Shamanic Practitioners and specializes in soul retrieval healing. Joan is a dancer, vocalist and musical director of Life Force Ensemble, a shamanic world music band and performing company. Please visit her website www.lifeforcearts.org.

Sally Mathews, MFA studied commercial art at the U. of Kansas, painting for a year and a half at the Instituto Allende in San Miguel de Allende, Mexico, and received certification to teach art from Carthage College and the U. of Wisconsin. She obtained a Master's of Art Ed. from the University of South Florida. She worked for Sacred Design Associates helping to design the Arch Book series for children published by Concordia, a Lutheran publishing house in St. Louis. Her book, *The Sad Night*, published by Clarion (Houghton-Mifflin) is a pictorial history book about the Aztecs, began as a Master's Degree Project in which she did both the art and the text. Mrs. Mathews, retired after twenty nine years of teaching art to elementary students, is now presenting lectures and art activities to adults citizens through the U. of South Florida "Senior" program, and has organized several artist and writer workshops for The National League of American PenWomen in San Miguel, Mexico.

Christine McCullough, MA received her Master of Arts in Holistic Counseling from Salve Regina University in 1997. Her undergraduate work in the area of Pre-literate art, culture, and religion brought her to the socio-spiritual study of The Goddess and Earth-Based Spirituality. She became a teacher of workshops and programs based on an exploration of The Sacred Feminine. She is a Certified Specialized Kinesiologist and holds certification in Mindfulness-based Stress Reduction Technique. She is apprenticed to Oh Shinnah Fast-Wolf and integrates her training in Shamanic healing techniques in her counseling practice. Artist, author, ceremonialist, and teacher, Chris was introduced to the magic of the labyrinth by Victoria Williams, MA, who was giving a workshop on this ancient tool at the second annual Women's Sacred Art Festival in Newport, RI. Together they formed the Labyrinth Ladies in 2005. You can visit her at www.thelabyrinthladies.com

Dr. Roger Millen, PhD currently directs Compassionate Counseling, an organization that facilitates growth in individuals, couples, groups, and organizations through counseling, consulting, training, and development. He received his PhD at Purdue University, majoring in Organizational Systems Analysis. He also trained with the National Training Laboratories of the Institute of Applied Behavioral Sciences. A Certified Master Practitioner and Trainer of Neuro-Linguistic Processing (NLP) and Ericksonian Hypnosis, he has also studied Gestalt, Jungian, and Process-

Oriented Psychology. Dr. Millen has been active in the New England Process-Oriented Psychology Society and the Association for Humanistic Psychology and President of the Healing Arts Alliance of Tampa Bay. Roger taught at the university graduate level for more than twenty years in the US and China. He has been a faculty member of several universities and lectured internationally. Roger is a longtime practitioner and teacher of T'ai Chi Ch'uan, Ch'I Kung, and meditation. He was ordained as a minister in the Universal Life Church and is actively involved in Twelve-Step Recovery Programs. Roger wants to send forth the following messages to the world: 'When the student is ready to learn, the teacher will come. The teacher can open the door, but the student must enter by himself. Tell me and I forget; show me and I remember; involve me and I understand." He is happily married and currently living in Gainesville, FL. He can be reached at rogermillen@bellsouth.net or 352-375-4391.

Dr. Poppy Moon, PhD, LPC, NCC has spent most of her adult life thinking about how to help children and adolescents blossom into unique socially and emotionally healthy individuals – and more importantly, how to teach adults tricks and techniques to assist in this process. It is rare to find Dr. Moon without some kind of puppet, magic trick, role-play costume, or crazy art project geared towards positive child development. Dr. Moon, a National Board Certified Licensed Professional Counselor and certified school counselor, works as an elementary school counselor, an adjunct professor at the University of West Alabama, and in private practice. She is a weekly columnist for the Northport Gazette, a monthly columnist for Kids Life Magazine, and a TV guest on Great Day Tuscaloosa. A dynamic speaker and presenter, Dr. Poppy Moon conducts high-energy hands-on workshops for counselors, teachers, mental health professionals, and other educators across the nation. She has published several peer-reviewed journal articles in the field of art-related play therapy. Contact: Dr. Poppy Moon, 1130 University Blvd., Ste B9, PMB 255, Tuscaloosa, AL 35401. poppymoon@gmail.com. Voice mail (205) 799-5661.

Vicki J. Morgan, MSW has a Bachelor of Science degree in Psychology with a minor in Special Education from Florida State University, and a Master's in Social Work from the University of South Florida. She has worked as a Behavioral Modification Specialist with Lee County Mental Health, FL, a Special Ed teacher (Learning Disabilities/Emotionally Handicapped) in Phoenix, AZ, and a Parent Educator in Independence, MO. She is a foster parent and has three children and five grandchildren. Currently Vicki spends her free time writing and painting. Visit her website at www.vickimorgan.com.

Alison Morrow is a mother and grandmother who is filled with delight, gratitude, and joy for life. She has enjoyed using the labyrinth for herself, and for leading workshops for several years. In creating finger labyrinths she has become interested in how they can be used to assist with healing. She is currently completing a Diploma in Spiritual Direction at Regis College, Toronto Schools of Theology at the University of Toronto, and is passionate about this ministry. She has a BA in Women's Studies and a Certificate of Adult and Continuing Education from the University of Calgary. Alison has studied Adult Education in the Master of Arts program at the Ontario Institute of Education at the University of Toronto.

Kay Plumb MA is an Expressive Artist and Healing Facilitator for groups and individuals. Intrigued by the experiential nature of the expressive arts process, its emphasis on the mind, body and spirit connections and especially its hands-on nature, she became interested in the unique connection between the arts and the healing process. As an expressive artist she works with visual art, mixed media, movement, and the writing modalities. The experiential work or process, together with intermodal media, allows for people to find their creativity. Kay obtained her MA in Liberal Arts and Expressive Arts in 2003, from Goddard College through its distance-learning program. She has been a volunteer for over six years in an Arts in Medicine Program helping in the planning and presenting of workshops and establishing a weekly "Night Out" Studio for patients, families and friends.

Lauren Lane Powell In love with the human voice since before she could speak, Lauren Lane Powell started teaching people how to sing in 1989. First in private vocal lessons, then full time for the last seven years, she reminds people how to use their 'authentic voice' naturally in workshops across the country. In 1992 she earned a degree in Voice and Music Education from Indiana University. Through her own vocal adventures and further studies, she rediscovered her own true authentic voice, a technique she continues to share with others. Early on, when her voice students started healing from all kinds of dis-ease, just by learning how to sing, she realized there is an important instrument of peace within our own bodies! "Sing For Your Soul!" & "Harmonies of Healing" came from her inner knowledge that vocalizing: singing, toning and speaking, is not some mysterious gift given to a chosen few! It is for Every Body!

Lauren's mission is to remind others how good it feels to SING and to help everyone rediscover the power of their own beautiful authentic healing voice! Find Lauren Lane Powell at singforyoursoul@aol.com or www.singforyoursoul.com.

Julia B. Riley, RN, MN, AHN-BC, REACE is a Certified Expressive Therapist, Registered Expressive Arts Consultant and Educator, Advanced Practice Board Certified Holistic Nurse, and a Complementary Therapist/Expressive Arts Facilitator with TideWell Hospice. As University of Tampa Adjunct Nurse Faculty, she teaches "Expressive Arts in Healing: Health Promotion through the Arts." She is author of *Communication in Nursing,* 5th edition, Mosby. Julie, an international speaker, is a member of the National Speakers Association and president of Constant Source Seminars. Her mission is to 'Re-spirit, Re-inspire, and Re-vitalize' nurses to give sensitive care and to find humor, joy, and meaning along the journey. Email Julia@constantsource.com. Visit her website at www.constantsource.com.

Dr. Kathleen Sands, Ed.D. is a writer, photographer, and teacher. A native New Yorker, she completed her undergraduate work at Marymount, Manhattan College. As a Canadian resident, Kathy earned both her master's and doctorate degrees at the University of Toronto. An example of arts-informed research and self-reflexive inquiry, her doctoral thesis explored the areas of trauma and creativity at midlife. Most recently, Arts Alive Project Manager for the City of St. Petersburg, Florida, Kathy divides her time between the United States and Canada. For information regarding her upcoming book, "My Buddha Wears Bifocals," she may be contacted at: kathleen.sands@alumni.utoronto.ca.

Carol Shore, MA, CET, is a practicing artist and an intermodal expressive arts facilitator. As visual Artist in Residence at a local hospital she engages patients, caregivers and staff in the positive, dynamic, and spontaneous creative process to explore its relationship to inner sources of meaning and potential energies for healing. She has worked with teens-at-risk for the Department of Juvenile Justice, participated in a team effort with World Relief Kosovo refugees, and helped design expressive opportunities for depotentiating the trauma of war. She is artist-publisher of a child's skillbook on body safety and abduction-prevention, providing safety strategies to more than one million families. Email: remotesea@gmail.com.

Elle Speed BFA, MA, is a Certified Sound Therapist. She completed this program at Globe Institute in San Francisco in 2008. It was a natural progression from her introduction to a toning group in 2003. Within a few years, she found herself as the facilitator of an ongoing group, Tones for Living, at Bayfront Medical Center, St. Petersburg, FL. Elle is a Music Practitioner, receiving her certification through the Music for Healing and Transition Program (MHTP) in 2006. In this capacity she has organized a volunteer program called " Music Rounds" which provides light-hearted, sometimes thought-provoking music to the patients at Bayfront Medical Center. Elle thinks sound and music are viable complementary techniques for healing because of their non-intrusive qualities and their financially competitive reality for the institution. Elle Speed received her BA in Music (voice, piano) with a minor in Education from Emmanuel College, Boston, MA. After developing a chronic illness, she looked to music as a tool for self-healing. Today she wishes to share the tools with everyone. Elle is a member of the non-profit organization, Institute for Healing through Sound and Music, whose mission is to make the general public aware of the power of sound and music as a self-help tool and also to provide certified sound and music practitioners to the medical institutions that have embraced this complementary therapeutic technique. Elle Speed can be contacted through www.IHSM.info.

Susan M. Stewart, RN, MA, CLL (Certified Laughter Leader) is an accomplished holistic educator and motivational speaker. A graduate of Mount Carmel School of Nursing and The Ohio State University, she is a Master Trainer and Coordinator of Integrative & Holistic Laughter Care with World Laughter Tour, Inc. She has a special interest in the application of laughter and movement for seniors, those facing the challenge of cancer & chronic health conditions and healthcare professionals. Her passion for laughter and movement is contagious; her mantra is "Get in your feel-good groove – ya gotta laugh, ya gotta move!" Contact Susan at LaughWalker@aol.com.

Annette Tewes, born in Germany in 1960, studied music as a child and as an exchange student to the US in her teens. She has been working on her voice for five years with the Method of Uncovering the Voice in various private lessons. Her university studies focused on Nature and Ecology. After graduation she worked for twenty years in a private business and as an expert witness in Northern Germany. As a mother of three children in a lively household and a passionate choir member, she never lost touch with her singing practice and will start music-therapy- and Kinesiology-training in 2009.

Joan Abrahamson Voyles, MS As a professional artist with a desire to grow through study of the relationship of artistic processes and healing, Joan Abrahamson Voyles completed the certificate program in Expressive Arts from the University of South Florida. She continued as a volunteer in a local arts in medicine program for over two years. She also was one of the first artists to work with Hospice Patients in what is now Tidewell Hospice based on the west coast of Florida. Voyles grew up in Griffith, Indiana, earned her BS in Art Education from Butler University, MS from Northern Illinois University and taught art in Indianapolis, Indiana, and Palatine, Illinois. In a subsequent career she had her own business as an executive recruiter with a special focus in nursing administration. Currently Voyles is a professional artist and leader in the Anna Maria Island and Bradenton area arts communities. She has a following of people who collect their favorites from her popular print series of local scenes (see: joanvoyles.com.) Most recently, Voyles completed the Botanical Art and Illustration Program in the Continuing Studies Program of the Ringling School of Art and Design in Sarasota, Florida, where she won blue ribbons in student shows. Five drawings are published in O. M. Bradia's *Ten Steps: A Course in Botanical Art and Illustration*, 2004-2006. Voyles is married to doctor, artist and author, Carl Voyles and has a son, Erik Abrahamson, a practicing attorney in Clearwater, Florida.

Rosemary Warburton, Sound Therapist and Licensed Massage Therapist, is Founder and Director of Sound Body Wholistic Health Center, a sound-healing center located in St. Petersburg, FL. She is also Vice-President and cofounder of the International Association for Sound, Breath and Healing, a non-profit organization dedicated to promoting personal and planetary health through the common language of music and sound. A student of Nada Yoga and Sanskrit, she has had a lifelong love of music and sound and has had a private sound healing practice since 1994. Contact: Rosemary Warburton: Sound Body Wholistic Health Center, 5530 1st Ave N, St. Petersburg, FL 33710. Contact: 727-388-1444
rosie@soundjourney.net.
www.soundbodycenter.com.
www.iasbh.org

Dr. Charles H. Ware, PhD, is an active chemical engineer at the age of 81 and currently Vice President of World Energy Systems, a technology development company. A lifelong philosopher and avid non-fiction reader, Charlie developed a particular interest in the mind-body connection. In the 1980's he became a student of *A Course in Miracles*, which profoundly influenced his thinking. In response to a challenge from a business associate in 1987, he created Charlie's Law™: "everything turns out right... when you let it." He later founded Charlie's Law Inc., publisher of posters, greeting cards, magnets, and a book entitled, *Murphy's Law Repealed!*

Rosemary J. Wentworth, MA, has done extensive work with incarcerated individuals and residential substance abuse treatment programs. She has also worked with children, the elderly, and women's group mentoring. Rosemary did her graduate work in holistic counseling from Salve Regina University, and holds a graduate certificate in expressive arts from the same. She directed the "Thea," Transformation Healing through the Expressive Arts, and is editor of a monthly poetry and art newsletter, "The Wentworth Wrinkle." She has had exhibits in pen & ink, pastels, and metal sculpture, and has had her poetry published in many places. Rosemary can be reached at celery4@cox.net.

Fay Wilkinson's passions are masks and stories. Through her expressive arts practice, at The Creative Cocoon, she explores the healing power of a playful approach to art-making, which invites authentic self expression and exploration. She has studied mask with Michael Chase in England and has worked with renowned storytellers and voice coaches in Canada. Fay works with kids at risk, the Canadian Mental Health Association, businesses and universities, plus people in transition. She instructs in the Expressive Arts Post-Graduate Certificate program at Sir Sandford Fleming College and serves as program coordinator. She gives talks, tells stories, and conducts workshops and retreats nationally and internationally. Contact: www.thecreativecocoon.com, fay@thecreativecocoon.com.

Dr Gary Wohlman, PhD, is presently a dual citizen of the USA and Australia, and is a permanent resident of Australia, where his approach to healing has become nationally accredited by the Department of Education & Training. Gary provides trainings and individual sessions all around the world with his unique method of body therapy. His multi-sensory approach to healing includes spoken affirmations in rhyme, integrated with deep stretching, breath, visualization, and sound. This approach is designed to transform lives through catalyzing maximum physical, emotional, communicative and creative release. His revolutionary "Wohlman Method for the Whole Person" has become government-endorsed in Australia. His nationally accredited programs are available — along with short courses for up-skilling holistic practitioners. Dr. Gary combines his skill as a transformational body therapist and presentation coach with a flair for the ridiculous, the absurd and the outrageous -- stemming from many moments over "many lifetimes" as a long-time "storytelling court jester." As a modern-day traveling troubadour, Gary (also known as Elijah in metaphysical circles) practices and teaches all over the world; he is dedicated to revitalizing physical, emotional and creative energies, and to transforming people's lives. He is a founding member of the Gaia-Oasis Centre for Vision, Meditation & Creativity in Bali, where over the last ten years he has pioneered "Awakening Creativity" retreats to assist people in renewing their 'passionate purpose and partnership with themselves,' and in living more expressive, joyful and fulfilling lives. For more in-depth information, visit: www.garywohlman.com

Carol A. Yancar, MA, LMFT, has a wide range of counseling skills and has had a private practice in the Seminole/Largo, FL, area for several decades, with a brief interruption of a few years as adjunct faculty at a community college in Morristown, TN. She is a trainer for Neuro-Linguistic Programming (NLP) and a Diplomat in Clinical Hypnotherapy. In addition to NLP, she uses techniques such as EMDR, Silva Mind Control, clinical hypnotherapy, and MARI Mandala in conjunction with her therapy. Carol's approach to change includes finding balance mentally, emotionally, physically, and spiritually in order for individuals to create choice in their lives. She is an ordained minister through the Lively Stones Healing Fellowship, and co-founded the Tampa Bay Energy Group, emphasizing the EFT (Emotional Freedom Technique) work of Gary Craig. She is a master level Reiki practitioner. Carol does consulting work, coaching, and teaching. Her publication, "Practitioner Manual for Introductory Patterns of Neuro-Linguistic Programming," and her CD set "Infinite Possibilities" are available. Contact: cyancar@msn.com.

INDEX

A

abreaction 298
acceptance 4, 7, 17, 34, 40, 41, 81, 83, 94, 97, 130, 227, 264, 306, 356, 403, 405
acrylics 282
active imagination 261, 268
Active Imagination 77
addictive 82
adolescents 178, 270, 284, 317, 318, 323, 442
adrenaline 93, 310
aesthetics 142, 285, 286, 288, 290, 291, 293, 294, 295, 326
affect regulation 83
Affect Regulation 150
affirmation 9, 34, 38, 116, 170, 179, 389, 390, 405
aggressive 96, 203, 341
aging 370, 371, 372, 375, 435, 437
Aging 371, 372, 374, 377
alchemical 84, 211, 257, 265
aliveness 8
allopathic 25, 414
allowing 16, 24, 36, 46, 62, 72, 74, 81, 82, 125, 156, 160, 168, 220, 303, 305, 306, 314, 406, 416
alter 9, 43, 332, 356, 363, 364, 365, 366
alternative 9, 27, 52, 241, 242, 279, 350, 414
ambivalence 83, 402
anchored 236
angel 11, 12, 387, 388, 389, 391, 392, 394, 395, 396, 397, 399, 402, 408
Anthroposophy 136, 138
anxiety 19, 43, 49, 60, 86, 94, 125, 131, 175, 197, 250, 251, 254, 281, 309, 310, 311, 313, 317, 332, 342, 372, 402, 403, 408, 439
aphasia 373
Archangel 12
archetypal 81, 206, 207, 218, 221, 272
Archetype 35, 36, 37, 208, 243
Aristotle 293, 295
art for art's sake 52, 287, 292
artist 4, 7, 8, 10, 11, 15, 16, 43, 46, 57, 64, 71, 128, 161, 196, 211, 212, 214, 215, 219, 220, 221, 224, 226, 227, 229, 230, 240, 245, 246, 289, 290, 292, 293, 294, 369, 371, 391, 392, 394, 395, 397, 399, 403, 413, 419, 421, 428, 434, 437, 441, 443, 444, 446
artistic intention 230
arts in medicine 2, 3, 5, 6, 10, 11, 71, 159, 250, 252, 253, 254, 255, 386, 387, 388, 389, 392, 394, 395, 400, 403, 404, 406, 434, 437, 440, 446
assess 282, 426, 427
assessment 80, 136, 237, 288, 330, 415
Assessment 42
attachment 81, 143, 261, 339, 340
attachments 56, 245
attending 4, 34, 35, 37, 46, 84, 141, 143, 198, 224, 227, 229, 281, 321, 328, 413
attunement 144
aural 141, 144, 145, 147
authentic 5, 10, 75, 115, 163, 447
authentic voice 7, 112, 113, 443
autism 99, 142, 438
automatic induction 147
avoidance behaviors 311

awakening 106, 165, 211, 245, 293, 299, 336, 399
Awakening 203, 205, 276, 374, 448
awareness 3, 7, 8, 9, 11, 31, 33, 34, 41, 43, 50, 59, 80, 81, 84, 85, 87, 96, 105, 111, 116, 117, 118, 128, 143, 144, 146, 147, 154, 155, 158, 160, 162, 163, 176, 183, 200, 208, 212, 217, 227, 235, 236, 237, 239, 242, 243, 244, 258, 286, 303, 304, 305, 306, 307, 310, 329, 350, 352, 374
awe 8, 36, 46, 84, 86, 186, 217, 218, 244, 301, 332, 392, 418, 419
Ayurvedic 103, 292

B

Baba Yaga 188
balance 10, 12, 18, 19, 36, 37, 41, 64, 65, 69, 70, 76, 97, 100, 101, 103, 104, 106, 127, 138, 140, 154, 155, 157, 190, 208, 211, 212, 218, 219, 220, 244, 258, 280, 283, 332, 348, 380, 429, 448
beauty 33, 36, 37, 56, 57, 58, 59, 60, 67, 70, 73, 74, 92, 123, 139, 159, 161, 211, 212, 217, 219, 220, 258, 266, 285, 286, 287, 288, 289, 290, 291, 294, 302, 351, 405, 407, 419
behavioral regulation 83
belief 37, 83, 92, 93, 95, 99, 216, 230, 244, 279, 288, 290, 305, 306
belief system 92, 95, 99, 306
belly laughter 175
biochemical 9, 83, 352
biofeedback 18, 30
biopsychosociocultural 241
blocked 165, 216, 299, 394, 418
blood flow 84, 175, 177
Blood pressure 93
body language 204
bodymind 64, 74, 84, 162, 163, 185, 208
bonding 175, 285, 326
borderline personality disorder 88
boundaries 61, 64, 82, 147, 158, 215, 298, 302, 321
brain chemistry 175
brain wave patterns 147
breakthrough 6, 410
breathe 21, 28, 70, 87, 101, 110, 112, 114, 117, 118, 120, 122, 125, 129, 156, 172, 234, 332
breathing 65, 84, 87, 101, 109, 110, 113, 116, 135, 141, 142, 145, 154, 156, 159, 178, 210, 235, 331, 332, 334, 335
broken 11, 68, 72, 153, 385, 406

C

cancer 6, 7, 9, 10, 12, 25, 93, 94, 163, 201, 240, 244, 251, 378, 397, 404, 411, 423, 438, 445
Candace Pert 9, 175, 224
cardiovascular 175, 178
career path 200
Cartesian 215, 258, 299
catalyst 141
catharsis 9, 293, 294, 340
cathartic 298
celebration 230, 263, 350, 439
Celebration 19, 346
centering 5, 14, 16, 18, 72, 84, 154, 155, 158, 159, 206, 212, 252, 409
chakras 103, 104, 225
chant 209, 292, 349
chaos 5, 51, 63, 64, 195, 219, 220, 235, 365, 417
Chartres 207, 347, 348
chicken dance 180
child within 8
childhood 27, 44, 135, 137, 142, 146, 224, 273, 298, 300, 301, 339, 356, 358, 378
childhood sexual abuse 298

children 24, 26, 38, 40, 41, 67, 120, 121, 122, 127, 135, 137, 138, 139, 145, 161, 178, 179, 223, 224, 225, 228, 230, 231, 232, 257, 266, 274, 281, 284, 293, 300, 301, 305, 312, 314, 315, 316, 328, 329, 331, 335, 336, 339, 340, 341, 342, 343, 344, 345, 363, 372, 378, 381, 383, 392, 419, 436, 440, 441, 442, 443, 445, 447
choices 33, 35, 41, 52, 60, 61, 68, 75, 81, 84, 120, 122, 141, 214, 237, 278, 280, 281, 282, 284, 346, 404, 405, 436
chronic pain 43, 44, 45, 46, 47, 48
circulation 154, 226, 371
clarity 75, 87, 153, 196, 208, 349, 350
clay 17, 185, 189, 281, 282, 431, 432
co-creation 67, 71, 75, 278, 302
Co-Creation 1
Code Blue 65
cognitive 81, 82, 154, 278, 299, 304, 305, 324, 344
cognitive distortion 299, 305
color 5, 8, 12, 15, 16, 44, 54, 65, 66, 70, 85, 118, 141, 161, 211, 212, 219, 233, 234, 237, 238, 239, 245, 270, 282, 283, 288, 303, 342, 359, 365, 389, 390, 393, 395, 398, 399, 404, 405, 413, 416, 420, 421, 427, 428
color diffusion paper 15
comfort 11, 38, 49, 65, 85, 123, 135, 195, 208, 211
comfort level 85
commitment 19, 60, 61, 64, 130, 238, 263, 430
community 8, 19, 51, 71, 127, 130, 145, 148, 177, 212, 214, 215, 235, 243, 244, 251, 252, 254, 276, 285, 289, 290, 291, 293, 326, 356, 371, 375, 376, 381, 401, 425, 434, 448

compassion 33, 34, 36, 38, 40, 56, 59, 60, 104, 123, 127, 128, 131, 218, 220, 243, 267, 278, 328, 378
compassion fatigue 56
complementary 2, 9, 174, 179, 218, 241, 391, 392, 445
complementary medicine 2
conditioned response 83
connectedness 52, 59, 160, 161
connection 4, 14, 15, 17, 19, 22, 25, 31, 32, 40, 41, 50, 52, 59, 71, 83, 84, 85, 86, 128, 142, 143, 148, 154, 159, 174, 178, 180, 208, 211, 212, 245, 275, 278, 302, 303, 305, 306, 347, 408, 443, 447
conscious thinking 76, 176
consciousness 9, 84, 103, 104, 117, 139, 159, 160, 208, 220, 227, 241, 242, 243, 271, 276, 291, 292, 307, 326, 388, 419
container 3, 4, 10, 80, 81, 85, 212, 233, 235, 236, 246, 258, 293, 422
containing 35, 235, 409
containment 234, 237
contemplation 131, 195, 196, 239, 242, 278, 322
control 10, 11, 20, 27, 30, 47, 61, 63, 68, 80, 83, 84, 86, 87, 92, 96, 99, 105, 120, 153, 188, 212, 270, 280, 281, 284, 311, 321, 362, 364, 366, 369, 370, 390, 400, 402, 403, 420, 423
coping skills 281, 311
core beliefs 84
cortical operations 80
cosmic 117, 231, 242, 245
cosmology 73, 216, 217, 241
courage 5, 33, 70, 122, 126, 128, 139, 375
craft 320, 321
crafted 189, 288
creation 15, 73, 75, 84, 86, 102, 107, 117, 138, 152, 155, 189,

195, 211, 220, 227, 235, 237, 239, 243, 245, 258, 260, 298, 314, 418, 422, 427, 432
creative process 3, 4, 5, 10, 11, 71, 83, 189, 214, 218, 219, 221, 240, 417, 419, 434, 444
Cretan 242, 347, 348
Crones 257
culture 2, 3, 7, 10, 52, 61, 64, 66, 94, 95, 96, 97, 98, 148, 174, 188, 206, 225, 227, 231, 241, 242, 244, 280, 290, 292, 294, 307, 399, 441
cure 2, 47, 276, 351

D

dance 2, 26, 32, 36, 69, 70, 71, 72, 75, 76, 96, 98, 99, 143, 158, 160, 161, 162, 164, 180, 182, 184, 187, 210, 237, 238, 252, 258, 263, 269, 273, 275, 283, 291, 292, 326, 327, 328, 330, 334, 337, 375, 376, 383, 390, 391, 417, 435
dance of life 160, 210
Deepak Chopra 49, 121, 152
deeper meaning 322
defense 174, 299
dementia 196, 372, 373, 374, 379, 437
depression 43, 45, 47, 67, 93, 95, 142, 175, 281, 282, 309, 310, 314, 317, 319, 320, 322, 351, 366, 372, 380, 413, 430, 438
Destiny 78
Developmental 43, 142, 147, 148, 317, 318, 384, 437
diabetes 178
diagnostic 4, 146, 234
diaphragm 112, 142
Diego Rivera 227
discipline 5, 63, 64, 65, 66, 67, 68, 69, 70, 73, 76, 154, 227, 331
disconnected 265, 279, 302

disease 2, 12, 25, 27, 30, 32, 162, 178, 197, 201, 254, 351, 372, 374, 381, 384, 385, 408, 435
disorder 93, 308, 309, 310, 351, 356, 367
dissociate 298, 310
Dissociation 89, 341, 367, 368, 436
dissociative spectrum 300
Distortions 265
distraction 83, 94, 116, 183, 210, 213, 392
distress 80, 117, 229, 230, 299, 311, 327, 349, 417
distrust 99, 301
diversion 3
doodle 224
Dr. Herbert Benson 8
dream 45, 80, 183, 184, 186, 187, 209, 211, 239, 251, 260, 270, 271, 272, 273, 274, 275, 326, 375
dreaming 212, 271, 272
dreams 2, 61, 70, 126, 236, 239, 270, 271, 272, 273, 274, 275, 311, 329
dressage 67, 69, 71, 72, 73
DSM 62, 310

E

earth soul retrieval 261, 268
echoes 73, 224
eco-feminism 260, 268
ego states 301, 367
Egyptian pyramids 226
electromagnetic energy 299
emotional intelligence 83
emotional numbing 311
emotional regulation 80
empathic 87, 143
empower 80, 244, 420, 428
empowering 4, 8, 62, 158, 227, 387
empowerment 43, 45, 96, 98, 152, 156, 157, 218, 258, 439
endorphins 8, 93, 114, 179

energies 3, 4, 5, 50, 165, 212, 299, 444, 448
energy 6, 20, 36, 46, 60, 61, 64, 67, 72, 84, 85, 97, 98, 101, 103, 104, 128, 134, 136, 138, 139, 148, 152, 154, 155, 156, 157, 165, 171, 176, 179, 180, 214, 215, 217, 218, 219, 220, 221, 240, 242, 244, 258, 274, 292, 293, 294, 295, 318, 334, 350, 351, 352, 372,453386, 404, 405, 409, 420, 421, 442
engage the body 175
enlightenment 98, 105, 307
ensouled 238
enthusiasm 179, 180
entrainment 147, 387
epic 241
Epidemic 177
equilibrium 154, 155
escapism 311
essence 7, 34, 52, 62, 75, 81, 120, 137, 153, 184, 187, 189, 217, 218, 252, 289, 292, 299, 302, 415
event related potential (ERP) 82
exercise 14, 43, 48, 97, 113, 161, 163, 164, 175, 178, 179, 180, 203, 230, 235, 238, 252, 333, 363, 371, 428, 429
experiential 50, 80, 81, 83, 84, 85, 159, 163, 219, 443
Exposure Therapy 309, 311, 313, 325
expression 3, 4, 7, 8, 9, 34, 45, 46, 51, 61, 72, 75, 81, 84, 87, 110, 116, 129, 139, 142, 144, 148, 158, 160, 161, 162, 163, 165, 195, 203, 204, 210, 211, 212, 214, 215, 216, 217, 220, 224, 225, 227, 234, 238, 242, 243, 285, 289, 290, 293, 305, 317, 341, 344, 394, 413, 416, 420, 435, 447
expressive 2, 3, 4, 5, 9, 14, 15, 17, 33, 34, 41, 43, 46, 48, 50, 56, 57, 59, 60, 61, 62, 63, 65, 66, 67, 70, 71, 72, 74, 75, 76, 80, 81, 82, 83, 84, 86, 87, 143, 161, 163, 183, 185, 187, 190, 191, 214, 215, 216, 217, 218, 220, 240, 250, 251, 254, 257, 279, 280, 282, 283, 284, 290, 318, 321, 323, 390, 391, 411, 413, 414, 426, 427, 433, 434, 436, 437, 440, 443, 444, 447, 448
expressive arts 2, 3, 4, 14, 17, 33, 34, 41, 43, 46, 48, 56, 57, 59, 60, 61, 62, 63, 65, 66, 67, 70, 71, 72, 74, 75, 76, 80, 81, 84, 86, 87, 161, 183, 185, 187, 190, 191, 214, 215, 216, 217, 218, 220, 240, 251, 254, 257, 279, 280, 282, 284, 411, 413, 414, 426, 427, 434, 436, 437, 440, 443, 444, 447
Expressive Therapies 23, 78
eye contact 15, 124, 144, 426

F

facilitate 43, 71, 83, 84, 147, 158, 162, 165, 246, 254, 278, 350, 416, 419, 426, 427, 437
fairy tales 257
fantasy 48, 55, 63, 259, 312, 333
fear networks 342
feel-good groove 179, 445
Filial Play Therapy 343
fitness 179
flashbacks 310
flat affect 142, 145, 373
flexibility 84, 167, 168, 264, 332, 415
flexible 167, 169, 170, 173, 212, 254, 326, 337, 375, 411
flow 5, 9, 16, 22, 34, 36, 46, 51, 54, 55, 57, 58, 61, 64, 65, 66, 70, 72, 76, 97, 98, 102, 110, 138, 141, 203, 212, 216, 219, 220, 221, 235, 237, 258, 306, 390, 397, 405, 413, 427, 433

focusing 72, 81, 84, 87, 214, 348, 373, 409, 435
folk wisdom 174
folklore 259
forgiveness 27, 28, 32, 303, 304, 306
freedom 4, 56, 60, 63, 70, 73, 100, 102, 110, 113, 162, 165, 168, 184, 216, 274, 279, 290, 300, 306, 307, 328, 335, 336, 349, 375
frequency 30, 100, 101, 102, 103, 105, 118, 208
fresh eyes 56
Frida Kahlo 227
frozen 162, 227, 300
frozenness 145
frustration 18, 82, 109, 111, 196, 197, 221, 280, 281, 283, 301, 306, 317, 366, 420
functional intervention 380, 383
Functional Intervention 380
functional magnetic resonance imaging (fMRI) 82
future pacing 152

G

Gaia 243, 258, 266, 448
Genes 10, 13
genetic 279
gestalt 73, 84
ghosts 80
gift 14, 37, 48, 73, 105, 139, 196, 213, 215, 231, 238, 246, 257, 381, 385, 391, 392, 395, 396, 406, 409, 412, 414, 415, 416, 417, 418, 419, 425, 433, 443
giggles 114, 176
Goddess 63, 79, 206, 207, 258, 263, 265, 266, 267, 268, 269, 438, 441
Golden Mean 58, 60, 72, 73
Graffiti 341
grateful 36, 40, 174, 231, 253, 254, 315, 366

gratitude 20, 33, 126, 176, 180, 231, 245, 352, 443
groove 92, 93, 94, 95, 96, 97, 98, 99
grounding 136, 141, 154, 155, 263
group processing 257
group rules 321
group therapy 50, 318
groups 39, 45, 58, 130, 145, 147, 159, 187, 212, 291, 318, 319, 321, 323, 326, 346, 351, 383, 386, 434, 441, 443
guided imagery 84, 196
guided prayer 302

H

Habits 23, 69
handwriting 358, 359, 365
harmonics 58
harmony 2, 36, 58, 69, 73, 74, 108, 109, 117, 131, 155, 162, 219, 244, 348
Healing Emotional/Affective Responses to Trauma (HEART) 304
healingspace 66, 76
healthy choices 178
heart 18, 25, 30, 34, 35, 37, 49, 54, 55, 64, 67, 70, 74, 84, 96, 102, 104, 108, 122, 125, 128, 129, 161, 163, 164, 168, 170, 174, 177, 185, 203, 204, 206, 209, 210, 214, 217, 220, 237, 238, 245, 254, 267, 273, 299, 300, 301, 310, 337
heart mapping 203
Heartnet 245
Herbert Benson 389
herstory 265
hidden 30, 86, 87, 137, 139, 146, 148, 226, 234, 401
Higher Power 302, 304, 306, 307
history 25, 80, 93, 95, 96, 129, 141, 146, 147, 152, 153, 196, 206, 231, 270, 285, 287, 289, 291,

293, 294, 324, 332, 348, 355, 356, 372, 375, 402, 429, 441
holistic 14, 18, 87, 165, 214, 241, 352, 434, 438, 445, 447, 448
holy ground 227
honeymoon 311
hope 5, 12, 19, 45, 63, 161, 163, 178, 198, 201, 211, 220, 229, 231, 246, 250, 280, 285, 303, 304, 306, 332, 352, 359, 366, 417
hormones 82
horse 57, 58, 64, 65, 66, 67, 68, 69, 70, 72, 74, 76, 188, 289, 389, 390
Hospice 11, 14, 128, 201, 203, 386, 392, 411, 412, 413, 414, 415, 417, 421, 422, 423, 424, 425, 426, 427, 430, 433, 435, 436, 444, 446
host 331, 356, 357
Human Growth Hormone (hGH)372
human potential 2, 218
humming 101, 113, 117, 122, 126, 135
hurry 5, 176
hypnosis 26, 305
hypnotic technique 302

I

I Ching 153, 154, 155, 157
Iatrogenic 305
iconic art 373
identity 47, 97, 147, 216, 245, 300
illusion 100, 126, 218, 271
imagery 15, 45, 87, 216, 261, 268, 271, 274
images 3, 4, 5, 8, 10, 43, 45, 46, 47, 57, 63, 66, 76, 84, 85, 118, 162, 182, 183, 184, 188, 206, 215, 217, 219, 220, 221, 224, 225, 227, 229, 231, 232, 233, 234, 237, 238, 244, 245, 265, 272, 274, 279, 283, 304, 306, 315, 334, 336, 369, 375, 389, 391, 392, 421
imaginal realm 294
imagination 7, 8, 36, 45, 48, 59, 102, 105, 138, 152, 160, 185, 191, 196, 214, 215, 217, 219, 220, 244, 251, 292, 293, 322, 369
imaging 80, 82, 131, 355
imagining 37, 82, 172, 230, 328
immune 9, 11, 82, 85, 175, 371, 388, 389, 403
Improvisation 23, 102, 129, 191, 408
Improvisational 161, 184, 189, 252, 434
impulse 216, 228, 388, 410, 419, 432
impulsion 72
impulsivity 80
inactivity 178, 281
incongruities 177
induction 147, 208
ineffective behaviors 278, 281
in-form 56
inner child 45, 303
inner critic 184
inner vision 4, 6, 103
insight 35, 36, 47, 59, 81, 84, 85, 86, 87, 92, 94, 97, 99, 153, 200, 209, 210, 219, 234, 298, 299, 304, 307
inspire 17, 20, 22, 212, 214, 293, 394, 419, 444
inspiring 177
instinct 390, 393, 397, 431
integral 3, 81, 161, 240, 241, 242, 435
integrity 5, 9, 38, 95, 98, 130, 131, 243, 340, 352
intention 10, 12, 14, 16, 18, 20, 36, 52, 81, 83, 84, 94, 98, 100, 104, 105, 106, 107, 135, 154, 161, 172, 179, 208, 212, 227, 238, 239, 258, 290, 346, 350, 389, 404, 423, 428

Intentionality 23
Intermodal 3, 13, 54, 78, 440
interpersonal 50, 279, 318, 321
intervention 2, 15, 16, 28, 282, 305, 317, 369, 370
Introspection 194, 195, 204, 435
intuition 5, 8, 16, 86, 96, 102, 218, 225, 226
inventive 375
invisible 3, 10, 12, 73, 81, 226, 356, 402, 413
invocation 263
I-Thou 16, 17, 19

J

jokes 176, 177
journaling 56, 80, 202, 210, 279, 355, 376
journey 48, 80, 92, 106, 107, 108, 125, 128, 135, 159, 161, 197, 203, 204, 206, 208, 209, 210, 212, 213, 218, 234, 238, 240, 242, 244, 245, 246, 264, 300, 302, 305, 307, 318, 346, 347, 348, 352, 375, 417, 422, 433, 444
joy 16, 35, 36, 57, 67, 70, 93, 98, 99, 108, 109, 123, 131, 134, 135, 136, 174, 178, 210, 250, 252, 301, 328, 329, 330, 335, 336, 350, 352, 366, 416, 421, 425, 443, 444
Judeo-Christian 61, 303
Jung 4, 7, 13, 35, 57, 77, 216, 234, 237, 239, 261, 268, 277
Jungian 272, 275, 276, 441

K

Kant 286, 287, 288, 295, 296
Karl Marx 291
kinesthetic 152, 153, 154, 155, 162, 279, 281
Knill 4, 13, 56, 78

L

labyrinth 206, 207, 211, 234, 241, 242, 243, 245, 246, 346, 347, 348, 349, 350, 351, 352, 441, 443
labyrinths 207, 346, 347, 348, 350, 351, 352, 443
Lakota 260
language of the unconscious 81
laugh 16, 36, 87, 113, 130, 174, 175, 176, 177, 179, 180, 223, 331, 379, 433, 445
laughing 16, 39, 126, 177, 179, 263, 333, 431
laughter 27, 36, 44, 45, 127, 174, 175, 176, 177, 178, 179, 422, 431, 433, 445
laughter classes 176, 178
laughter library 177
layers 37, 55, 81, 206, 265, 343, 394, 427
left brain 59
legacy 16, 165
leisure 380, 383
letting go 5, 17, 25, 29, 32, 55, 65, 67, 139, 171, 185, 210, 219
liberation phase 375
LifeDance 241, 242, 245, 246
lifestyle 178, 371
lifestyles 176, 178, 372
lighten-up 177
Liminality 293
Line of Our Life 230
linguistic components 341
living image 4, 6
loss of identity 43
love 16, 18, 34, 36, 38, 39, 41, 54, 55, 58, 59, 62, 65, 73, 94, 104, 109, 118, 123, 126, 131, 141, 185, 217, 221, 227, 236, 240, 254, 257, 262, 266, 267, 270, 279, 282, 299, 306, 307, 320, 328, 334, 335, 336, 361, 366, 372, 384, 385, 404, 406, 416,

417, 421, 424, 432, 433, 443, 446

M

magic 44, 45, 127, 160, 185, 191, 251, 267, 272, 281, 317, 328, 355, 358, 361, 405, 406, 407, 411, 412, 427, 431, 441, 442
magic 44, 69, 152, 182, 189, 269, 439
maintenance 80, 227, 407, 429
mandala 6, 21, 36, 61, 233, 234, 235, 236, 237, 238, 239, 242, 389, 436
mantra 7, 8, 94, 99, 127, 209, 211, 261, 349, 445
mapping 357, 358, 363
maps 234, 263
masks 80, 182, 183, 185, 186, 187, 189, 190, 192, 292, 323, 447
matriarchal 261, 268
meaning 2, 3, 4, 12, 17, 19, 35, 40, 57, 59, 61, 66, 81, 84, 85, 147, 159, 183, 195, 208, 212, 215, 229, 232, 236, 239, 242, 243, 245, 265, 269, 275, 279, 286, 287, 288, 386, 387, 444
medicine wheel 234
meditation 5, 6, 9, 51, 80, 81, 82, 86, 87, 88, 117, 154, 162, 163, 186, 203, 208, 209, 212, 234, 238, 239, 254, 257, 263, 350, 351, 396, 404, 423, 442
memory 74, 83, 92, 93, 94, 96, 135, 137, 158, 161, 195, 196, 197, 219, 224, 252, 264, 265, 270, 298, 302, 303, 304, 305, 306, 329, 339, 341, 344, 361, 369, 373, 374, 379, 381, 384, 390, 410, 437
merging 306
messy 7, 319
metanoia 300

metaphor 57, 61, 66, 67, 81, 155, 159, 161, 162, 206, 210, 240, 242, 271, 349, 390, 403
Mexican pyramids 226
military veterans 312
mindful 24, 85, 210, 261, 352
mindfully 81, 176, 195
mindfulness 80, 81, 82, 83, 86, 87, 160, 163, 209, 213, 217, 242
Mindfulness 80, 81, 83, 88, 89, 158, 441
miniatures 309, 312, 313, 315, 325
miracle 47, 49, 65, 94, 385
mirror 177, 257, 265, 272, 429
mobilize 167, 293
monoprints 224
mood 8, 55, 80, 81, 83, 162, 175, 177, 179, 253, 313, 315, 390, 397, 402, 439
mood logs 80
mood-food 179
motherhood 138, 139
mourning 38, 56, 253
movement 2, 5, 7, 9, 54, 55, 56, 57, 63, 64, 70, 72, 73, 85, 94, 96, 102, 103, 104, 106, 141, 143, 144, 145, 146, 154, 157, 158, 159, 161, 162, 163, 167, 175, 178, 179, 180, 182, 183, 184, 185, 187, 190, 191, 210, 212, 235, 237, 253, 258, 294, 330, 331, 333, 335, 338, 348, 350, 352, 409, 421, 436, 439, 443, 445
multiple intelligences 278, 284
multiplicities 301
music 2, 6, 7, 15, 16, 26, 32, 36, 44, 49, 50, 51, 52, 53, 56, 58, 64, 65, 71, 75, 93, 94, 103, 106, 109, 111, 117, 118, 119, 121, 122, 123, 128, 129, 130, 133, 134, 135, 139, 141, 142, 145, 148, 160, 163, 166, 180, 182, 184, 216, 221, 223, 228, 250, 252, 253, 275, 302, 320, 326, 327, 330, 331, 337, 349, 351, 370,

371, 372, 374, 376, 381, 384, 404, 405, 409, 419, 435, 436, 438, 441, 445, 446
music instinct 148
music making 50, 51, 52, 371, 372
mystery 8, 10, 76, 160, 208, 217, 218, 219, 220, 258, 266, 276, 413
mythology 85, 246, 259, 292

N

Native 11, 12, 135, 289, 444
natural 3, 4, 7, 17, 26, 34, 58, 63, 68, 72, 83, 84, 85, 86, 95, 102, 108, 109, 110, 111, 112, 113, 114, 115, 135, 136, 137, 153, 160, 174, 179, 201, 235, 272, 288, 299, 312, 338, 355, 415, 445
needs 2, 3, 6, 19, 50, 59, 62, 68, 72, 93, 96, 121, 127, 139, 143, 154, 187, 209, 212, 215, 227, 231, 246, 252, 255, 278, 279, 280, 281, 282, 283, 284, 301, 303, 305, 313, 314, 318, 350, 386, 394
nepios 301
nervous energy 72
neural pathways 373
neurobiological reorganization 88
Neuro-Linguistic Programming (NLP) 448
neuroplasticity 81
neurotransmitters 85, 160
nightmares 68, 239, 310, 311
Noh Theatre 187
Norman Cousins 175, 179
notice 34, 41, 52, 66, 87, 101, 102, 110, 113, 114, 137, 204, 234, 235, 237, 273, 327, 407, 408
noticing 33, 34, 54, 234, 238
not-knowing 6, 55
numinous 56, 265
nurtured 127, 215, 243, 301
nurturing 84, 96, 97, 243

O

obesity 178
observer 80, 195, 198, 201, 206, 287, 288, 293
opening 4, 7, 8, 35, 103, 131, 155, 226, 251, 272, 283, 349, 389, 409, 440
opiate receptors 83
optimal well-being 174
order 34, 35, 44, 50, 56, 57, 64, 66, 70, 71, 73, 74, 80, 97, 121, 143, 163, 196, 204, 208, 210, 211, 219, 227, 242, 246, 251, 253, 275, 278, 279, 281, 287, 298, 303, 323, 333, 343, 344, 366, 394, 409, 424, 448
overtones 58, 263
OZ 33, 34, 37, 42

P

pacing 39
pageant 263
pain 10, 11, 24, 25, 26, 29, 31, 32, 39, 40, 43, 44, 45, 46, 47, 48, 69, 83, 85, 115, 118, 126, 131, 172, 175, 227, 250, 274, 286, 298, 301, 305, 365, 371, 388, 401, 403, 412, 413, 415, 416, 421, 423, 424, 430
pain medication 371
paint 6, 10, 11, 15, 16, 36, 44, 54, 65, 184, 186, 189, 211, 230, 235, 237, 238, 239, 254, 282, 294, 302, 319, 320, 323, 355, 374, 376, 381, 385, 389, 390, 393, 394, 395, 396, 398, 405, 411, 412, 417, 418, 420, 428, 431
painterly 54, 56
Paolo 4, 13, 56, 78
paradigm 3, 34, 214, 241, 259, 267, 300, 303, 306
paradox 5, 10, 62, 83, 183, 234, 246, 293
parallel process 82
partnership 259, 267, 373, 374, 448

pas de deux 73
passionate 167, 171, 246, 263, 371, 435, 443, 445, 448
pastels 184, 189, 233, 320, 355, 358, 392, 427, 447
patience 12, 36, 251, 318, 326, 337
pation 301
pattern 60, 97, 162, 207, 208, 212, 224, 226, 228, 262, 306, 311, 347, 375, 391, 395, 400, 407, 413, 416, 425, 426
peace 33, 49, 69, 74, 76, 79, 100, 106, 115, 123, 131, 195, 206, 233, 235, 237, 238, 239, 341, 349, 350, 366, 424, 443
peptides 9
perception 3, 10, 11, 43, 62, 83, 103, 179, 212, 280, 281, 299, 300, 333
perceptions 3, 83, 87, 212, 280, 293, 306, 311
permanence 314
perpetrator 298, 303, 305
personal symbols 80, 85
perspective 2, 27, 85, 120, 163, 175, 176, 180, 182, 196, 199, 201, 202, 218, 219, 244, 245, 279, 280, 304, 310, 394, 400, 404, 422
Pert 7, 9, 13, 84, 89, 181, 232
Phenomenological 85, 147, 219
photo collage 203
photo collages 80
photographs 17, 105, 194, 195, 197, 198, 202, 313
pictorial 197, 203, 441
pilgrimage 238, 347
placebo 46, 48
Plato 291, 296
play 5, 6, 7, 8, 9, 17, 21, 27, 32, 35, 48, 51, 68, 75, 81, 95, 96, 103, 109, 117, 122, 127, 129, 130, 143, 161, 163, 171, 172, 182, 183, 188, 210, 215, 219, 238, 243, 252, 255, 272, 279, 281, 285, 288, 290, 294, 295, 306,
309, 312, 313, 314, 316, 324, 327, 343, 344, 372, 374, 375, 376, 404, 406, 422, 425, 428, 430, 432, 442
playback theatre 252, 253
poetry 16, 35, 47, 56, 62, 129, 188, 238, 250, 252, 253, 254, 275, 435, 436, 447
poetry magnets 16
polarized 236
portals 239, 263
possession 62, 67, 228, 293
possibilities 33, 50, 51, 58, 60, 61, 64, 118, 195, 197, 218, 237, 258, 352
post-modern 240, 241
postures 153, 154, 155
power 4, 5, 12, 26, 34, 36, 43, 47, 51, 54, 57, 58, 59, 60, 61, 62, 63, 66, 67, 70, 72, 73, 74, 75, 76, 97, 102, 104, 106, 126, 127, 134, 137, 144, 160, 174, 183, 185, 186, 196, 198, 206, 210, 212, 213, 214, 218, 219, 220, 230, 241, 251, 258, 267, 279, 280, 282, 284, 286, 292, 294, 298, 304, 314, 332, 333, 339, 342, 352, 370, 389, 390, 392, 394, 395, 412, 413, 437, 444, 445, 447
power of naming 258
power of suggestion 196
practice 2, 3, 4, 14, 17, 18, 19, 20, 22, 24, 25, 26, 37, 47, 50, 51, 52, 56, 58, 64, 65, 66, 80, 103, 109, 117, 136, 138, 142, 145, 146, 155, 162, 175, 177, 217, 218, 219, 233, 234, 235, 236, 237, 239, 261, 268, 284, 286, 291, 292, 318, 327, 369, 420, 424, 426, 429, 434, 436, 439, 441, 442, 446, 447, 448
prayerful intentions 306
presence 12, 14, 16, 17, 18, 36, 41, 42, 70, 73, 144, 161, 166, 195, 196, 202, 208, 232, 237, 244,

246, 270, 303, 306, 330, 346, 351, 360, 387, 407, 408, 416
present 2, 6, 10, 14, 17, 18, 19, 20, 22, 26, 38, 40, 41, 45, 50, 51, 52, 55, 56, 67, 73, 80, 81, 83, 99, 103, 135, 144, 149, 152, 154, 160, 176, 184, 187, 195, 196, 209, 210, 218, 221, 226, 227, 230, 241, 246, 253, 254, 275, 278, 280, 283, 298, 303, 304, 305, 306, 307, 319, 321, 336, 344, 386, 387, 390, 412, 415, 425, 431
process 3, 4, 5, 6, 7, 8, 10, 16, 17, 20, 26, 29, 30, 35, 36, 45, 46, 47, 50, 51, 56, 57, 59, 60, 61, 63, 65, 66, 67, 71, 72, 73, 74, 76, 81, 84, 85, 86, 94, 95, 97, 99, 100, 101, 128, 131, 134, 137, 139, 147, 152, 153, 154, 157, 158, 159, 160, 163, 183, 185, 186, 190, 195, 198, 203, 204, 208, 209, 210, 211, 212, 214, 216, 217, 218, 219, 221, 224, 226, 227, 233, 237, 238, 239, 240, 241, 246, 250, 252, 254, 271, 272, 282, 289, 293, 298, 300, 301, 302, 303, 304, 305, 306, 307, 313, 318, 322, 326, 339, 340, 343, 344, 348, 351, 364, 370, 373, 387, 389, 390, 391, 392, 393, 394, 397, 399, 400, 401, 402, 403, 405, 406, 407, 409, 410, 412, 413, 415, 419, 420, 421, 423, 424, 425, 426, 427, 428, 429, 430, 431, 432, 433, 435, 438, 442, 443
progressive illness 175
psychiatric nursing 14
psychic discharge 271
psychodrama 252, 355
PTSD 145, 309, 310, 311, 315, 316, 317, 324, 339, 340, 341, 342, 344, 345
pulse 30, 93, 97, 147
Puppetry 339, 340

purpose 2, 18, 40, 46, 52, 72, 98, 100, 102, 112, 167, 171, 209, 214, 219, 243, 285, 286, 287, 289, 290, 291, 292, 294, 295, 298, 299, 303, 304, 305, 307, 316, 321, 350, 448
purpose in life 299, 303, 307
purposeful 180, 279, 280

Q

qualities 61, 62, 66, 103, 139, 147, 159, 221, 239, 300, 306, 323, 330, 445
quality of life 158, 372, 412
quantum physics 10, 299
quest 59, 138, 259
Quest 57

R

rape 310
reactive 120, 152
rebound 175
reclaim 126, 127, 263
reconciling 85
recovery 26, 47, 49, 145
reflective 17, 80, 208, 238, 287
refresh 5
regressive techniques 305
regret 305, 399
rehabilitation 175, 374
relatedness 73, 218
relaxation 5, 44, 45, 72, 83, 84, 92, 101, 145, 208, 242, 303, 355
release 45, 81, 82, 85, 94, 95, 101, 112, 115, 118, 125, 131, 156, 162, 166, 167, 168, 169, 172, 179, 209, 210, 219, 293, 300, 332, 333, 391, 399, 448
remaking 85, 258
remembered wellness 9
rename 263
repertoire 33, 163, 375
repressed 33, 298, 300, 303
resilience 5, 84
resonate 9, 37, 56, 64, 103, 121, 227

respite 127, 176, 355
restorative 5
restores 3, 4, 8, 158, 176, 218
reverence 214, 258, 267
right brain 59, 82, 83
risk factors 80
rites of passage 122, 212, 263
ritual 10, 56, 63, 65, 165, 212, 258, 261, 263, 268, 269, 285, 290, 291, 293, 294, 295, 334, 350, 439, 440
roots 8, 25, 36, 146, 148, 194, 198, 332, 384
Rumi 182, 221, 222, 276
ruminative thinking 83

S

sacred 14, 17, 18, 19, 20, 45, 48, 99, 100, 161, 195, 206, 208, 216, 218, 220, 233, 234, 236, 239, 242, 258, 260, 261, 266, 268, 270, 314, 351, 425, 426
sacrifice 226, 274
safe 3, 4, 52, 80, 85, 87, 93, 95, 96, 99, 116, 122, 196, 203, 220, 246, 257, 273, 278, 291, 304, 309, 313, 317, 318, 319, 321, 344, 363
safety 4, 8, 27, 60, 61, 97, 126, 127, 141, 258, 278, 282, 287, 305, 314, 321, 340, 424, 444
salvific 217
Sand Tray 309, 311, 313
Sand Tray Exposure Therapy 309
Sand Tray Exposure Therapy (STET) 309
savoring 176, 234
scapegoating 321
scarves 159, 160, 161, 163, 252, 253
seasons 95, 201, 235
Secondary emotions 82
seed banks 260, 268
self-care 14, 17, 43
self-condemnation 305

self-discovery 106, 141, 195, 246, 329
Self-Discovery 100, 106
self-efficacy 62, 80
self-soothing 282, 351
sense of self 6
senses 7, 33, 55, 83, 97, 160, 162, 163, 197, 258, 286, 304, 305
sentinel event 56
sexual abuse 111
sexual orientation 146
shaman 12, 294
shapeshifter 185
shared cultural voice 227
sharing 25, 51, 59, 60, 73, 74, 93, 99, 130, 203, 204, 231, 263, 313, 317, 326, 328, 329, 335, 391, 394, 398, 401, 405, 412, 413, 415, 416, 419, 422, 423, 424, 425, 427, 429, 430, 432, 433
ShiBaShi 158, 159
shift 3, 5, 10, 11, 18, 34, 116, 156, 158, 161, 162, 163, 167, 176, 197, 204, 218, 293, 295, 303, 332, 352, 411, 422, 424
shoulding 55
sign language 10, 253
simplicity 187, 189
sing 16, 35, 36, 66, 101, 108, 109, 110, 111, 112, 113, 114, 115, 122, 124, 129, 135, 137, 141, 143, 144, 145, 146, 147, 148, 149, 166, 191, 219, 252, 349, 373, 376, 443
sixth sense 306
smile 61, 177, 180, 327, 344, 397, 399, 408
Snow White 265, 272, 273, 274
social/interpersonal skills 318
somatic 83, 141, 147, 152, 153, 281
sonic acupuncture 117
soothe 143, 147
Soul 13, 23, 62, 77, 78, 107, 108, 109, 111, 191, 206, 214, 221, 222, 247, 268, 272, 276, 277, 284, 443

sparklers 312
spectroscopy 82
spiral 207, 208, 244, 263, 264, 269, 299, 347
spiritual 20, 46, 47, 52, 53, 56, 60, 66, 69, 73, 75, 84, 85, 103, 105, 136, 137, 138, 147, 158, 180, 208, 214, 215, 216, 217, 218, 219, 220, 221, 238, 239, 255, 285, 292, 293, 294, 295, 298, 299, 300, 303, 304, 305, 306, 312, 347, 350, 351, 358, 441
spiritual practice 20, 180
Spiritual Practice 180, 181
spirituality 52, 207, 214, 215, 217, 221, 240, 241, 243, 245, 290, 302, 351, 358, 366, 434, 437
spontaneity 5, 64, 121, 306
spontaneous 9, 83, 130, 145, 159, 184, 195, 219, 237, 238, 333, 336, 355, 365, 373, 391, 395, 398, 399, 412, 413, 427, 430, 444
state dependency 82
still 2, 16, 18, 30, 34, 43, 45, 46, 47, 48, 49, 60, 65, 66, 68, 71, 73, 74, 76, 101, 105, 108, 109, 113, 114, 116, 120, 123, 125, 127, 128, 161, 189, 195, 197, 200, 204, 207, 208, 215, 234, 257, 270, 272, 300, 310, 319, 332, 333, 362, 369, 374, 391, 395, 396, 397, 398, 399, 401, 416, 429, 431
stillpoint 154
stimulate 101, 104, 143, 178, 196, 212, 338, 379
story 10, 12, 27, 28, 36, 37, 38, 49, 57, 62, 65, 66, 67, 74, 95, 160, 162, 164, 182, 183, 184, 185, 187, 188, 189, 190, 196, 197, 203, 204, 211, 218, 220, 230, 241, 242, 243, 251, 252, 253, 254, 263, 266, 270, 272, 273, 283, 311, 342, 345, 362, 363, 378, 379, 380, 381, 382, 384, 385, 391, 398, 399, 403, 407, 410, 417, 419, 425
storytelling 2, 148, 161, 189, 250, 254, 263, 291, 344, 378, 448
stress 25, 82, 83, 84, 85, 87, 93, 96, 101, 103, 110, 113, 119, 126, 131, 158, 159, 162, 174, 175, 177, 310, 350, 351, 352, 371, 372, 388, 389, 390, 391, 392, 395, 399, 400, 401, 402, 403, 408, 412, 438
stress hormones 174, 177
stretching 165, 168, 170, 178, 200, 448
stuck 63, 67, 69, 154, 167, 224, 236, 312
subconscious 9, 56, 95, 299
Sufi 259, 267
suppressed 85, 404
surrendering 238
survival 38, 43, 63, 83, 92, 93, 94, 95, 97, 104, 142, 145, 175, 182, 201, 225, 226, 279, 282, 294, 301
survivor 43, 340
symbol 57, 58, 59, 70, 73, 206, 207, 288, 347, 390, 391, 392
symbolism 57, 198, 201, 204, 406
Symbols 13, 307
synaesthesia 54
synergy 81, 241
systems approach 290

T

Tai Chi 159
talk therapy 67, 318, 319
Tao 70, 127
Taoist 58, 153
teens 136, 233, 281, 282, 317, 318, 319, 320, 321, 322, 323, 436, 444, 445
temperament 72
the deep 56, 57, 92, 234
the lived moment 81
the mass 135

Healing with Art and Soul   463

thread 62, 74, 207, 257, 321, 424
thresholds 2, 265
Tibetan singing bowl 139
timeless 5, 8, 212, 220, 384
tinnitus 117
Tolstoy 288, 296
tone deaf 124, 125
Tone Deafness 119
touching 15, 17, 73, 190, 253, 359, 406, 407, 417, 425
traditional 2, 3, 50, 96, 106, 128, 174, 221, 223, 233, 234, 238, 241, 261, 290, 291, 313, 343, 413, 417
trance 40, 92, 93, 97, 98, 147, 152, 261, 355
transcendence 152, 299
transformation 43, 45, 47, 69, 70, 75, 85, 100, 107, 217, 218, 220, 241, 242, 293, 294, 302, 307, 370, 387, 434
Transpersonal 23
trauma 6, 56, 82, 93, 94, 95, 96, 98, 145, 162, 298, 299, 300, 301, 303, 304, 305, 306, 310, 313, 339, 340, 341, 342, 343, 344, 361, 395, 396, 397, 438, 440, 444
traumatic 7, 38, 95, 145, 298, 309, 310, 311, 312, 324, 333, 340, 341, 342, 343, 365
tree-hugging 263
truth 6, 7, 8, 35, 37, 50, 68, 98, 104, 112, 129, 130, 168, 170, 171, 182, 186, 187, 204, 218, 252, 263, 363

U

unblock 138
unconscious 34, 35, 37, 56, 82, 84, 85, 86, 93, 96, 120, 136, 168, 214, 218, 224, 227, 229, 230, 342, 391
unicursal 206, 207, 346
uninhibited 224, 230

unity 2, 73, 104, 146, 206, 218, 234, 276
universal language 85
universal meanings 231
Universal Music Day 119, 123, 128, 129, 131
universal truths 188
Universe 32, 106, 121, 125, 215, 217, 219, 220, 232, 242, 248, 277
unstruck sound 117
user-friendly 16, 377

V

vagus nerve 142
validate 2, 5, 174, 195, 223, 332
validation 196, 389, 413, 428
van der Kolk 145, 150
verbalization 344
vibration 101, 106, 114, 117, 118, 125, 139, 242
victim 43, 68, 253, 280, 303, 332
victory 152, 226, 306
Visionary 35, 36, 42
visual arts 56, 60, 61, 62, 250, 369
visualization 9, 84, 152, 165, 196, 220, 298, 302, 303, 304, 306, 448
visualizations 85, 165, 166
vital 61, 165, 185, 214, 215, 217, 220, 254, 307, 329, 375
vitality 138, 165, 372
voicing 229

W

wake up 101, 124, 261
warm fuzzies 203
watercolor 15, 56, 61, 219, 230, 252, 320, 355, 359, 376, 390, 404, 416, 419, 427, 428, 432, 434
well-being 11, 49, 53, 96, 102, 119, 143, 160, 178, 216, 281, 438
wellness center 241
what emerges 74, 238

wheels 280, 284
white moment 66
whole person 2, 3, 255, 366
wholistic 63
WISC-R 342
wisdom 8, 9, 36, 73, 95, 98, 126, 134, 135, 153, 158, 160, 183, 185, 186, 198, 215, 217, 218, 219, 220, 224, 257, 261, 266, 408
wonder 8, 36, 86, 102, 109, 112, 126, 139, 160, 174, 179, 217, 220, 301, 337, 351, 382, 403, 409, 419
wounded healers 263
Writings for Alters 355, 365

Y

Yin and Yang 59, 153, 155
yin-yang design 229

Z

zeitgeist 56